Decision Making
in
Dental Treatment Planning

Decision Making
in
Dental Treatment Planning

WALTER B. HALL, D.D.S., M.S.D.

Professor,
Department of Periodontics,
University of the Pacific School of Dentistry,
San Francisco, California

ALAN H. GLUSKIN, D.D.S.

Professor and Chairperson,
Department of Endodontics,
University of the Pacific School of Dentistry,
San Francisco, California

W. EUGENE ROBERTS, D.D.S., Ph.D.

Professor,
Department of Orthodontics,
University of Indiana School of Dentistry,
Indianapolis, Indiana

EUGENE E. LaBARRE, D.M.D., M.S.

Associate Professor and Chairman,
Department of Removable Prosthodontics,
University of the Pacific School of Dentistry,
San Francisco, California

SECOND EDITION
with 254 illustrations

Ⓜ Mosby

St. Louis Baltimore Boston Carlsbad Minneapolis New York Philadelphia
London Milan Sydney Tokyo Toronto

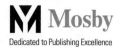
Mosby
Dedicated to Publishing Excellence

A Times Mirror
Company

Publisher: John Schrefer
Editor: Penny Rudolph
Associate Developmental Editor: Kimberly Frare
Project Manager: Dana Peick
Senior Production Editor: Dottie Martin
Designer: Renée Duenow
Manufacturing Supervisor: Don Carlisle
Cover Designer: Liz Rudder

Printed in the United States of America
Composition by Accu-color, Inc.
Printing/binding by Maple-Vail Book Manufacturing Group

Mosby–Year Book, Inc.
11830 Westline Industrial Drive
St. Louis, Missouri 63146

Library of Congress Cataloging-in-Publication Data

Decision making in dental treatment planning/[edited by]
    Walter B. Hall...[et al.].—2nd ed.
      p. cm.
      Includes bibliographic references and index.
      ISBN 0-8151-4194-7
      1. Dental therapeutics—Planning. 2. Dental therapeutics—
    Decision making. I. Hall, Walter B.
      [DNLM: 1. Dental Care. 2. Patient Care Planning. 3. Decision Trees.
WU 29 D294 1998]
RK318.D43 1998
617.6—dc21
DNLM/DLC
for Library of Congress   98-13366
                               CIP

98 99 00 01 02 / 9 8 7 6 5 4 3 2 1

Contributors

†Gordon R. Arbuckle, D.D.S., M.S.D.
Associate Professor, Orthodontics,
University of Indiana, School of Dentistry,
Indianapolis, Indiana

James J. Baldwin, D.D.S., M.S.D.
Associate Professor, Orthodontics,
University of Indiana, School of Dentistry,
Indianapolis, Indiana

Maria Antonia Barcalo Puig, M.D., D.D.S.
Private Practice, Orthodontics,
Barcelona, Spain

Roberto Barone, M.D., D.D.S.
Department of Periodontology,
University of Siena School of Dentistry,
Siena, Italy

Burton E. Becker, D.D.S.
Private Practice, Periodontics,
Tucson, Arizona

William Becker, D.D.S., M.S.D.
Private Practice, Periodontics,
Tucson, Arizona

David C. Brown, B.D.S., M.D.S., M.S.D.
Assistant Professor, Endodontics,
University of the Pacific School of Dentistry,
San Francisco, California

W. Paul Brown, D.D.S.
Assistant Professor, Endodontics,
University of the Pacific School of Dentistry,
San Francisco, California

Gretchen J. Bruce, B.S., D.D.S.
Assistant Professor, Periodontics,
University of the Pacific School of Dentistry,
San Francisco, California

Pedro Buitrago Vera, M.D., D.D.S., M.S.
Section of Periodontics,
School of Stomatology,
University of Oviedo,
Oviedo, Spain

Jordi J. Cambra, M.D., D.D.S.
Private Practice, Periodontics,
Barcelona, Spain

David B. Clark, D.D.S., M.S.D.
Assistant Professor, Orthodontics,
University of Indiana, School of Dentistry,
Indianapolis, Indiana

Carlo Clauser, M.D.
Private Practice, Maxillo-Facial Surgery,
Florence, Italy

A. Scott Cohen, D.D.S.
Assistant Professor, Endodontics,
University of the Pacific School of Dentistry,
San Francisco, California

Pierpaolo Cortellini, M.D., D.D.S.
Periodontology,
University of Siena, Dental School,
Siena, Italy

Mithridade Davarpanah, M.D., D.M.D.
Clinical Assistant Professor,
Department of Periodontology,
University of Paris,
Paris, France

Francisco Enrile de Rojas, M.D., D.D.S., M.S.
Section of Periodontics,
School of Stomatology,
University of Oviedo,
Oviedo, Spain

Daniel Etienne, D.C.D., M.S.
Associate Professor,
Department of Periodontology,
Faculty of Dental Surgery,
Université Paris VII,
Paris, France

Hipolito Fabra-Campos, M.D., D.D.S.
Private Practice, Endodontics,
Valencia, Spain

---

†Deceased.

James A. Garibaldi, D.D.S., M.A.
Associate Professor, Oral Surgery,
University of the Pacific School of Dentistry,
San Francisco, California

Timothy F. Geraci, D.D.S., M.S.D.
Private Practice, Endodontics,
Oakland, California

Alan H. Gluskin, D.D.S.
Professor and Chairperson,
Department of Endodontics,
University of the Pacific School of Dentistry,
San Francisco, California

†William W. Y. Goon, D.D.S.
Professor of Endodontics,
University of the Pacific School of Dentistry,
San Francisco, California

Gene A. Gowdey, D.D.S.
Assistant Professor, Diagnostic Sciences,
University of the Pacific School of Dentistry,
San Francisco, California

William Grippo, D.D.S.
Private Practice,
Napa, California

Walter B. Hall, D.D.S., M.S.D.
Professor,
Department of Periodontics,
University of the Pacific School of Dentistry,
San Francisco, California

William F. Hohlt, D.D.S.
Associate Professor, Orthodontics,
University of Indiana, School of Dentistry,
Indianapolis, Indiana

John Kwan, D.D.S.
Private Practice, Periodontics,
Oakland, California

---

†Deceased.

Eugene E. LaBarre, D.M.D., M.S.
Associate Professor and Chairman,
Department of Removable Prosthodontics,
University of the Pacific School of Dentistry,
San Francisco, California

Casimir Leknius, D.D.S., M.S.
Associate Professor, Fixed Prosthodontics,
University of the Pacific School of Dentistry,
San Francisco, California

Larry G. Loos, D.D.S., M.E.
Professor and Chairman,
Department of Fixed Prosthodontics,
University of the Pacific School of Dentistry,
San Francisco, California

William P. Lundergan, D.D.S.
Associate Professor and Chair,
Periodontics,
University of the Pacific School of Dentistry,
San Francisco, California

Alex McDonald, D.D.S., Ph.D.
Assistant Professor, Oral Surgery,
University of the Pacific School of Dentistry,
San Francisco, California

Kathy I. Mueller, D.D.S., D.M.D.
Private Practice,
San Francisco, California

Neal Murphy, D.D.S., M.S.
Lecturer, Orthodontics and Periodontics,
University of California, Los Angeles,
School of Dentistry,
Los Angeles, California

I. E. Naert, D.D.S.
Lecturer, Prosthetic Dentistry,
Catholic University of Leuven,
School of Dentistry,
Leuven, Belgium

Arun Nayyar, D.M.S., M.S.
Associate Professor and Director, Fixed Prosthodontics,
Medical College of Georgia,
School of Dentistry,
Augusta, Georgia

Michael Newman, B.A., D.D.S.
Professor, Periodontics,
University of California, Los Angeles,
School of Dentistry,
Los Angeles, California

Raphael Pasalodos-Gibert, D.D.S.
Private Practice, Orthodontics,
Barcelona, Spain

Joan Pi Urgell, M.D., D.D.S.
Private Practice, Implantology,
Barcelona, Spain

Giovan Paolo Pini-Prato, M.D., D.D.S.
Professor and Chairman, Periodontology,
University of Siena, School of Dentistry,
Siena, Italy

W. Eugene Roberts, D.D.S., Ph.D.
Professor,
Department of Orthodontics,
University of Indiana School of Dentistry,
Indianapolis, Indiana

Jose Manuel Roig-Garcia, M.D., D.D.S.
Private Practice, Endodontics,
Valencia, Spain

Mariano Sanz, M.D., D.D.S.
Associate Professor and Chairman, Periodontology,
University of Madrid, School of Dentistry,
Madrid, Spain

Robert Sarka, B.S., D.D.S., M.S.
Professor, Removable Prosthodontics,
University of the Pacific School of Dentistry,
San Francisco, California

Joseph H. Schulz, D.D.S.
Associate Professor, Endodontics,
University of the Pacific School of Dentistry,
San Francisco, California

Alberto Sicilia, M.D., D.D.S.
Associate Professor, Periodontology,
University of Oviedo, School of Dentistry,
Oviedo, Spain

E. Robert Stultz, Jr., D.M.D., M.S.
Private Practice,
San Raphael, California

Charles F. Sumner III, D.D.S., J.D.
Associate Professor, Periodontics,
University of the Pacific School of Dentistry,
San Francisco, California

Maurizio Tonetti, D.D.S., M.S.
Department of Periodontics,
University of Bern School of Dentistry,
Bern, Switzerland

Chi Tran, D.D.S.
Assistant Professor, Fixed Prosthodontics,
University of the Pacific School of Dentistry,
San Francisco, California

Steven A. Tsurudome, D.D.S., M.S.
Assistant Professor, Department of Periodontics,
University of the Pacific School of Dentistry,
San Francisco, California

Galen W. Wagnild, D.D.S., M.S.
Private Practice,
San Francisco, California

Borja Zabelegui, M.D., D.D.S.
Private Practice, Endodontics,
Bilbao, Spain

Jon Zabelegui, M.D., D.D.S.
Private Practice, Endodontics,
Bilbao, Spain

Mark Zablotsky, B.S., D.D.S.
Assistant Professor, Periodontics,
University of the Pacific School of Dentistry,
San Francisco, California

Giliana Zuccati, M.D.
Department of Periodontics,
University of Siena School of Dentistry,
Siena, Italy

For their love, support, and understanding
during the preparation of this text,
we dedicate it to our wives and children:
Francella, Scott, and Greg Hall
Riitta, Adam, and Suvi Gluskin
Cheryl, Carrie, and Jeffery Roberts
Denise, Elizabeth, Andrew, and Suzanne LaBarre

Preface

This second edition of *Decision Making in Dental Treatment Planning* is an effort to illustrate the thought processes of dentists in several of the clinical specialties when their specific aspect of care is involved in complex dental cases. It is a logical progression from an earlier text, *Decision Making in Periodontology*, wherein the decision making process in only one field was presented. In complex cases, the periodontist would not attempt to dictate the whole treatment plan. The treatment plan would be correlated with what those performing other aspects of care believed would work best; thus in complex case treatment planning, the difficulties that a general dentist tackles daily confront the specialist but in an even more complex way. The dentist must work with the decisions made by others and sequence the treatment to achieve an end result agreed upon by the patient and all of those treating. The general dentist often must make all of these decisions alone, sometimes a daunting task and one in which the dentist should know when to seek help from the appropriate specialists.

This text presents decision making for treatment planning complex and interdisciplinary cases as viewed by specialists in periodontics, endodontics, orthodontics, prosthodontics, and oral surgery. Conflicting viewpoints among specialists will be evident to the reader. As one must do in practice, the individual dentist must resolve these differences to present treatment plan options to the patient. This text should be helpful to the dentist in comprehending how various experts "think" in their decision making processes. Readers can weigh the merits of any conflicting approaches presented by various contributors and arrive at their own conclusions while better understanding how others may arrive at different conclusions.

As new treatment approaches are presented and validated in practice, decision making in treatment planning changes, often becoming more complex. In the last decade, implants and guided tissue regeneration have greatly altered the options available for treatment. Some older approaches to treatment can be replaced with far superior new ones (e.g., rather than extracting or maintaining teeth that in the past were labeled "hopeless," such as second molars with large three-walled distal defects, guided tissue regeneration can totally change their prognosis with a high level of predictability). The cost of some newer approaches can be high (e.g., implants) or can greatly reduce the cost of options such as bridge construction (e.g., regenerating a severe Class II furca defect on an endangered tooth rather than extracting it and placing a bridge). Patients have a right to know the pros and cons of each of these approaches. The dentist must be able to verbalize the deductive process used to arrive at appropriate treatment options. This text should be helpful to the practicing dentist in improving skills in this aspect of daily practice. For the student, it should be helpful in teaching how what has been learned will be used.

Our thanks go to the editors at Mosby, Penny Rudolph and Kimberly Frare, for their expertise and patience; to Elizabeth Carpenter, Katherine Martin, Maria Co Viray, Teresa Kuhlman, and Page Marshall for typing the manuscript; to our many contributors who made the text possible; to Eric Curtis for his illustrations; and to our families for their support and encouragement in preparing this book.

Walter B. Hall
Alan H. Gluskin
W. Eugene Roberts
Eugene E. LaBarre

CONTENTS

---

†Deceased.

†Deceased.

How to Use This Book

Each two- to four-page chapter in this text consists of an algorithm or decision tree, appearing on the right-hand page, and a brief explanatory text with illustrations and references, appearing on the left-hand page. The decision tree is the focus of each chapter and should be studied in detail first. The letters on the decision tree refer the reader to the text, which provides a brief explanation of the basis for each decision. Boxes have been used on the decision tree to indicate invasive procedures or the use of drugs. Dotted-line boxes indicate the nature of major decisions that must be made. A combination of line drawings and half tones were selected to clarify the text. Cross references have been inserted to avoid repeating information given in other chapters. References that are readily available to the practitioner have been selected.

For reader convenience, the text has been divided into sections from the following specialty areas: periodontics, endodontics, orthodontics, prosthodontics, and oral surgery. An index is included to facilitate the location of specific information.

The decisions outlined here relate to typical situations. Unusual cases may require the clinician to consider alternatives; however, in every case, the clinician must consider all aspects of an individual patient's data. The algorithms presented here are not meant to represent a rigid guideline for thinking but rather a skeleton to be fleshed out by additional factors in each individual patient's case. Because different specialty areas may view a problem in different ways, the reader must evaluate each of these differing views to arrive at the appropriate treatment plan for each individual patient.

PART ONE

Periodontics

Walter B. Hall, Editor

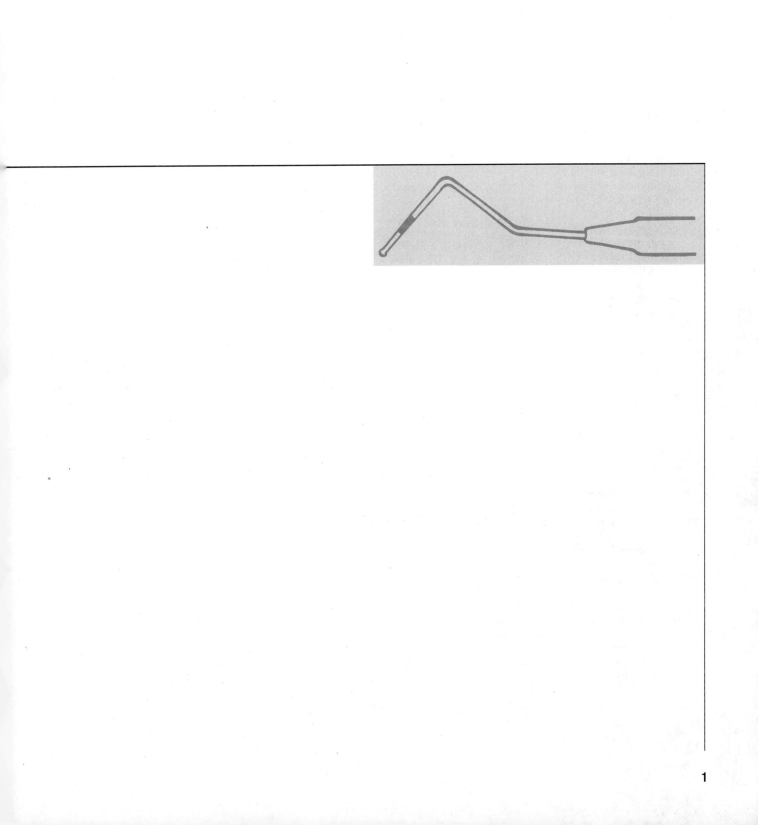

1 Sequence of Periodontal Treatment

Walter B. Hall

When a patient has a periodontal problem, a typical sequence of examination and diagnosis should precede treatment planning. The patient's medical, dental, and plaque-control histories should be recorded and amplified upon during clinical and radiographic examinations. From these data, diagnoses and prognoses can be developed.

A For purposes of treatment planning, periodontal problems are divided into acute (symptomatic) problems, in which symptoms are present, and asymptomatic problems, in which no acute problems are present. Symptomatic problems require prompt treatment, usually at the diagnostic visit. Only the four most common symptomatic problems are outlined here. The more common periodontal diseases usually are asymptomatic, and treatment can be planned on a more orderly basis that best fits into the patient's and dentist's schedules.

B Herpetic gingivostomatitis usually is managed with palliative care (mild pain killers, a topical anesthetic mouthwash), prophylaxis, and instruction about the infectious nature of the problem.

C Necrotizing ulcerative gingivitis and necrotizing ulcerative periodontitis are handled by instrumentation alone or in conjunction with an oral antibiotic, usually penicillin.

D Periodontal abscesses usually are handled by incision and drainage along with antibiotic therapy.

E Therapy for human immunodeficiency virus (HIV) periodontitis requires close collaboration with the patient's physician in developing a palliative treatment plan (see Chapter 48). Acute or severe episodes of HIV periodontitis in which tissue necrosis is rapid and painful should be treated initially with povidone iodine (Betadine) and if bone is exposed, applied several times a day; after 1 week, prescribe chlorhexidine rinses morning and night until the necrosis is controlled. Extremely severe episodes may be treated with metronidazole (Flagyl) as the physician directs. If an HIV-infected patient is or becomes stable, as is true in many cases today, dental treatment should be handled as with noninfected patients. Even guided tissue regeneration (GTR), using resorbable membranes, may become feasible (see Chapter 21).

F Gingivitis of the typical type probably is the most prevalent disease affecting humans, and most people experience at least localized inflammations of this type in any given year. Its subgroupings are related to host factors. Gingivitis usually responds favorably to prophylaxis (or root planning, if roots are exposed) and to thorough plaque-removal practices by the patient. In the absence of daily, thorough plaque removal, it will return. Desquamative gingivitis is far less common and usually is the gingival expression of dermatologic diseases. Prophylaxis (or root planing), regular plaque removal (often difficult), and topical steroid applications are common treatments.

G Adult periodontitis is the current name for typical, slowly progressive periodontitis. Its treatment (see Chapter 10) usually consists of initial therapy (root planing, oral hygiene training, occasionally occlusal adjustment, and occasionally temporary splinting or minor tooth movement). After several weeks or months of patient effort, the response is evaluated, and decisions are made regarding the comparative value of surgery or continued maintenance.

H Juvenile periodontitis, mixed dentition periodontitis, and rapidly progressive periodontitis are discussed elsewhere.* Although different bacteria appear to predominate as etiologic agents with these diseases, they are treated in a similar manner. A regimen of tetracycline (250 mg four times daily) or metronidazole (Flagyl) is used for 3 weeks, during which all root planing is accomplished. This regimen is repeated several times during the first year to contact the virulent bacteria. Often, only regular maintenance or localized surgery is required once this control is established. Such cases are best referred to dental schools or to periodontists.

I Gingival enlargements (often called hyperplasias) may result from drug therapy (diphenylhydantoin, cyclosporine, or nifedipine treatment)* or from poor oral hygiene during orthodontic treatment in the pubertal years. They are treated with initial therapy, surgery if the deformities interfere with adequate plaque removal, occlusion, or regular maintenance. Stopping the use of the medication or removing the orthodontic bands is necessary in few cases.

---

*See Hall WB: *Decision making in periodontology*, ed 3, St Louis, 1998, Mosby.

References

Barsh LI: *Dental treatment planning for the adult patient*, Philadelphia, 1981, WB Saunders, p 152.

Carranza FA, Newman MG: *Clinical periodontology*, ed 8, Philadelphia, 1996, WB Saunders, p 399.

Genco RJ, Goldman HM, Cohen DW: *Contemporary periodontics*, St Louis, 1990, Mosby, p 359.

Grant DA, Stern IB, Listgarten MA: *Periodontics*, ed 6, St Louis, 1988, Mosby, p 592.

Schluger S, Yuodelis R, Page RC, Johnson RH: *Periodontal diseases*, ed 2, Philadelphia, 1990, Lea & Febiger, p 331.

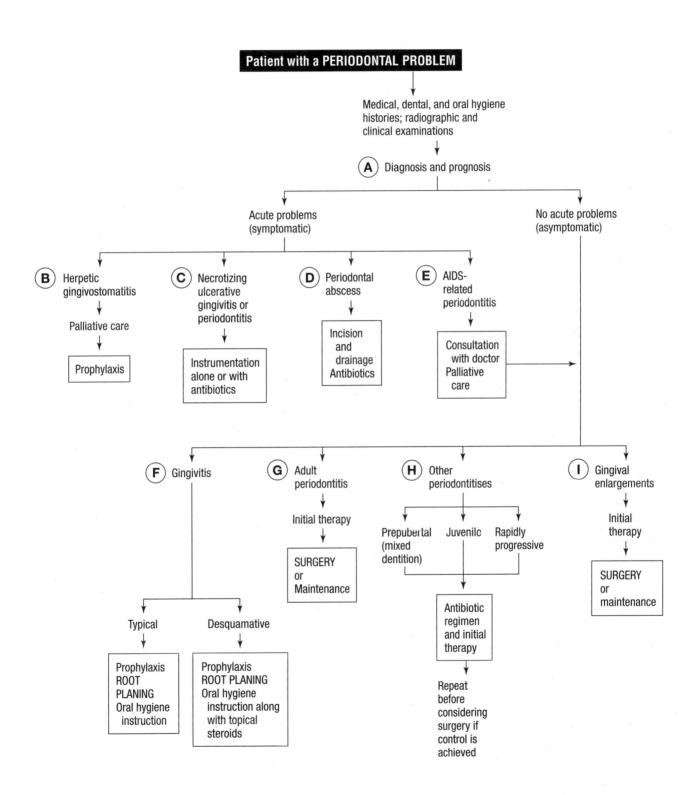

Patient with a PERIODONTAL PROBLEM

Medical, dental, and oral hygiene histories; radiographic and clinical examinations

(A) Diagnosis and prognosis

Acute problems (symptomatic)

No acute problems (asymptomatic)

(B) Herpetic gingivostomatitis

Palliative care

Prophylaxis

(C) Necrotizing ulcerative gingivitis or periodontitis

Instrumentation alone or with antibiotics

(D) Periodontal abscess

Incision and drainage Antibiotics

(E) AIDS-related periodontitis

Consultation with doctor Palliative care

(F) Gingivitis

(G) Adult periodontitis

Initial therapy

SURGERY or Maintenance

(H) Other periodontitises

Prepubertal (mixed dentition)   Juvenile   Rapidly progressive

Antibiotic regimen and initial therapy

Repeat before considering surgery if control is achieved

(I) Gingival enlargements

Initial therapy

SURGERY or maintenance

Typical

Prophylaxis ROOT PLANING Oral hygiene instruction

Desquamative

Prophylaxis ROOT PLANING Oral hygiene instruction along with topical steroids

2 Referral to a Periodontist

Walter B. Hall, Charles F. Sumner III

When there is a periodontal component to the treatment plan for a complex dental problem, several factors determine the need or desirability to refer the patient to a periodontist. Some dentists have mastered many aspects of periodontal care. Dentists must have a realistic concept of their own abilities and limitations. In some states a quasilegal requirement for referral or offer of referral of complex cases has been developed. A patient with a complex problem needs to know that specialists in periodontics exist and may be consulted. If a case has complexities involving multiple specialized areas, referral is especially desirable.

A If there are no significant periodontal aspects in the treatment plan, referral is not necessary.[1]

B If the treatment plan has a significant periodontal component, dentists must decide whether they have the required skills to treat the periodontal problem or if better care could be provided by a specialist. If the dentist does not have the skills necessary, the patient must either be referred to a periodontist or refused treatment. General practitioners who have additional training may treat cases that are no longer in the earliest stages. Should the general dentist decide that the level of disease is within the ability to treat, however, the patient must still be informed of the periodontal disease and what its extent is and that there are specialists in the treatment of this dental disease. To fail to inform the patient would be to render care without a complete informed consent.[2,3]

C If the dentist believes that he or she has the necessary skill to provide the periodontal treatment, it must be decided whether referral would be in the best interest of the patient or whether it is required by practice concepts in his or her area to refer the case. The dentist must make the patient aware that a specialist—the periodontist—is available for consultation. If the dentist feels capable of handling the case and if the patient selects treatment by the dentist, the dentist must decide whether to treat the case or to refuse to accept the person as a patient. The general practitioner who performs the necessary treatment with the patient's informed consent is legally bound to disclose to the patient if the treatment is not successful.[4] The patient must be referred to a specialist as soon as the dentist becomes aware or should have become aware that the initiated therapy is not proving to be as effective as could be expected in the hands of a specialist.

D If the dentist feels that he or she has the skill to manage the periodontal care, but that better care could be provided by a periodontist, he or she must determine whether the patient is likely to accept the referral and can afford treatment by a specialist. If so, the patient should be referred. If not, the dentist may consider altering the plan so that the patient can be managed or refuse to accept the person as a patient. If the patient declines to be referred, the informed consent aspects of the discussion should be recorded in the chart.

A suggestion that the patient seek the care of a specialist is not enough. The practitioner is obliged to adequately inform the patient about the extent of the disease and the consequences if he or she fails to follow through with the referral.[5] Courts have found dentists negligent in cases in which patients have asserted that they were not made aware of the consequence of a dentist failing to seek care. Thus it would be prudent to follow up on each referral and not simply dismiss the patient who apparently has not taken the advice.

Some courts have held a referring dentist liable for not having warned the patient of the extent and type of care that would be given by the specialist.[6] However, in most instances it is the primary obligation of the specialist or a member of the dentist's staff to properly inform the patient and obtain a satisfactory informed consent.[7,8]

Patients are at a disadvantage should they need to rely only on their own resources when choosing a specialist. Once having informed the patient of the need for special care, the dentist is obliged to assist the patient in making a prudent choice. Having fulfilled the obligation of referring the patient to a specialist who is reasonably believed to be competent, the referring dentist is not held liable for the negligent acts of the specialist. An exception exists to this rule when there is a partnership or fiduciary relationship between the general practitioner and the specialist.

Having entered into a joint relationship with the patient in the care and treatment of that patient's periodontal disease, it is essential that some agreement be reached as to the responsibility of follow-up care once the case has been referred to a specialist. Furthermore, it is equally essential that the patient be made aware, and consents to, these plans.

Periodontal disease is more frequently controlled than cured. Having taken on the responsibility of care, both the general practitioner and the specialist must meet a community standard in all aspects of determining a diagnosis, planning treatment, and providing maintenance care. Both parties have a duty to inform the patient of their plans, their prognoses, and the consequences of not following the plans. They must also offer the patient an alternative plan, if available, describing its advantages and disadvantages. Only then can the patient make an informed decision and the dentist proceed with an informed consent.[9,10,11]

References

Grant DA, Stern IB, Listgarten MA: *Periodontics*, ed 6, St Louis, 1988, Mosby, p 605.

Hall WB: *Pure mucogingival problems*, Berlin, 1984, Quintessence Publishing, p 169.

Zinman EJ: Common dental malpractice errors and preventive measures, *J West Soc Periodont* 23:149, 1976.

Legal References

1. *Helling v Carey*, Wash, 519 P 2d 981, 1974.
2. *Canterbury v Spence*, 464 F2d 772, 1972.

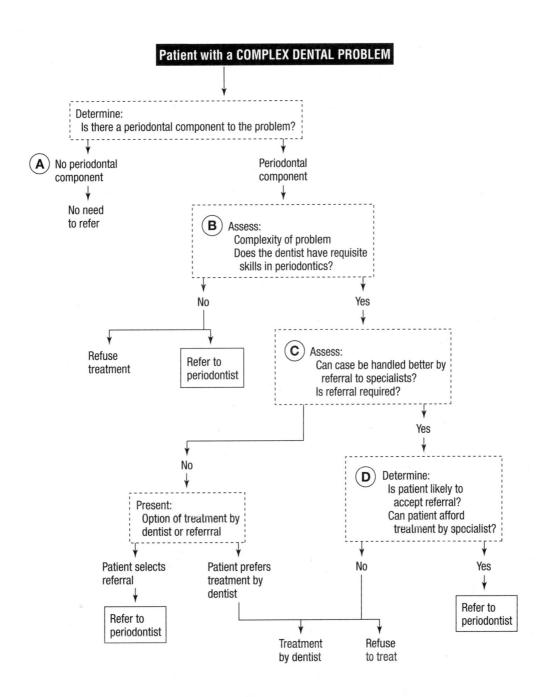

Patient with a COMPLEX DENTAL PROBLEM

Determine:
Is there a periodontal component to the problem?

A No periodontal
component

Periodontal
component

No need
to refer

B Assess:
Complexity of problem
Does the dentist have requisite
skills in periodontics?

No

Yes

Refuse
treatment

Refer to
periodontist

C Assess:
Can case be handled better by
referral to specialists?
Is referral required?

Yes

No

Present:
Option of treatment by
dentist or referrral

D Determine:
Is patient likely to
accept referral?
Can patient afford
treatment by specialist?

Patient selects
referral

Patient prefers
treatment by
dentist

No

Yes

Refer to
periodontist

Treatment
by dentist

Refuse
to treat

Refer to
periodontist

3. *Cobbs v Grant*, 104 Cal Rptr 505, 1972.
4. *Baldor v Roger*, 81 S Rptr 2d 660, 1955.
5. *Moore v Preventive Medicine Medical Group, Inc.*, 178 Cal App 3d 728;
   223 Cal Rptr 85, 1986.
6. *Llera v Wisner*, 557 P 2d 805, 1976.

7. *Mustacchio v Parker*, 535 So 2d 833, La App 2Cir, 1988.
8. *Bulman v Myers*, DDS, 467 A 2d 1353, Pa Super, 1983.
9. *Kennedy v Gaskell*, 274 CA 2d 244; 78 Cal Rptr 753, 1969.
10. *Mayer v Litow*, 154 CA 2d 413; 316 P2d 351, 1957.
11. *Wolfsmith v Marsh*, 51 C 2d, 832; 337 P 2d 70, 1959.

3 Hopeless Teeth

Walter B. Hall

Hopeless teeth are those that cannot be treated with reasonable expectations of eliminating or even controlling their dental problems. Such teeth are not always extracted but in some situations may be maintained, occasionally for years, with full recognition that no means of treating them or stopping their loss of attachment exist. For example, such patients may have lost 50% or more of the attachment on all their remaining teeth. Pocket elimination surgery might be ruled out on the basis of leaving inadequate support to keep the teeth at all with any reasonable degree of comfort or function. A Widman flap might be used to débride the area once fully, but neither the patient nor the dentist could expect to control the disease process with root planing, even with use of antibiotics. Such teeth might be maintained, if the patient demanded, for some time before abscesses and pain might necessitate their removal. Such patients should proceed with full knowledge that their prognosis is hopeless and be aware of the risks of abscesses and the possible danger to their general health. The concept of hopeless teeth, therefore, should be explained fully when such a prognosis is used so that the patient not only assumes all the attendant risks of keeping such teeth but also is fully informed in the legal sense (see Chapter 2).

Today many teeth previously regarded as hopeless are salvageable by means of guided tissue regeneration (GTR). Badly involved Class II furcation involvements, large three-walled infrabony defects, and osseous craters that were nontreatable have become predictably treatable. Significant numbers of formerly hopeless teeth can be saved by this means today. Recent advances with extensive GTR procedures (see Chapter 31) have made most two-walled infrabony defects routinely treatable. Multiple tooth GTR procedures (see Chapter 13) are becoming increasingly successful; even groups of teeth with more than 50% loss of attachment (LOA) can be made maintainable with regenerated support. Mobility does not limit the potential for success.

A Some teeth must be regarded as hopeless because they are not restorable, because they are malposed to an extent not correctable orthodontically, or because of vertical or spiral cracks that extend apically down their roots.

Some teeth may not be amenable to GTR. Root proximity (less than 1 mm between roots) may make GTR impossible because proximal root surfaces, especially those with furcas (maxillary molars or first premolars), may not be accessible to instrumentation.

Cracked tooth problems can make a tooth's prognosis hopeless. If cracked tooth syndrome exists and the symptoms are bothersome to the patient, the tooth may have to be removed if the crack extends vertically down the root. If the crack is essentially in the crown, placing a restorative crown may control the symptoms and restrict further crack spreading so that the prognosis for the tooth could be improved. Vertical cracks in the root of the tooth, however, are not treatable, and the prognosis is hopeless.

B Next, assess the endodontic health of a severely periodontally involved tooth. If a tooth is not endodontically treatable (i.e., calcified canals, roots too crooked to be obturated, severely internally or externally resorbed or perforated), it should be regarded as hopeless.

If the tooth is a molar with a Class III furcation involvement, determine its endodontic status. If endodontic therapy is needed and can be performed, the prognosis for the tooth would be greatly improved. If not, the possibilities of improving the molar's prognosis would be dependent upon the possibility of root amputation or hemisection being used to eliminate the furcation involvement and to create a maintainable situation on the remaining portion of the tooth. If this could not be done (because of root form or fusion), the prognosis would be hopeless unless GTR is feasible.

C If the tooth is nonrestorable because of the caries or fracture status of its remaining portion, it should be viewed as hopeless even if it is maintained and the periodontal treatment continues.

If the tooth is not endodontically involved or is endodontically treatable, the next step would be to determine whether it is treatable periodontally.

D Usually, a tooth with less than 50% LOA is treatable by frequent root planing (see Chapter 10) or with mucogingival osseous surgery (see Chapter 14). Teeth with more than 50% LOA usually will require more extensive treatment if they are to be saved.

E Some teeth with more than 50% LOA may be salvaged by GTR with highly predictable success. Teeth with Class II or III furcation involvement (see Chapter 30) may be treatable. Most Class II furcation involvements with greater than 3 mm of horizontal loss into the furca but not "through-and-through" problems are good candidates for GTR. Teeth with Class III furcation involvements may be treatable by GTR or by root amputation, hemisection, or a tunnel operation. If the roots are fused too far apically or are apically fused, such approaches cannot be used, and the tooth should be regarded as hopeless. Teeth with three-walled defects, even of severe depth, will routinely regenerate if the defect is narrow, no more than 1 mm horizontally from tooth to crest of bone. If the three-walled defects are wider, GTR can be expected to be routinely successful. Teeth with a two-walled infrabony crater can be successfully treated by GTR unless their roots are less than 1 mm apart or the proximal furcas are too severely involved to be instrumented owing to restricted access, in which case they should be regarded as hopeless unless root amputation, hemisection, or extraction of one of the involved teeth makes the defect on the remaining tooth treatable. A tooth with more than 50% LOA that is not amenable to GTR today may still be maintained if it can be splinted to other less involved teeth. If such splinting is not possible, the tooth should be regarded as hopeless.

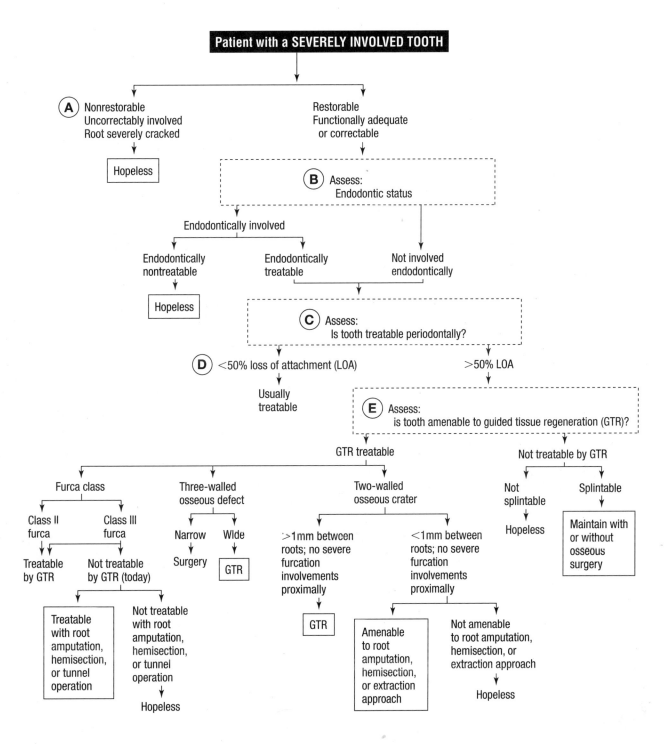

References

Corn H, Marks MA: Strategic extractions in periodontal therapy, *Dent Clin North Am* 13:817, 1969.

Eakle WJ, Maxwell EH, Braly BV: Fractures of posterior teeth in adults, *J Am Dent Assoc* 112:215, 1986.

Everett FG, Stern IB: When is tooth mobility an indication for extraction? *Dent Clin North Am* 13:791, 1969.

Maxwell EH, Braly BV: Incomplete root fracture: predictions and prevention, *Cal Dent Assoc J* 5:51, 1977.

Schluger S, Yuodelis R, Page RC, Johnson RH: *Periodontal diseases*, ed 2, Philadelphia, 1990, Lea & Febiger, p 341.

4 Periodontal Reasons to Extract a Tooth

Walter B. Hall

When a patient with a complex dental problem has a periodontally badly involved tooth, one with 50% or more loss of attachment (LOA), a decision must be made regarding the consequences of extracting the tooth. Assessment of the value of the individual tooth to the overall treatment plan is the first step in deciding whether to extract or to attempt to retain the tooth.

A If the tooth has no critical importance to the overall treatment plan, it should be extracted rather than maintained because it may compromise the success of the overall restorative plan.

B If the tooth is critically important to the overall treatment plan, how the tooth would be used in that plan must be determined. If it will not be a critical abutment tooth, extraction may be the best option. If it might add to the likelihood of success of the treatment plan, its retention would not compromise other critical teeth, and a "strategic retreat" (should it fail) is planned, surgical treatment may be a valid approach. Maintenance with a poor-to-hopeless prognosis may be considered if its retention does not jeopardize the overall plan or the chances for retaining it for a significant portion of the patient's remaining life seem good.

C If the tooth is a critical abutment, the chances of treating it periodontally with reasonable likelihood of retaining it for a significant period should be assessed. If the prognosis does not appear good, the possibility of replacing the tooth with an implant should be considered. If this cannot be done because of the anatomy of the area (see Chapter 36) or because the patient is unable or unwilling to consider an implant, the tooth should be extracted and a removable prosthetic replacement plan devised.

D If the tooth can be treated periodontally with a reasonable chance of maintaining it for a significant time, a decision should be made on the need for splinting before surgery. If needed, temporary or provisional splinting should be performed before surgery.

E If splinting is not needed, the possibility of successful regeneration of lost attachment should be considered. If guided tissue regeneration (GTR) can be performed predictably (see Chapter 22), it should be done and its success evaluated after 6 months. If the tooth is not amenable to GTR, the tooth has a guarded prognosis and may be treated by other surgical means; the success of the procedure should be evaluated 2 to 6 months later. If treatment is successful in improving the prognosis of the tooth, restoration may be instituted at this time. If the tooth's prognosis does not merit its inclusion in the plan at the times of reevaluation, it should be extracted and an alternative plan instituted.

References

Hall WB: Periodontal preparation of the mouth for restoration, *Dent Clin North Am* 24:195, 1980.

Hall WB: Removal of third molars: a periodontal viewpoint. In McDonald RE, Hart WC, Gilmore HW, Middleton RA, editors: *Current therapy in dentistry*, St Louis, 1980, Mosby, p 225.

Laskin DM: Evaluation of the third molar problems, *J Am Dent Assoc* 82:824, 1971.

Schluger S, Yuodelis R, Page RC, Johnson RH: *Periodontal diseases*, ed 2, Philadelphia, 1989, Lea & Febiger, p 346.

Sorrin S, Burman LR: A study of cases not amenable to periodontal therapy, *J Am Dent Assoc* 31:204, 1944.

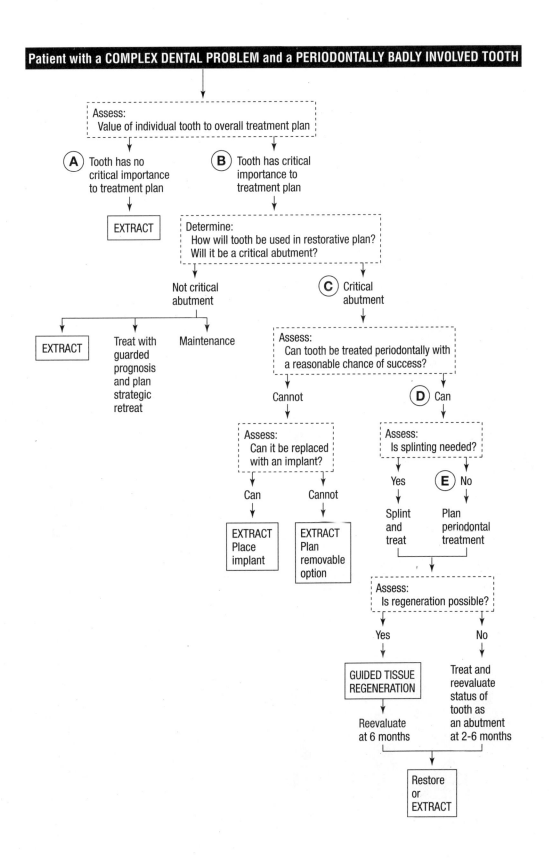

Patient with a COMPLEX DENTAL PROBLEM and a PERIODONTALLY BADLY INVOLVED TOOTH

Assess:
Value of individual tooth to overall treatment plan

(A) Tooth has no critical importance to treatment plan

EXTRACT

(B) Tooth has critical importance to treatment plan

Determine:
How will tooth be used in restorative plan?
Will it be a critical abutment?

Not critical abutment

EXTRACT

Treat with guarded prognosis and plan strategic retreat

Maintenance

(C) Critical abutment

Assess:
Can tooth be treated periodontally with a reasonable chance of success?

Cannot

Assess:
Can it be replaced with an implant?

Can

EXTRACT
Place implant

Cannot

EXTRACT
Plan removable option

(D) Can

Assess:
Is splinting needed?

Yes

Splint and treat

(E) No

Plan periodontal treatment

Assess:
Is regeneration possible?

Yes

GUIDED TISSUE REGENERATION

Reevaluate at 6 months

No

Treat and reevaluate status of tooth as an abutment at 2-6 months

Restore or EXTRACT

5 Cracked Tooth Syndrome

Walter B. Hall

When a patient with a periodontal problem complains of pain localized to one tooth, especially if this is triggered by heavy function, investigate the possibility that the tooth may be cracked (Figs. 5-1 to 5-3). If a tooth is cracked superficially, the symptoms may be controlled by crowning that tooth. Selective grinding may be helpful temporarily, but fractures tend to spread within teeth, making crowning the safest long-term solution to controlling these problems. If the crack is symptomatic, it may be extending to involve the pulp. If the crack is deep already, endodontics may be helpful. If the tooth has been treated endodontically and now is symptomatic, the crack may be affecting the periodontal ligament. When a crack is contiguous with a deep pocket, the prognosis for the tooth is guarded at best, and therapy should be planned with this in mind.

A When a tooth with a periodontal pocket is painful, an endodontic involvement must be ruled out before proceeding with any periodontal surgery. Whether or not the tooth is vital or nonvital to electrical pulp testing or to hot and cold, new periapical radiographs should be obtained and evaluated for evidence of periapical radiolucencies. They should be evaluated visually and with a fiberoptic light source for cracks. The fiberoptic light will stop at the plane of a crack where the light is refracted, and no glow of light will extend to other parts of the tooth if the crack extends to the pulp. If an intraoral television system is available, this device may visualize the crack even better (Fig. 5-4). The tooth should be tapped and pressed in various directions against each cusp in an attempt to elicit the sharp, brief twinge of pain that is symptomatic of a cracked tooth.

B If a symptomatic tooth tests vital, a radiograph may still suggest an endodontic problem. If no evidence of a crack (either visual or symptomatic) can be elicited, use selective grinding to minimize trauma. The tooth should be observed for several months to determine that symptoms have disappeared before any periodontal surgery is undertaken. If evidence of a crack can be elicited, an

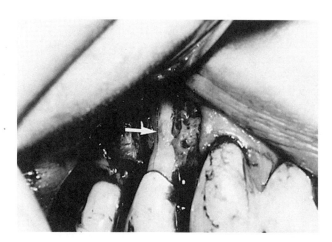

Fig. 5-1 An endodontically treated first premolar with a vertical crack and a resulting deep periodontal defect.

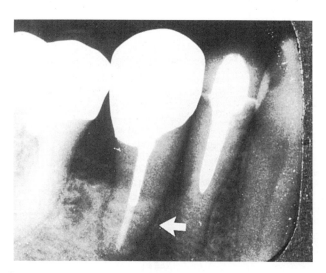

Fig. 5-2 Vertical periodontal defect resulting from a cracked tooth.

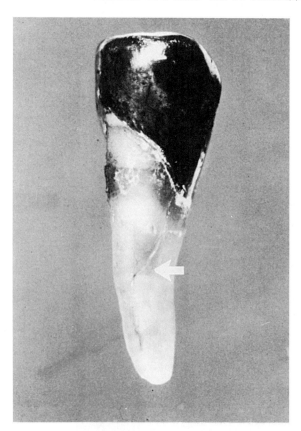

Fig. 5-3 Spiral fracture.

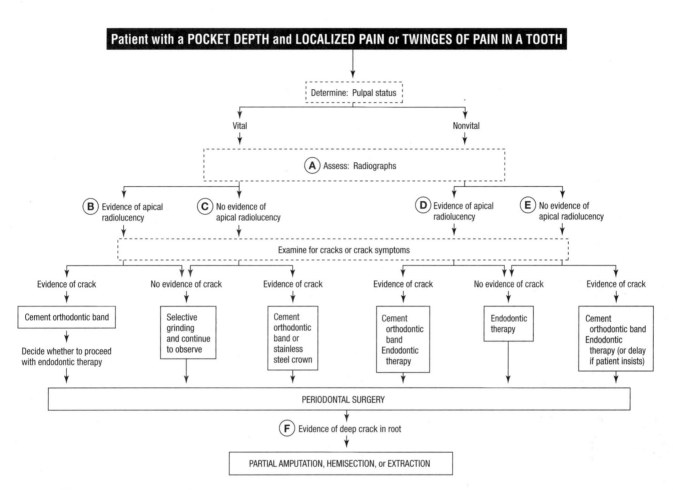

Patient with a POCKET DEPTH and LOCALIZED PAIN or TWINGES OF PAIN IN A TOOTH

Determine: Pulpal status

Vital — Nonvital

A Assess: Radiographs

B Evidence of apical radiolucency | **C** No evidence of apical radiolucency | **D** Evidence of apical radiolucency | **E** No evidence of apical radiolucency

Examine for cracks or crack symptoms

Evidence of crack | No evidence of crack | Evidence of crack | Evidence of crack | No evidence of crack | Evidence of crack

Cement orthodontic band → Decide whether to proceed with endodontic therapy | Selective grinding and continue to observe | Cement orthodontic band or stainless steel crown | Cement orthodontic band Endodontic therapy | Endodontic therapy | Cement orthodontic band Endodontic therapy (or delay if patient insists)

PERIODONTAL SURGERY

F Evidence of deep crack in root

PARTIAL AMPUTATION, HEMISECTION, or EXTRACTION

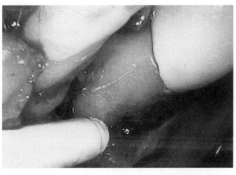

Fig. 5-4 Intraoral fiberoptic video picture of a tooth with a clearly visible vertical crack.

orthodontic band should be cemented to minimize the likelihood of the crack's spreading. The dentist and patient should decide together either to perform endodontic therapy promptly or to "wait and see" whether symptoms subside before undertaking any periodontal surgery.

C If a symptomatic tooth tests vital and has no evidence of periapical radiolucency, examine it for cracks or crack symptoms. If no evidence of a crack is elicited, use selective grinding and observation for several months before any periodontal procedures are undertaken. If evidence of a crack can be elicited, cement an orthodontic band or stainless steel crown to minimize fracture spread before any periodontal surgery.

D If a symptomatic tooth tests nonvital, this may be confirmed by a radiographic periapical radiolucency. If so, examine the tooth for cracks. If no evidence of a crack can be elicited, complete endodontic treatment promptly before any periodontal surgery is undertaken. If evidence of a crack is found, cement an orthodontic band to its crown to minimize fracture spreading. A decision by the dentist and patient to initiate endodontic treatment promptly or to "wait and see" should be agreed upon by both. If symptoms do not subside, endodontics should be undertaken before any periodontal surgery. If symptoms subside, periodontal surgery could be undertaken with full recognition that an endodontic flair up could be precipitated, necessitating prompt treatment.

E If a symptomatic tooth tests nonvital and radiographic evidence of a periapical radiolucency is not found, evaluate the tooth for evidence of a crack. If no evidence of a crack can be elicited, the tooth should be treated endodontically before any periodontal surgery is performed. If evidence of a crack can be elicited, cement an orthodontic band to the crown and perform endodontic treatment before any periodontal surgery is undertaken.

F When periodontal treatment is undertaken in any of these situations, a crack extending down the root where attachment has been lost may become visible. Once the area has been débrided, use the fiberoptic light source or intraoral television to search for cracks. If a deep crack is found, the tooth may have to be extracted or possibly one root of a multirooted tooth may be amputated (in maxillary molars) or the tooth hemisected (in mandibular molars). If a patient elects not to have such a tooth extracted, the dentist should carefully document the patient's choice and the advice that keeping the tooth is risky.

References

Cameron CE: The cracked tooth syndrome: additional findings, *J Am Dent Assoc* 93:971, 1976.

Eahle WS, Maxwell EH, Braly BV: Fractures of posterior teeth in adults, *J Am Dent Assoc* 112:215, 1986.

Hiatt WH: Incomplete crown-root fracture, *J Periodontol* 44:369, 1973.

Maxwell EH, Braly BV: Incomplete tooth fracture: prediction and prevention, *Cal Dent Assoc J* 5:51, 1977.

Ritchey B, Mendenhall R, Orban B: Pulpitis resulting from incomplete tooth fracture, *Oral Surg Oral Med Oral Pathol* 10:665, 1957.

6 When to Use Microbial Tests for Specific Periodontal Pathogens in Diagnosis and Treatment Planning

Mariano Sanz, Michael G. Newman

The etiologic role of specific bacteria in destructive periodontal diseases is established. Although many of the microorganisms found in deep periodontal pockets are part of the resident oral flora, a limited number of bacterial species are considered as etiologically relevant. These bacteria, so called periodontal pathogens, fulfill well-defined etiology criteria (Haffajjee and Socransky, 1994) that include: (1) association between the pathogen and presence of disease, (2) elimination of the pathogen after therapy or in absence of disease, (3) cause of a specific host response against the pathogen, (4) the presence of well-defined virulence factors, and (5) the presence of disease when the pathogen is inoculated in animal models. Only three species, *Actinobacillus actinomycetemcomitans, Porphyromonas gingivalis,* and *Bacteroides forsythus,* clearly fulfill these criteria and are considered true periodontal pathogens. There are also a limited number of bacteria that partially fulfill Socransky's criteria and are considered to be etiologically relevant. These include: *Prevotella intermedia, Fusobacterium nucleatum, Campylobacter rectus, Eikenella corrodens, Peptostreptococcus micros, Selenomonas* sp., *Eubacterium* sp., spirochetes, and *S. intermedius.* Therefore the detection of these potential periodontal pathogens may have an important role in the diagnosis and treatment of certain forms of periodontal diseases.

In treating complex dental problems with a periodontal component, types of periodontitis that have severe or rapid onset or do not respond well to conventional periodontal therapy, are significant determinants of treatment planning. Clinical measurements, radiographic evaluation, and monitoring for progression of disease must be assessed to determine whether microbial tests can be useful. In many such cases these tests determine the type and magnitude of the entire treatment plan. The following factors are applicable to all patients.

A The age of the patient may determine the potential usefulness of microbial tests. In early-onset periodontitis, when periodontal disease is usually severe, identification of specific pathogens such as *A. actinomycetemcomitans* or *P. gingivalis* is often valuable information that can be used to guide treatment. Elimination of these and other periodontopathic bacteria through adequate periodontal or antimicrobial therapy can be associated with improved clinical outcomes and a better periodontal prognosis.

B In adult forms of periodontitis, the severity of the problem is assessed clinically and radiographically. For individual adults, the future course of the disease can be anticipated by knowing whether the patient is either a heavy smoker (greater than 20-pack years) or has a genetic predisposition to severe disease. Heavy smokers have a 4.2 times greater risk of severe disease, and those who have the IL 1 genetic predisposition have an 18.9 times greater risk for severe disease.

C Less severe adult patients, or genotype negative individuals, should be treated by conventional periodontal therapy. In most of these cases the disease can be arrested and the patient successfully treated, however a minority of cases do not respond adequately to conventional methods despite good levels of oral hygiene. These patients may also benefit from microbial testing and, based on these results of testing, use of microbially-targeted periodontal therapy.

D In adult patients, it is also important to assess their systemic health status. Patients with associated systemic disease may have an altered host response. Impaired healing, inability to tolerate certain treatments, potential drug interactions, or compromised immune systems may all cause opportunistic infections to appear in patients. In these patients, it is of increased importance to perform a microbial test to ensure that the appropriate antimicrobial therapy is prescribed.

References

Carranza FA, Newman MG: *Clinical periodontology,* ed 8, Philadelphia, 1996, WB Saunders, p 714.

Haffajjee A, Socransky SS: Microbial etiological agents of destructive periodontal diseases, *Periodontology 2000* 5:78, 1994.

Kornman KS, Crane A, Wang H-Y, di Giovine FS, Newman MG, Pirk FW, Wilson, Jr, TT, Higginbottom FL, Duff GW: The interleukin 1 genotype as a severity factor in adult periodontal disease, *J Clin Periodontol* 22:258, 1995.

Lang NP, Karring T: *Proceedings of the 1st European workshop in periodontology,* London, 1994, Quintessence Publishing.

Newman MG, editor: World workshop in clinical periodontics, *Ann Periodontol,* 1:84, 1996.

Van Winkelhoff AJ, Rams TE, Slots J: Systemic antibiotic therapy in periodontics, *Periodontology 2000* 10:45, 1996.

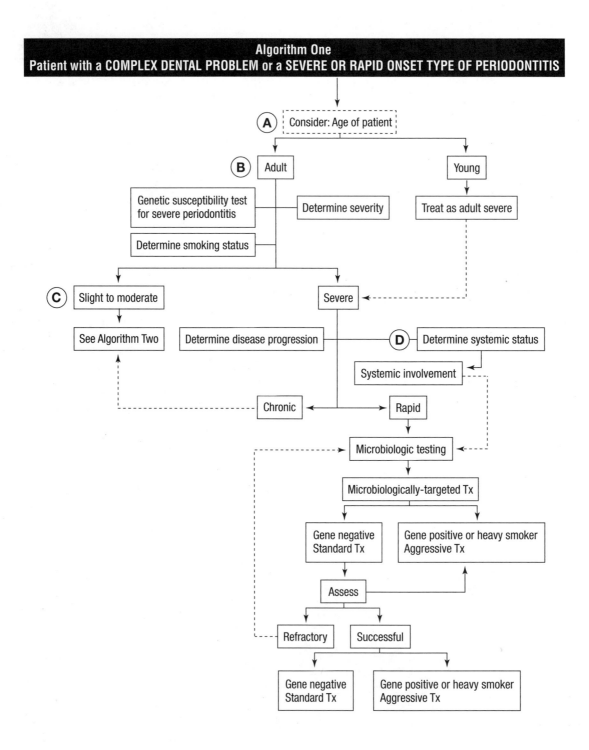

**Algorithm One
Patient with a COMPLEX DENTAL PROBLEM or a SEVERE OR RAPID ONSET TYPE OF PERIODONTITIS**

A · Consider: Age of patient

B · Adult

Young

Genetic susceptibility test for severe periodontitis

Determine severity

Treat as adult severe

Determine smoking status

C · Slight to moderate

Severe

See Algorithm Two

Determine disease progression

D · Determine systemic status

Systemic involvement

Chronic

Rapid

Microbiologic testing

Microbiologically-targeted Tx

Gene negative Standard Tx

Gene positive or heavy smoker Aggressive Tx

Assess

Refractory

Successful

Gene negative Standard Tx

Gene positive or heavy smoker Aggressive Tx

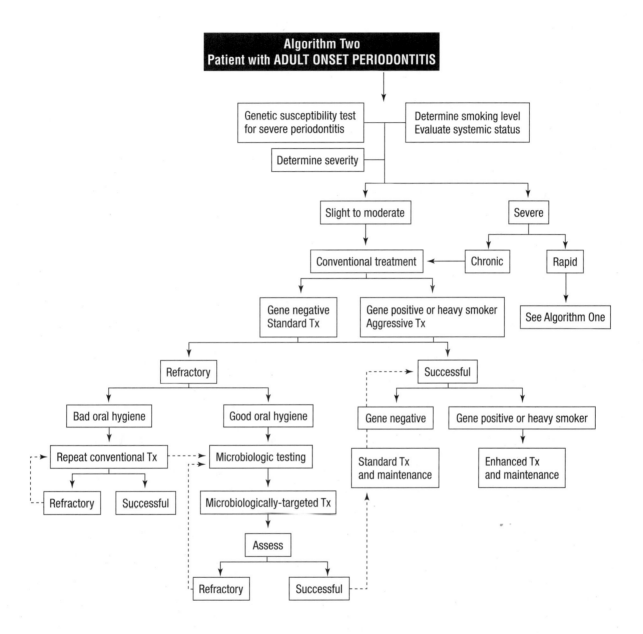

Algorithm Two
Patient with ADULT ONSET PERIODONTITIS

Genetic susceptibility test for severe periodontitis

Determine smoking level
Evaluate systemic status

Determine severity

Slight to moderate

Severe

Conventional treatment

Chronic

Rapid

See Algorithm One

Gene negative
Standard Tx

Gene positive or heavy smoker
Aggressive Tx

Refractory

Successful

Bad oral hygiene

Good oral hygiene

Gene negative

Gene positive or heavy smoker

Repeat conventional Tx

Microbiologic testing

Standard Tx
and maintenance

Enhanced Tx
and maintenance

Refractory

Successful

Microbiologically-targeted Tx

Assess

Refractory

Successful

7 Periodontally Compromised Potential Abutment Teeth

Walter B. Hall

One of the most complex decisions that a dentist must make regularly involves determining the adequacy of periodontally involved teeth to function as abutments in a restorative treatment plan. The dentist must decide by weighing the pros and cons of each of the many factors involved. The patient must be informed of, and able to cope with, various degrees of uncertainty in such complex decisions and must be able to afford the cost of the whole treatment plan before proceeding. If the patient elects not to proceed, the dentist must advise the patient of the probable consequences of this decision. Such complex situations require careful documentation.

A The status of the attachment of the potential abutment tooth is important. A tooth that has lost more than half of its attachment is a poor risk as an abutment; however, if that tooth has a narrow, three-walled osseous defect, it is a candidate for a bone regeneration procedure, and there is a reasonable likelihood of success sufficient to change the prognosis for the tooth. In situations in which guided tissue regeneration (GTR) has a strong probability of success (see Chapter 13) a tooth that would be a poor abutment can be converted to one that may make a good-to-excellent abutment (see Chapter 7). If this situation does not exist and the tooth has lost more than half of its support, it is unlikely to be a good abutment risk. If the tooth has moderate loss of attachment (LOA), it has a reasonable prognosis for successful use as an abutment. If it has little LOA, it is a good candidate.

B Root form is another important factor to assess. Several radiographs of the tooth can be used to give an important conceptualization of the form for the root (Fig. 7-1). Exploration of furcations on a multirooted tooth can provide useful information on its potential cleansability. Teeth with small or cone-shaped roots are poor abutments when compared with those with large roots (or flared ones on multirooted teeth). If a molar has a Class II furca involvement that is involved 3 mm or more horizontally, it is a good candidate for GTR with eventual use as an abutment (see Chapter 30). If a molar has a "through-and-through" involvement, GTR may be used, or root amputation or hemisection may make its remaining parts useful as an abutment if that approach can be afforded by the patient (see Chapter 72). A molar with minimal furcation involvement and flared roots, however, is a good abutment candidate, even where pocket elimination surgery is used.

C The status of the crown of the potential abutment area is important. If it is badly broken down, it is a poorer candidate than if it can be restored readily. Crown lengthening can improve the potential restorability of some poorer candidates (see Chapter 11).

D The pulpal status affects the potential of a tooth to be used as an abutment. If the tooth has been endodontically treated but either requires further treatment (i.e., apicoectomy) or retreatment or appears to have a cracked root, its usefulness as an abutment depends upon the likelihood of success of the additional treatment. If its root is cracked or it cannot be retreated, it is not a potential abutment. If the earlier endodontic procedure appears satisfactory, the tooth usually is a good potential abutment. If the tooth has an untreated pulpal problem, its potential for use as an abutment depends upon factors affecting the probability for successful endodontic treatment (i.e., accessibility of root canals, presence of pulp stones internal resorption). If it is treatable, it has good potential as an abutment. A tooth with a healthy pulp, however, is almost always a better abutment candidate than an endodontically treated one because endodontically treated teeth become more brittle and more susceptible to fractures.

E The alignment of a tooth affects its usefulness as an abutment. A significantly malposed tooth that cannot be orthodontically moved into good alignment is a poor potential abutment. Some periodontally involved teeth are good candidates for orthodontic movement (see Chapter 84) and can become fair-to-good candidates for use as abutments—but only at considerable cost to the patient in both time and money. A tooth already in normal or usual alignment is always a better candidate for use as an abutment.

F The number of other abutment teeth and their periodontal statuses affect the potential usability of the tooth in question as an abutment. If few other potential abutments are present and they have much LOA, the tooth in question is a poorer candidate for use as an abutment

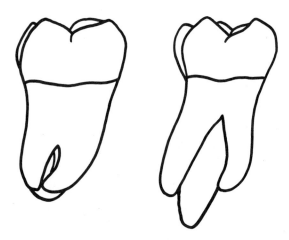

Fig. 7-1 Molar teeth may have fused or spread roots. The spread type usually provides better support as an abutment for a restoration replacing a missing tooth.

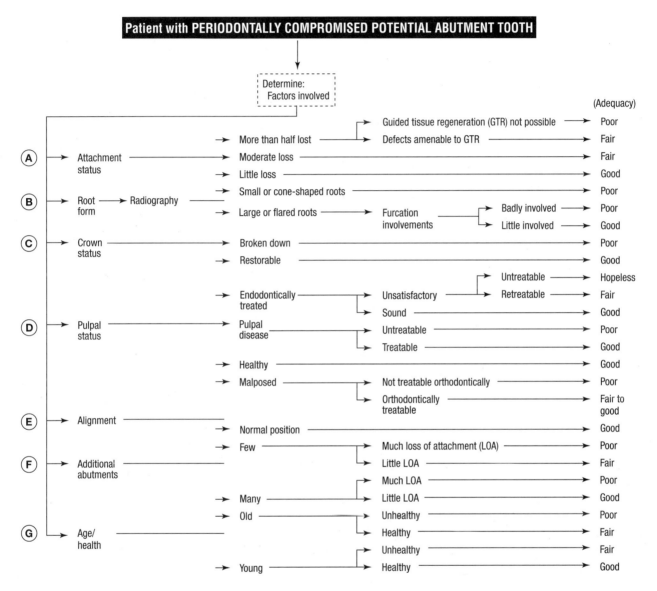

Patient with PERIODONTALLY COMPROMISED POTENTIAL ABUTMENT TOOTH

because more will be demanded of it. If the other potential abutments, though few in number, have little LOA, the tooth in question is a better candidate. If there are many additional potential abutment teeth, but all or most have significant LOA, the potential use of the tooth in question is less. If the other potential abutments have little LOA, the tooth in question has better possibilities for use as an abutment, too.

G Other factors (such as plaque removal skills of the patient and regularity of dental care) must be weighed by the dentist and patient in deciding upon the potential for a periodontally involved tooth to be used as an abutment. Age and health are two essential factors, however. In one sense, older patients have poorer prognoses than younger ones because their healing capabilities may be lower. In

another sense, older patients have better prognoses in that their teeth and dental work will not have to last as long, on the average. A potential abutment tooth that is periodontically compromised in an otherwise healthy patient has a better prognosis, in general, than one in an unhealthy mouth.

References

Grant DA, Stern IB, Listgarten MA: *Periodontics*, ed 6, St Louis, 1988, Mosby, p 982.

Hall WB: Periodontal preparation of the mouth for restoration, *Dent Clin North Am* 24:195, 1980.

Schluger S, Yuodelis R, Page RC, Johnson RH: *Periodontal diseases*, ed 2, Philadelphia, 1990, Lea & Febiger, p 341.

8 Canine Disclusion (Cuspid Rise) Versus Group Function

Walter B. Hall

After deciding that a patient may benefit from selective grinding during treatment for periodontitis, the dentist must decide whether establishing canine disclusion (cuspid rise) or group function in lateral movements is best (Fig. 8-1). Canine disclusion may provide a "cuspid-protected" occlusion in parafunctional lateral movements that may be beneficial if posterior teeth have significant bone loss, considerable occlusal wear, or a number of cracks, and if the patient clenches or grinds the teeth. Canine disclusion is preferable to group function of weakened posterior teeth, but if canine disclusion cannot be used, group function is preferred.

A If both of the canines on one side have little or no bone loss, the first condition for the use of canine disclusion is met. The radiographs should show normal-sized maxillary and mandibular canine roots that have little radiographic evidence of bone loss. Probing should confirm that little attachment has been lost. If the canines occlude in lateral movement toward the side in which these teeth are present, canine rise is a logical objective of selective grinding. If sound maxillary and mandibular canines do not occlude in lateral movement, canine disclusion cannot be attained. If the posterior teeth have little or no bone loss, group function is the objective. If the posterior teeth have moderate-to-severe bone loss and

the canines are essentially sound, however, either the canines may be restored to create canine disclusion or orthodontic positioning of the canines can be used to permit it.

B If one or both canines on one side have moderate-to-severe bone loss and guided tissue regeneration is not feasible, canine disclusion should be discarded as an objective. If the adjacent posterior teeth have little or no bone loss, group function is the logical objective. If the adjacent posterior teeth have moderate-to-severe bone loss, as do the canines, splinting to distribute the loading more evenly is necessary, especially if the teeth are mobile. If mobility is minimal, selective grinding to "smooth out" the group function may suffice.

References

D'Amico A: The canine teeth: normal functional relation of the natural teeth of man, *Cal Dent Assoc J* 26:6, 1958.

Grant DA, Stern JB, Listgarten MA: *Periodontics,* ed 6, St Louis, 1988, Mosby, p. 986.

Ramfjord S, Ash MM: Occlusion, ed 3, Philadelphia, 1983, WB Saunders, p 370.

Schluger S et al: *Periodontal diseases,* ed 2, Philadelphia, 1990, Lea & Febiger, p 392.

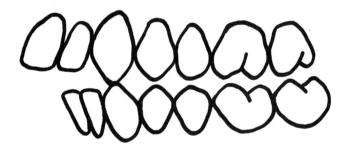

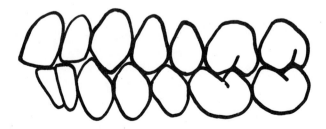

Fig. 8-1 Working side contacts in canine disclusion or group function situations.

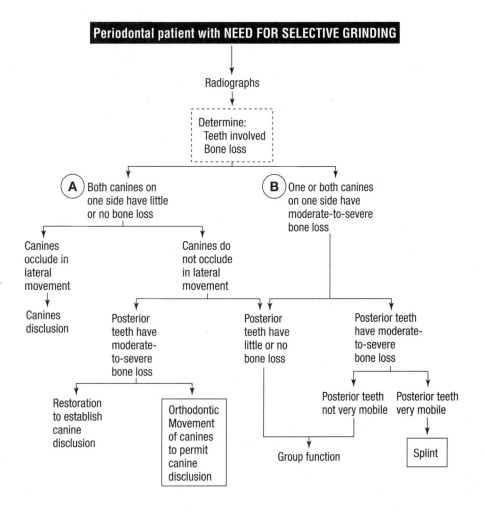

Periodontal patient with NEED FOR SELECTIVE GRINDING

Radiographs

Determine:
Teeth involved
Bone loss

A Both canines on one side have little or no bone loss

B One or both canines on one side have moderate-to-severe bone loss

Canines occlude in lateral movement

Canines do not occlude in lateral movement

Canines disclusion

Posterior teeth have moderate-to-severe bone loss

Posterior teeth have little or no bone loss

Posterior teeth have moderate-to-severe bone loss

Restoration to establish canine disclusion

Orthodontic Movement of canines to permit canine disclusion

Posterior teeth not very mobile

Posterior teeth very mobile

Group function

Splint

9 Periodontal Reasons to Extract a Tooth

Walter B. Hall

A patient planning to have orthodontic treatment may have pure mucogingival problems. The dentist must be aware of the relationship of, and the correct sequence of treatment for, orthodontic and pure mucogingival problems when they occur together. Orthodontic and pure mucogingival problems are related but not in a cause-and-effect manner. A tooth that erupts in a position in which it is in prominent version and thus prone to occlusal trauma also is likely to have erupted with minimal attached gingiva. Both relate to the prominent eruptive position of the tooth. Understanding this relationship is most important in planning therapy for these cases.

A The age of the patient is important in deciding how to sequence treatment of combined pure mucogingival and orthodontic problems.

B If the patient is young and has an overbite-overjet discrepancy that would prohibit free gingival grafting on mandibular incisors before some orthodontic movement, proceed with some orthodontic treatment in the maxillary arch before grafting so that the graft will not be disturbed directly when the patient closes in centric relation. Adult patients in good periodontal health should be treated similarly.

C If a young patient does not have an overbite-overjet problem but has pure mucogingival problems, consider grafting before beginning orthodontic treatment because the placement of a vestibular arch wire will alter the approach to brushing. Once the arch wire is placed, the brush must be placed apical to it and turned so that the bristle tips contact the teeth and gingiva. The bulkiness of the brush thus positioned causes the lip to press the brush heavily against prominent root surfaces, especially in areas where frena are present. These are the same areas where minimal attached gingiva is present. The patient who struggles to meet the orthodontist's requests for especially good daily plaque removal may injure these predisposed areas, producing recession (Fig. 9-1). The dentist and patient (and patient's parent when appropriate) should consider gingival grafting of mandibular incisors and all canines that have pure mucogingival problems before initiating orthodontic treatment. The option of waiting and augmenting gingiva if recession does occur must be considered with the patient (and parent), as well. The same considerations apply for those patients who have completed correction of overbite-overjet discrepancy problems.

D In the case of predisposed first premolars, another aspect of orthodontic therapy must be considered. In many orthodontic cases four first premolars or two first premolars are extracted to create space for realigning the remaining teeth. If a first premolar has minimal attached gingiva and is going to be extracted, there is no pure mucogingival concern. If the predisposed tooth is to be retained, however, the need to consider grafting before orthodontic treatment is most important.

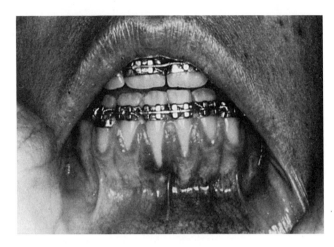

Fig. 9-1 A patient with inadequate attached gingiva who has experienced recession since starting orthodontic treatment.

E If periodontitis is present in the adult patient, the status of potential anchor teeth must be considered first. A molar with a definite furcation involvement or worse (see Chapter 25) is not a good candidate to serve as an anchor tooth without prior successful guided tissue regeneration (GTR). Some teeth with deep pockets may have to be extracted; others may be moved into, or out of, periodontal defects once inflammation is controlled and prognoses have improved (see Chapter 84). If both mucogingival-osseous and pure mucogingival problems exist, their surgical treatment usually is accomplished at the same time. In adult orthodontic cases for which one objective is to move a periodontally involved tooth into, or out of, an osseous defect before surgery, the pure mucogingival grafting procedure may be delayed until after the orthodontic goal has been achieved. Then the mucogingival-osseous and pure mucogingival problems can be treated together surgically, if indicated. If there are no periodontitis problems requiring uprighting and no orthodontic movement into defects is being considered, mucogingival-osseous surgery may be used to correct pocketing and pure mucogingival problems by using an apically positioned flap (see Chapter 23). If problems amenable to GTR exist (see Chapter 14), that approach should be used before or after orthodontic treatment as a means of regaining lost attachment and creating a greater band of attached gingiva.

References

American Academy of Periodontology: *World workshop in clinical periodontics*, VII-2, Chicago, 1989, American Academy of Periodontology.

Boyd RL: Mucogingival considerations and their relationship to orthodontics, *J Periodontol* 49:67, 1978.

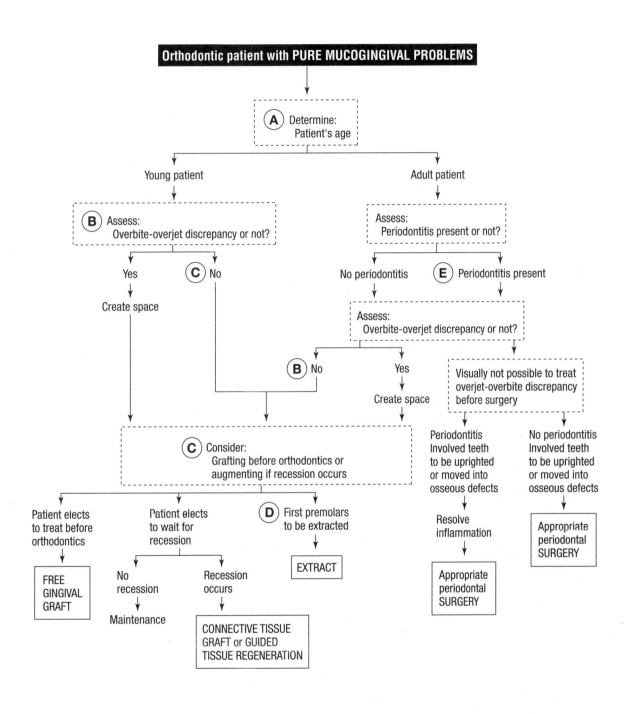

Orthodontic patient with PURE MUCOGINGIVAL PROBLEMS

(A) Determine: Patient's age

Young patient — Adult patient

(B) Assess: Overbite-overjet discrepancy or not?

Assess: Periodontitis present or not?

Yes — (C) No

No periodontitis — (E) Periodontitis present

Create space

Assess: Overbite-overjet discrepancy or not?

(B) No — Yes

Create space

Visually not possible to treat overjet-overbite discrepancy before surgery

(C) Consider: Grafting before orthodontics or augmenting if recession occurs

Periodontitis Involved teeth to be uprighted or moved into osseous defects

No periodontitis Involved teeth to be uprighted or moved into osseous defects

Patient elects to treat before orthodontics

Patient elects to wait for recession

(D) First premolars to be extracted

Resolve inflammation

Appropriate periodontal SURGERY

FREE GINGIVAL GRAFT

No recession — Recession occurs

EXTRACT

Appropriate periodontal SURGERY

Maintenance

CONNECTIVE TISSUE GRAFT or GUIDED TISSUE REGENERATION

Coatoam GW, Behrents RG, Bissada NF: The width of traumatized gingiva during orthodontic treatment, *J Periodontol* 52:307, 1981.

Dorfman HS: Mucogingival changes resulting from mandibular incisor tooth movement, *Am J Orthod* 74:286, 1978.

Hall WB: Can attached gingiva be increased non-surgically? *Quint Int* 13:455, 1982.

Hall WB: Pure mucogingival problems, Berlin, 1984, Quintessence Publishing, p 44.

10 Surgery Versus Repetitive Root Planing

Walter B. Hall

At the time of initial therapy evaluation, the dentist's greatest concern is what to do next. Broadly speaking, the options are either to perform surgery or to maintain the patient with repetitive root planing. The dentist must decide which approach is indicated, but the patient may choose the less desirable option because of reasons such as cost or fear. Esthetics become a concern when surgery appears to be a reasonable option in maxillary anterior regions. If the probable esthetic result of surgery, even if therapeutically successful, would be unacceptable to the patient, maintenance would be a reasonable alternative. In cases in which deep and inaccessible pocket areas would remain, the use of a modified Widman flap might be desirable to permit thorough, one-time débridement while minimizing postsurgical exposure. Guided tissue regeneration (GTR) may permit significant restitution of periodontal support on teeth with deep osseous defects, making surgery of this type a most desirable option for a patient with localized severe defects.

A. The success of the patient's plaque control efforts is an important factor in deciding whether a patient "merits" surgery. A patient who has been unable to clean the supragingival portions of the teeth before surgery is not a promising candidate to do well with the more tortuous and minimally accessible areas usually exposed following osseous surgery. A patient who has cleaned these areas well is more likely to be able and willing to clean well after surgery. GTR, if even partially successful, facilitates plaque control.

B. A patient who has removed plaque well usually has a good response to initial therapy. Signs of inflammation are diminished or absent, and both pocket depth and mobility are likely to have decreased. Occasionally, however, a patient's response is not good, despite efforts at plaque control; surgery for such a patient is less likely to be a good alternative.

C. If the patient's response is exceptionally good and there are no requirements that surgery be considered (i.e., pure mucogingival problems, inadequate crown exposure), the patient may do well with only repetitive planing rather than surgery. If there are restorative demands for a surgical approach, however, one should consider surgery unless the esthetic results would be unacceptable. If the patient has localized areas that are inaccessible to root planing, consider surgery. When esthetic concerns exist, a modified Widman flap approach would permit a one-time, thorough débridement, which might be advantageous. A patient whose response has been poor despite good plaque control is not a promising candidate for surgery. If there are no restorative demands for surgery, place the patient on regular, repetitive root planing and evaluation. If there are demanding restorative needs, consider surgery unless the esthetic results would be unacceptable. If the patient has localized, inaccessible pockets, GTR could be used when esthetics are important, or pocket elimination might be used when esthetics are not a concern or will be minimized restoratively.

D. A patient who has done poorly in plaque control usually shows a poor response to initial therapy; occasionally, however, good responses may occur despite the patient's efforts. For patients with poor oral hygiene who exhibit a good response, surgery may be a practical option if they have restorative needs that would be benefited by surgery. If a patient has no esthetic concerns, surgery can be done. If the patient does have esthetic concerns, maintenance root planing would be a better choice. If the patient with good response but poor oral hygiene has no demanding restorative needs, repeat root planing and evaluate again. If the patient has localized, inaccessible pocket areas, GTR is indicated. If the patient with poor oral hygiene has the expected poor response to initial therapy and no restorative requirements to consider surgery, the patient should be placed on a repetitive root planing program. If there are restorative requirements, repeat the root planing, and evaluate again to see if the patient can improve the oral hygiene to a level at which surgery would be reasonable. If the patient has localized, inaccessible pocket areas, a modified Widman flap approach would permit a one-time, thorough débridement. GTR could be considered, despite poor oral hygiene, if a very critical tooth can be saved and the patient recognizes the risk of continued poor oral hygiene.

References

Carranza FA, Newman MG: *Clinical periodontology,* ed 8, Philadelphia, 1996, WB Saunders, p 565.

Genco RJ, Goldman HM, Cohen DW: *Contemporary periodontics,* St Louis, 1991, Mosby, p 626.

Grant DA, Stern IB, Listgarten MA: *Periodontics,* St Louis, 1988, Mosby, p 602.

Hall WB: Clinical practice. In Steele PF, editor: *Dimensions in dental hygiene,* ed 3, Philadelphia, 1982, Lea & Febiger, p 143.

Hall WB: Procedure code 452: eliminating the confusion, *Cal Dent Assoc J* 11:33, 1983.

Lindhe J: *Textbook of clinical periodontology,* ed 2, Copenhagen, 1989, Munksgaard, p 328.

Schluger S, Yuodelis R, Page RC, Johnson RH: *Periodontal diseases,* ed 2, Philadelphia, 1990, Lea & Febiger, p 461.

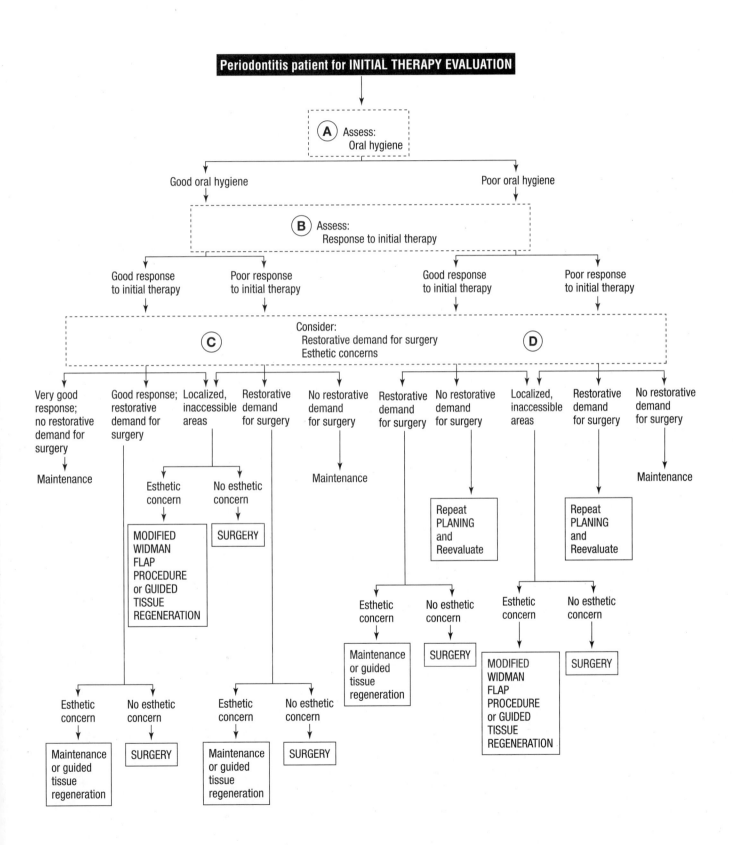

Periodontitis patient for INITIAL THERAPY EVALUATION

(A) Assess:
Oral hygiene

Good oral hygiene — Poor oral hygiene

(B) Assess:
Response to initial therapy

Good response to initial therapy — Poor response to initial therapy — Good response to initial therapy — Poor response to initial therapy

Consider:
(C) Restorative demand for surgery
Esthetic concerns (D)

Very good response; no restorative demand for surgery → Maintenance

Good response; restorative demand for surgery

Localized, inaccessible areas

Restorative demand for surgery

No restorative demand for surgery → Maintenance

Restorative demand for surgery

No restorative demand for surgery

Localized, inaccessible areas

Restorative demand for surgery

No restorative demand for surgery → Maintenance

Esthetic concern → MODIFIED WIDMAN FLAP PROCEDURE or GUIDED TISSUE REGENERATION

No esthetic concern → SURGERY

Esthetic concern → Maintenance or guided tissue regeneration

No esthetic concern → SURGERY

Esthetic concern → Maintenance or guided tissue regeneration

No esthetic concern → SURGERY

Repeat PLANING and Reevaluate

Esthetic concern → Maintenance or guided tissue regeneration

No esthetic concern → SURGERY

Repeat PLANING and Reevaluate

Esthetic concern → MODIFIED WIDMAN FLAP PROCEDURE or GUIDED TISSUE REGENERATION

No esthetic concern → SURGERY

11 Crown Lengthening

Gretchen J. Bruce

One of the challenges of restorative dentistry is the restoration of teeth with insufficient supragingival tooth height. Clinical situations that require a decision to restore or extract such a tooth are (1) short clinical crown, (2) root caries, (3) subgingival perforation, (4) fractures, (5) retrograde wear, and (6) altered passive eruption. When teeth are restored without regard to biologic principles, the periodontium may develop increased probing depths, problems with respect to plaque control, and a swollen cyanotic appearance.

"Biologic width" has been described as the space occupied by the junctional epithelium and connective tissue attachment coronal to the alveolar crest. This dimension is approximately 2.04 mm (Fig. 11-1). An additional millimeter representing the gingival crevice is combined with this measurement to permit the establishment of an intracrevicular restorative margin. A minimum of 3 mm of sound tooth above the alveolar process is necessary when a restoration or fracture approaches the crest. Violation of the biologic width may result in inflammation and bone resorption. Surgical procedures such as gingivectomy or an apically positioned flap, with or without osseous surgery, can be used to increase the clinical crown length.

A If the tooth is periodontally healthy or affected by gingivitis only, crown lengthening can be accomplished by gingivectomy in cases of excess gingiva. This approach requires an adequate zone of attached gingiva with at least 3 mm of sound tooth structure above the crest of bone. If a mucogingival problem is anticipated, use an apically positioned flap to retain the available gingiva and lengthen the crown. A gingival graft is performed in instances of inadequate attached gingiva. Electrosurgery and laser surgery alternatives to gingivectomy are quick methods for reducing excess tissue and providing good control of hemorrhage. Care must be taken to avoid contact with the bone. Even minimal contact with the alveolar process may result in overcoagulation, necrosis, resorption of bone, and gingival recession. In most circumstances use of a blade is preferable to an electrosurgical unit.

B If the bone level is normal with no root fracture, use mucogingival-osseous surgery to expose at least 3 mm of root beyond where the restorative margin is to be placed. If a fracture extends into the root, assess the prognosis, accessibility, and esthetics before proceeding further. When a fracture compromises a furcation, root resection is a consideration. Extraction is indicated if the fracture extends to the middle third of the root or jeopardizes the support of the adjacent teeth. If the root fracture occurs in a more favorable location (coronal to the mid-third of the root), use a gingival flap with osseous surgery to expose the fractured area and create the appropriate biologic width.

Maintenance of esthetics is a major concern in the anterior and premolar region. Orthodontics–forced eruption is a treatment option that allows extrusion of the fractured tooth with conservation of bone and esthetics; however, the need for periodontal surgery is not necessarily elimi-

nated. Minimal crown lengthening to correct osseous contours then may be confined to the extruded tooth.

C If the tooth requiring crown lengthening has a periodontal pocket, assess the degree of periodontal support, strategic value, and prognosis using the same criteria as in section *B*. Initial therapy is performed before crown lengthening to decrease inflammation and promote better hemostasis. Use mucogingival-osseous surgery to eliminate the periodontal pockets and to lengthen the crown.

References

Johnson RH: Lengthening clinical crowns, *J Am Dent Assoc* 121(4):473, 1990.

Pruthi VK: Surgical crown lengthening in periodontics, *J Can Dent Assoc* 53(12):911, 1987.

Rosenberg M, Kay H, Keough B, Holt R: *Periodontal and prosthetic management for advanced cases*, 1988, Quintessence, p 164.

Sivers JE, Johnson GK: Periodontal and restorative considerations for crown lengthening, *Quintessence Int* 16(12):833, 1985.

Wagenberg B, Eskow R, Langer B: Exposing adequate tooth structure for restorative dentistry, *Int J Periodontol Restor Dent* 9(5):323, 1989.

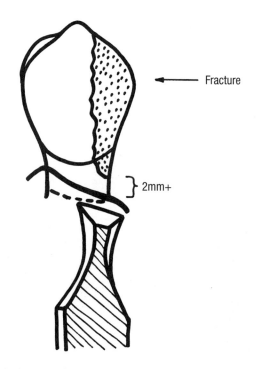

Fig. 11-1 When crown lengthening is performed where a fracture extends apically into the root, bone must be removed to expose a minimum of 2 mm of root structure apical to the ultimate margin of the restoration.

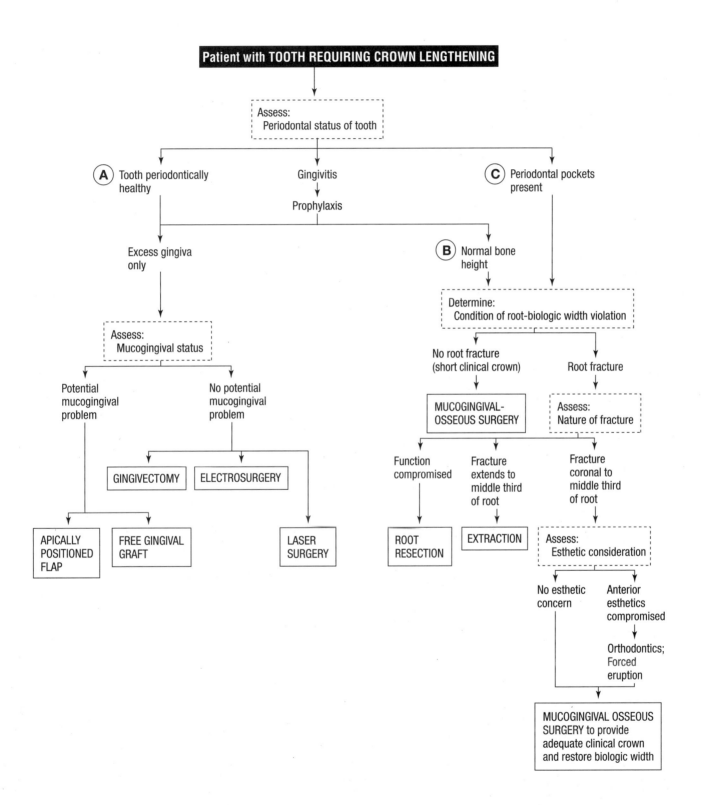

Patient with TOOTH REQUIRING CROWN LENGTHENING

Assess:
Periodontal status of tooth

Ⓐ Tooth periodontically healthy

Gingivitis

Prophylaxis

Ⓒ Periodontal pockets present

Excess gingiva only

Ⓑ Normal bone height

Determine:
Condition of root-biologic width violation

Assess:
Mucogingival status

No root fracture (short clinical crown)

Root fracture

Potential mucogingival problem

No potential mucogingival problem

MUCOGINGIVAL-OSSEOUS SURGERY

Assess:
Nature of fracture

GINGIVECTOMY

ELECTROSURGERY

Function compromised

Fracture extends to middle third of root

Fracture coronal to middle third of root

APICALLY POSITIONED FLAP

FREE GINGIVAL GRAFT

LASER SURGERY

ROOT RESECTION

EXTRACTION

Assess:
Esthetic consideration

No esthetic concern

Anterior esthetics compromised

Orthodontics;
Forced eruption

MUCOGINGIVAL OSSEOUS SURGERY to provide adequate clinical crown and restore biologic width

12 Ridge Augmentation

Walter B. Hall

Periodontal surgery may be used to improve the form of an edentulous ridge to permit placement of a more esthetic and cleansable fixed bridge on an area where the loss of teeth has resulted in a grossly deficient or grotesquely malformed ridge. Such problems often occur when teeth are lost as a result of an accident or severe abscessing. Fracture of a cortical plate during extraction of teeth also may create such defects. Either the ridge may be contorted in a manner that makes the bridge construction difficult to clean and unesthetic, or the ridge may be so deficient that excessively long, ugly pontics have been or would be placed in fixed-bridge construction.

A When a patient has an edentulous ridge area, both adequate proximal and distal abutment teeth must be present for ridge augmentation to be necessary.

B Determine the amenability of the site for fixed-bridge construction. If the edentulous area is too lengthy to permit fixed-bridge construction, either a removable denture approach or implants are indicated (see Chapters 104-108).

C If the edentulous site is amenable to fixed-bridge construction, assess the form of the edentulous ridge area to decide whether an esthetic, cleansable bridge can be constructed using the ridge as it exists. If no augmentation is needed, but the ridge is grotesquely formed or so shaped that an esthetic, cleansable bridge cannot be constructed, one should consider ridge augmentation.

D The approach to ridge augmentation is selected by assessing the availability of a soft-tissue donor site for an inlay or overlay approach. If a good donor site is available, that approach may be offered to the patient. When no adequate donor site is available, only the guided bone augmentation (GBA) approach or use of a synthetic bone fill material can be presented to the patient.

References

Abrams L: Augmentation of the deformed residual edentulous ridge for fixed prosthesis, *Compend Contin Ed Dent* 1:205, 1980.

Bohannon HM: Studies in the alterations in vestibular depth 1: complete denudation, *J Periodontol* 33:120, 1962.

Carranza FA, Jr: *Glickman's clinical periodontology*, ed 7, Philadelphia, 1990, WB Saunders, p 890.

Genco RJ, Goldman HM, Cohen DW: *Contemporary periodontics*, St Louis, 1990, Mosby, p 643.

Hall WB: *Pure mucogingival problems*, Berlin, 1984, Quintessence Publishing, p 161.

Lindhe J: *Textbook of clinical periodontology*, ed 2, Copenhagen, 1989, Munksgaard, p 433.

Rosenberg S: Use of ceramic material for augmentation of the practically edentulous ridge: a case report, *Compend Contin Ed Dent* 77(3):20, 1984.

Schluger S, Yuodelis R, Page RC, Johnson RH: *Periodontal diseases*, ed 2, Philadelphia, 1990, Lea & Febiger, pp 563, 632.

Seibert J: Reconstruction of the deformed partially edentulous ridges using full-thickness overlay grafts, Parts 1 and 2, *Compend Contin Ed Dent* 4(5):437, 1983.

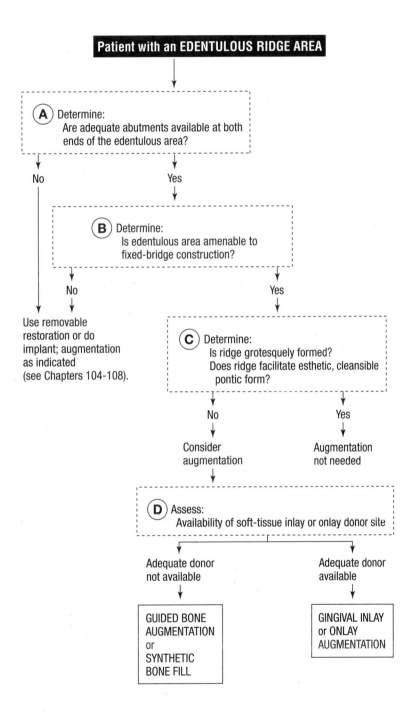

Patient with an EDENTULOUS RIDGE AREA

(A) Determine:
Are adequate abutments available at both ends of the edentulous area?

No

Yes

(B) Determine:
Is edentulous area amenable to fixed-bridge construction?

No

Yes

Use removable restoration or do implant; augmentation as indicated (see Chapters 104-108).

(C) Determine:
Is ridge grotesquely formed?
Does ridge facilitate esthetic, cleansible pontic form?

No

Yes

Consider augmentation

Augmentation not needed

(D) Assess:
Availability of soft-tissue inlay or onlay donor site

Adequate donor not available

Adequate donor available

GUIDED BONE AUGMENTATION or SYNTHETIC BONE FILL

GINGIVAL INLAY or ONLAY AUGMENTATION

13 A New Classification of Indications for Periodontal Surgery and Augmentation

Walter B. Hall

The Miller Classification for determining the level of root coverage attainable in treating marginal recession was devised before the use of guided tissue regeneration (GTR) as it is performed today. The height of interproximal papillae and bone no longer limits the amount of new attachment and root coverage that can be obtained, as was the case with the Miller Classification. A newer system of classification of indications for periodontal surgery and augmentation was presented by Hall et al. (1996).

Complete root coverage with new connective tissue attachment is the primary objective of pure mucogingival and mucogingival-osseous surgery. Though it may not always be attainable, this objective guides the selection of the most desirable surgical approach.

A The first decision to be made when surgery is being considered for a patient is whether root exposure is present or not. If root exposure is present, whether the problem is a pure mucogingival one, a mucogingival-osseous one only, or a combined one, a decision must be made to determine whether full root coverage is a reasonable goal or not.

B If no root exposure has occurred, the need for more attached gingiva should be evaluated. If more attached gingiva is desirable, in the opinion of the dentist, a free gingival graft is the treatment of choice before other treatment. If more attached gingiva is not needed, periodontal maintenance should suffice.

C If root exposure has occurred, a decision must be made whether the problem is one of recession only or a combined pure mucogingival–mucogingival-osseous problem.

D If the problem is a pure mucogingival one only, the adequacy of a donor site for a connective tissue graft must be determined (see Chapter 20). If an adequate donor site is present, a connective tissue graft would be the treatment of choice for teeth with single surface areas of recession. In all other cases GTR would be the treatment of choice.

E If the problem is a combined pure mucogingival–mucogingival-osseous one or only a mucogingival-osseous one, the extent of the loss of attachment (LOA) must be assessed. If the loss does not include interproximal attachment loss and if an adequate donor site for a connective tissue graft is present, a connective tissue graft would be the treatment of choice. If not, GTR should be used.

If interproximal LOA has occurred, the extent of the LOA would determine what surgery is appropriate. If the LOA is minimal (e.g., less than 5 mm), mucogingival-osseous surgery for pocket elimination may be used. If the LOA is greater than 5 mm on any surface of a tooth, GTR is the better approach, and full root coverage may be attempted.

Reference

Hall WB, Sutter M, Williams C, Lundergan WP: Aktueller Stand der Andwendung Freler Gingiva Transplantate, *Phillip Journal* 12:457, 1996.

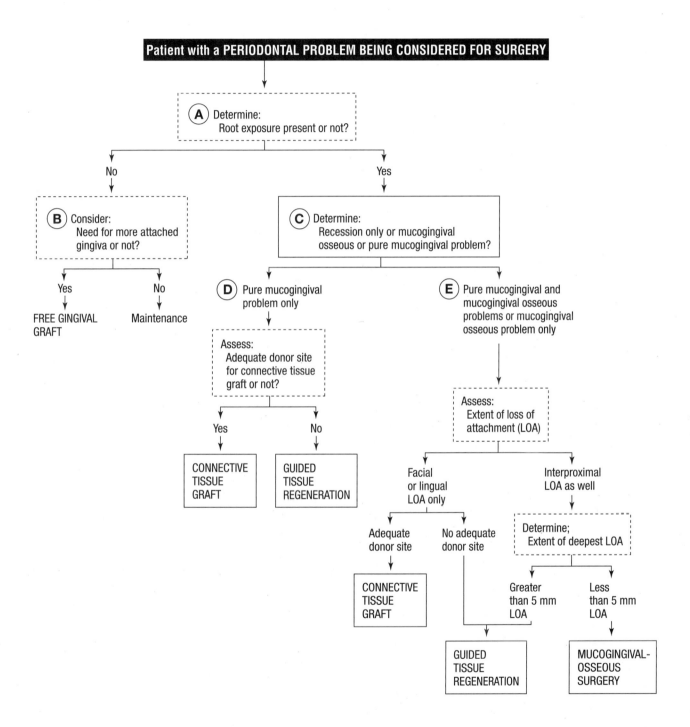

Patient with a PERIODONTAL PROBLEM BEING CONSIDERED FOR SURGERY

A Determine:
Root exposure present or not?

No — **B** Consider:
Need for more attached gingiva or not?

Yes → FREE GINGIVAL GRAFT

No → Maintenance

Yes — **C** Determine:
Recession only or mucogingival osseous or pure mucogingival problem?

D Pure mucogingival problem only

Assess:
Adequate donor site for connective tissue graft or not?

Yes → CONNECTIVE TISSUE GRAFT

No → GUIDED TISSUE REGENERATION

E Pure mucogingival and mucogingival osseous problems or mucogingival osseous problem only

Assess:
Extent of loss of attachment (LOA)

Facial or lingual LOA only

Adequate donor site → CONNECTIVE TISSUE GRAFT

No adequate donor site → GUIDED TISSUE REGENERATION

Interproximal LOA as well

Determine;
Extent of deepest LOA

Greater than 5 mm LOA → GUIDED TISSUE REGENERATION

Less than 5 mm LOA → MUCOGINGIVAL-OSSEOUS SURGERY

14   Selection of the Appropriate Periodontal Surgical Technique

Walter B. Hall

When the dentist has determined that periodontal surgery is needed, the dentist or the periodontist (to whom the patient may have been referred) must first determine the nature of the surgical problem. Periodontal surgical procedures may be regarded as pure mucogingival procedures or mucogingival-osseous procedures, though the differences are less important today.

A Pure mucogingival procedures include those whose goals are gingival augmentation when inadequate attached gingiva is present. These procedures (from most versatile to least) include the following: connective tissue graft, free gingival graft, and pedicle grafts. Ridge augmentation is a procedure used when no teeth are involved to create a better formed, more esthetic ridge on which to construct a bridge.

    The dentist must determine if recession is active in an area of inadequate gingiva, especially areas with less than 2 mm of attached gingiva. Earlier recordings, photographs, and old study models are more useful than the patient's impressions, though the latter may be all that is available. If recession can be documented as active, gingival augmentation is recommended. If not, the dentist must decide whether proposed orthodontic or restorative treatment will require gingival augmentation. If so, the advantages and disadvantages of augmentation must be discussed with the patient and the decisions recorded. If the patient decides not to undergo gingival augmentation or if the orthodontic or restorative treatment does not indicate an immediate need for augmentation, the area may be maintained, and a connective tissue graft for root coverage should be used should recession occur.

B Mucogingival-osseous problems are the result of inflammatory periodontal diseases that cause loss of attachment (LOA), bone loss, and pocket formation. These problems demand attention before restoration orthodontics. Regaining lost attachment therefore is the most desirable goal.

C Guided tissue regeneration (GTR) has been demonstrated to be a predictable procedure in the presence of Class II furcas more than 3 mm horizontally between roots (less so for through and through or Class III furcas) three-walled osseous defects, or osseous craters (two-walled defects). Recently, extensive procedures using partially impermeable membranes have been used successfully for treating multiple tooth problems, even those with horizontal bone loss (see Chapter 13).

D When lesions not predictably amenable to new attachment procedures are present, the dentist should consider the desirability of pocket elimination surgery before restoration or orthodontics (or in some cases [e.g., uprighting a tooth] after orthodontics). GTR often is a better alternative. If the problem is relatively minimal and the patient demonstrably motivated, maintenance with frequent root planing alone may be the best option.

References

Carranza FA, Jr, Newman MG: *Clinical periodontology*, ed 8, Philadelphia, 1996, WB Saunders, p 568.

Genco RJ, Goldman HM, Cohen DW: *Contemporary periodontics*, St Louis, 1990, Mosby, p 554.

Pihlstrom BL, Ortiz Campos C, McHugh RB: A randomized four year study of periodontal therapy, *J Periodontol* 52:227, 1981.

Waerhaug J: Healing of the dento-epithelial junction following subgingival plaque control, I: as observed on extracted teeth, *J Periodontol* 49:119, 1978.

Weeks PR: Pros and cons of periodontal pocket elimination procedures, *J West Soc Periodontol* 28:4, 1980.

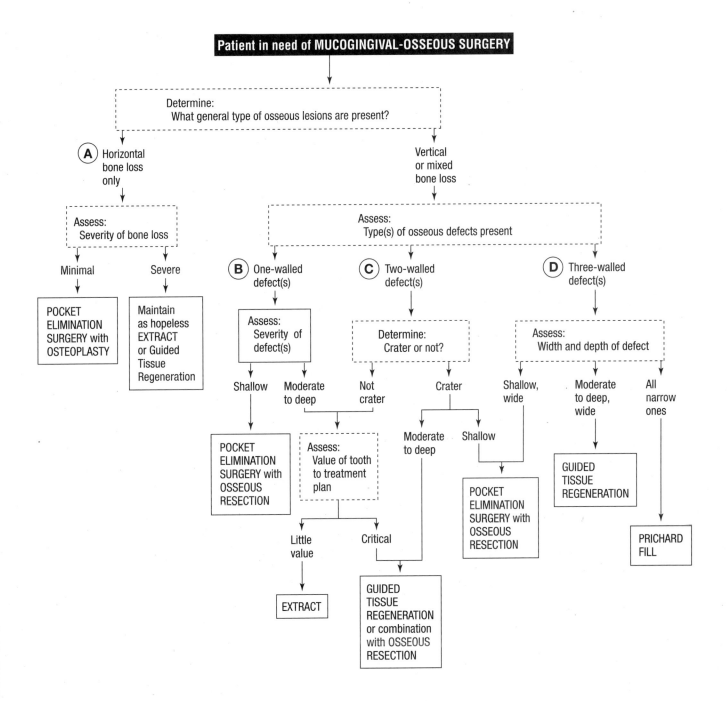

Patient in need of MUCOGINGIVAL-OSSEOUS SURGERY

Determine:
What general type of osseous lesions are present?

(A) Horizontal bone loss only

Vertical or mixed bone loss

Assess:
Severity of bone loss

Minimal

Severe

POCKET ELIMINATION SURGERY with OSTEOPLASTY

Maintain as hopeless EXTRACT or Guided Tissue Regeneration

Assess:
Type(s) of osseous defects present

(B) One-walled defect(s)

(C) Two-walled defect(s)

(D) Three-walled defect(s)

Assess:
Severity of defect(s)

Determine:
Crater or not?

Assess:
Width and depth of defect

Shallow

Moderate to deep

Not crater

Crater

Shallow, wide

Moderate to deep, wide

All narrow ones

POCKET ELIMINATION SURGERY with OSSEOUS RESECTION

Assess:
Value of tooth to treatment plan

Moderate to deep

Shallow

GUIDED TISSUE REGENERATION

PRICHARD FILL

POCKET ELIMINATION SURGERY with OSSEOUS RESECTION

Little value

Critical

EXTRACT

GUIDED TISSUE REGENERATION or combination with OSSEOUS RESECTION

15 Selection of Gingival Augmentation Techniques

Walter B. Hall

Once the dentist has decided that a pure mucogingival problem requires surgery to create a broader band of attached gingiva, he or she must select the technique most likely to achieve root coverage to just a broader band of attached gingiva to minimize recession in the future. Esthetics is a prime consideration. Connective tissue grafts and guided tissue regeneration (GTR) are more likely than free grafts to be successful in covering roots and in matching the appearance of adjacent gingiva. Connective tissue grafting appears to be more successful than GTR; therefore, when root coverage is a goal, the connective tissue graft would be preferable to any other graft procedure unless an adequately thick donor site for a connective tissue graft is not available (see Chapter 20).

A If no esthetic concern exists, as in most mandibular areas and in maxillary molar areas, a free gingival graft is one option. When no existing recession requiring root coverage is present, a free gingival graft is an acceptable choice and the easiest to perform.

Free gingival grafts for covering roots have long been a desired goal of those practicing pure mucogingival surgery. The predictability to success with a free graft is not great, although claims for improved success through root treatment either with citric acid or complicated suturing have been made. The free gingival graft usually is taken from the palate, which may be of a markedly different color than the gingiva adjacent to the area to be grafted. If the donor gingiva is such a poor color match that it would create a greater esthetic problem, if successful, than that created by root exposure, free gingival grafting for root coverage should not be attempted.

B When no esthetic problem exists but recession requiring root coverage is present, or when an esthetic problem is present, use a connective tissue graft or GTR for root coverage and for a better esthetic result. Connective tissue grafts have a higher degree of predictability of success; therefore, they are the first choice.

C The optimal donor site for a connective tissue graft is in the anterior palatal area beneath the rugae, where the submucosa is fatty (see Chapter 20).

If finger pressure suggests that little spongy feeling submucosa is present, GTR as a means of augmentation and root coverage is the alternative choice.

If the area of recession is so great (more than 6-8 mm from cementoenamel junction to bony crest) that excision of a donor specimen would extend close to the anterior palatine artery, GTR would be a safer approach.

References

American Academy of Periodontology: *World workshop in clinical periodontics,* VII-1, Chicago, 1989, American Academy of Periodontology.

Carranza FA, Newman NG: *Glickman's clinical periodontology,* ed 8, Philadelphia, 1996, WB Saunders, p 651.

Hall WB: *Pure mucogingival problems,* Berlin, 1984, Quintessence Publishing, p 129.

Langer B, Langer L: Subepithelial connective tissue graft technique for root coverage, *J Periodontol* 56:175, 1983.

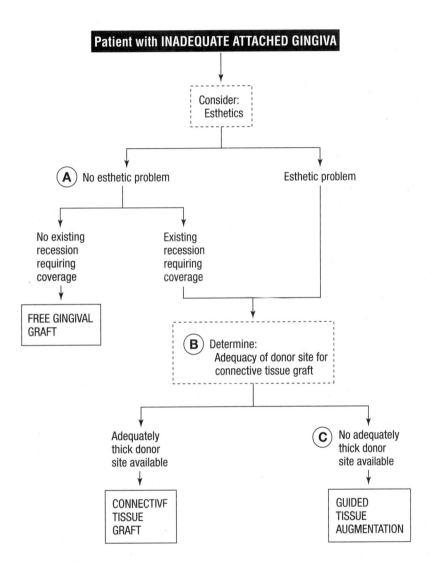

16 Recession Treatment: Root Coverage or Not?

Walter B. Hall

When a patient has a root or roots exposed by recession, esthetic needs and restorative needs will influence the need for grafting in an interrelated manner. If the band of attached gingiva is adequate but recession has occurred, surgery may be used to cover exposed roots if an esthetic need exists. If no esthetic need exists and no restoration affecting the gingival margin is planned, maintenance care alone should suffice. If the band of attached gingiva is "inadequate" in the dentist's opinion, the need to consider gingival augmentation will be greater (Figs. 16-1 to 16-5).

A First decide upon the "adequacy" of the existing band of attached gingiva. An adequate band of attached gingiva is one that is sufficient to prevent initial or continued recession. The patient's age, other dental needs, oral hygiene status, caries activity, and esthetic needs are some factors that would influence a decision that treatment is needed if

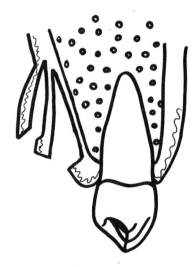

Fig. 16-3 Sagittal view of the palatal donor area showing the primary and secondary (CT graft) flaps prepared.

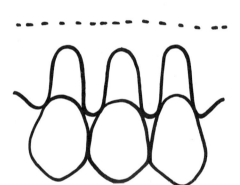

Fig. 16-1 Multiple adjacent teeth with gingival recession to be treated with a subepithelial connective tissue (CT) graft.

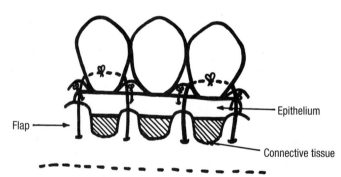

Fig. 16-4 The CT graft sutured to cover the exposed roots with the receptor site flap positioned covering much of the connective tissue.

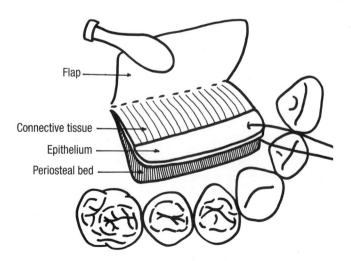

Fig. 16-2 Obtaining the CT graft from the palate.

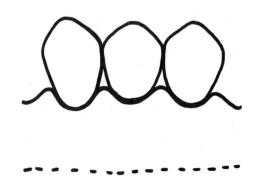

Fig. 16-5 The healed area with full root coverage.

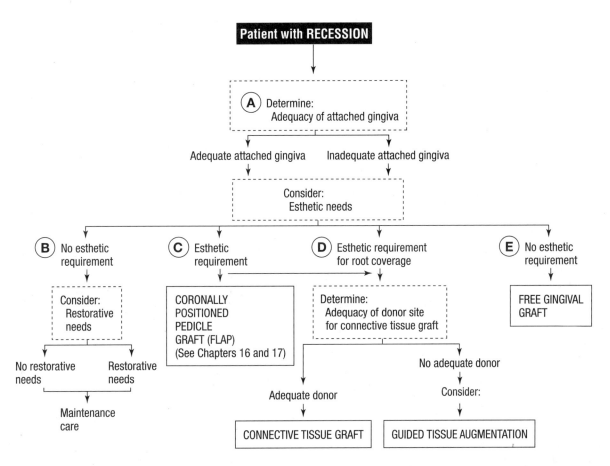

the band of attached gingiva is judged to be "inadequate" to prevent initial or continued recession when resolving the overall dental needs.

B If the patient has an adequate band of attached gingiva and no cosmetic or esthetic need to attempt root coverage exists, dental health should be maintainable with regular oral hygiene effort, prophylaxis, or root planing. If a Class V restoration or crown is to be placed, the apical margin of the restoration may be placed within the gingival crevice without strong likelihood of inducing recession. The apical margin could also be placed supragingivally if root sensitivity, caries activity, or other restorative requirements (i.e., crown length) are not involved; then maintenance care should suffice.

C If root coverage is necessary to meet esthetic or cosmetic goals and the band of attached gingiva on the tooth or teeth with recession is adequate, a coronally positioned pedicle graft or flap (see Chapters 16 and 17) could be the treatment; however, a connective tissue graft or guided tissue regeneration (GTR) should be considered (see Chapter 34).

D When an inadequate band of attached gingiva is present and esthetic, cosmetic, or restorative goals indicate the need for root coverage, a connective tissue graft would be most

appropriate, particularly if several teeth are involved. If an adequate donor site for such a graft is not available (i.e., the donor site in the rugae area is insufficiently thick), then GTR would be the choice for augmentation (see Chapter 20).

E If the patient has "inadequate" attached gingiva to meet his or her dental needs without initiating recession or further recession and no cosmetic or esthetic concern exists, a free gingival graft without root coverage may be performed for stabilization.

References

Allen EP, Miller PD: Coronal positioning of existing gingiva: short-term results in the treatment of shallow marginal tissue recession, *J Periodontol* 60:316, 1989.

American Academy of Periodontology: *World workshop in clinical periodontics,* VII-1, Chicago, 1989, American Academy of Periodontology.

Hall WB: *Pure mucogingival problems,* Berlin, 1984, Quintessence Publishing, p 61.

Langer B, Langer L: Subepithelial connective tissue graft technique for root coverage, *J Periodontol* 56:715, 1985.

Matter J: Free gingival grafts for the treatment of gingival recession—a review of some techniques, *J Clin Periodontol* 9:103, 1980.

17 Root Coverage in Cases of Localized Recession

Giovan Paolo Pini-Prato, Carlo Clauser, Pierpaolo Cortellini

A Miller has divided recession into four classes according to the prognosis for healing in terms of root coverage. Classes I and II (no loss of interdental bone or soft tissue) allow for complete root coverage; the reference point for measuring the recession is the cementoenamel junction. Classes III and IV (with interdental bone loss) do not guarantee 100% root coverage (see Chapter 13).

B Guided tissue regeneration (GTR) proved to be effective in the treatment of recession in animals (Cortellini et al, 1991) and in humans (Tinti and Vincenzi, 1990; Cortellini et al, 1991; Tinti et al, 1992). A comparative study was made on GTR in the treatment of gingival recession (Pini-Prato et al).

   Mucogingival surgery (MGS) yielded better results in terms of root coverage when the recession was less than 4.98 mm (Fig. 17-1), whereas greater root coverage was achieved with membranes when the recession was deeper than 4.98 mm (Fig. 17-2). In either case the membrane procedure resulted in a significantly greater gain in clinical attachment and a reduction in probing depth.

C The 3-mm threshold was selected on the basis of the results obtained by Allen and Miller (1989). These results showed an average of 97.8% root coverage using coronally positioned flaps to treat shallow recessions when at least 3 mm of keratinized gingiva (KG) was available apical to the exposed root.

D A free gingival graft (FGG) may consist of connective tissue only or of both epithelial and connective tissue (Fig. 17-3). No comparative study has been published to assess the appropriateness of either technique; therefore the choice of graft type is left to the discretion of the individual clinician.

E GTR has been tested with no gingival augmentation, even when less than 1 mm of KG was present. The procedure requires designing a large and thick flap that can provide an abundant blood supply and be coronally positioned to cover the membrane entirely with no pulling. A slight increase in the amount of keratinized tissue is expected at the end of the treatment (Tinti et al, 1992; Pini-Prato et al), although a shallow vestibule may result, therefore a FGG before the regenerative procedure is advisable to prevent the reduction of the vestibule and to facilitate surgery.

F In cases of interdental bone loss, use the adjacent teeth as reference points. The area to be covered may be measured as the distance between the gingival margin (GM) of the

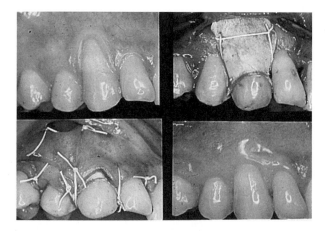

Fig. 17-2 Guided tissue regeneration procedure on a maxillary right canine with a 6-mm recession.

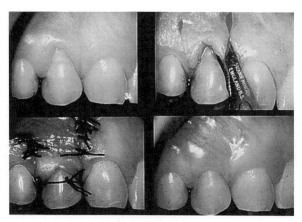

Fig. 17-1 A shallow recession (4 mm) on a maxillary right first premolar is treated by a coronally positioned flap. 3 mm of keratinized gingiva were available apical to the recession.

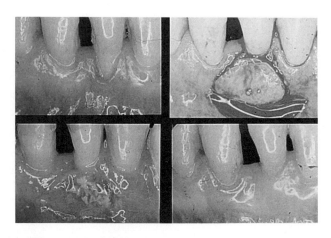

Fig. 17-3 A recession associated with interdental bone resorption is treated by a free gingival graft. The final level of the gingival margin is consistent with the adjacent teeth.

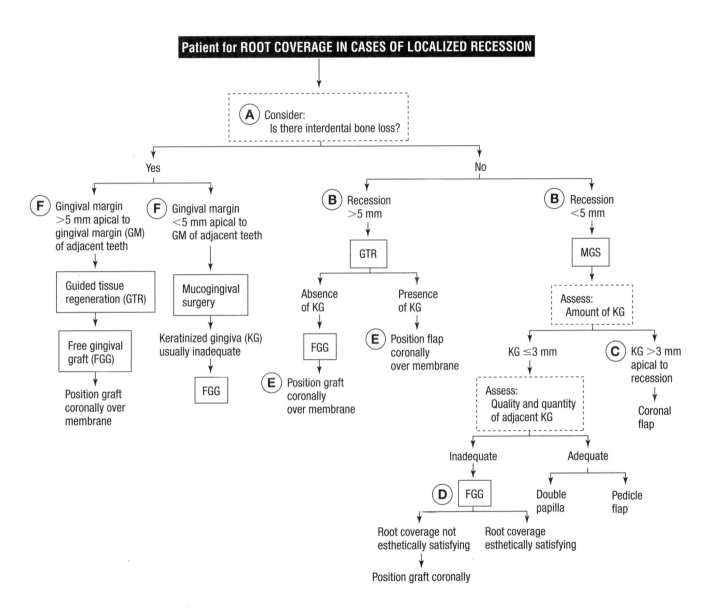

Patient for ROOT COVERAGE IN CASES OF LOCALIZED RECESSION

A Consider:
Is there interdental bone loss?

Yes — No

F Gingival margin >5 mm apical to gingival margin (GM) of adjacent teeth

F Gingival margin <5 mm apical to GM of adjacent teeth

B Recession >5 mm

B Recession <5 mm

Guided tissue regeneration (GTR)

Mucogingival surgery

GTR

MGS

Free gingival graft (FGG)

Keratinized gingiva (KG) usually inadequate

Absence of KG — Presence of KG

Assess: Amount of KG

Position graft coronally over membrane

FGG

FGG

E Position flap coronally over membrane

KG ≤3 mm — **C** KG >3 mm apical to recession

E Position graft coronally over membrane

Assess: Quality and quantity of adjacent KG

Coronal flap

Inadequate — Adequate

D FGG

Double papilla — Pedicle flap

Root coverage not esthetically satisfying — Root coverage esthetically satisfying

Position graft coronally

area to be treated and the line that connects the most apical levels of the GMs of the adjacent teeth. This may be considered the most coronal level able to be reached with a covering procedure.

References

Allen EP, Miller PD: Coronal positioning of existing gingiva: short-term results in the treatment of shallow marginal tissue recession, *J Periodontol* 60:316, 1989.

Cortellini P, De Sanctis M, Pini-Prato GP et al: Guided tissue regeneration procedure in the treatment of a bone dehiscence associated with a gingival recession: a case report, *Int J Periodont Restor Dent* 11(6):472, 1991.

Cortellini P, De Sanctis M, Pini-Prato GP, et al: Guided tissue regeneration procedure using a fibrin-fibronectin system in surgically induced recessions in dogs, *Int J Periodont Restor Dent* 11(6):151, 1991.

Miller PD: A classification of marginal tissue recession, *Int J Periodont Restor Dent* 5:9, 1985.

Pini-Prato GP, Tinti C, Vincenzi G et al: Guided tissue regeneration versus mucogingival surgery in the treatment of human buccal recessions, *J Periodontol* 63:919, 1992.

Tinti C, Vincenzi G: Il trattamento delle recessioni gengivali con la tecnica di "rigenerazione guidata dei tessuti" mediante membrane Gore-Tex (R), variante clinica, *Quintessence Int* 6:465, 1990.

Tinti C, Vincenzi G, Cortellini P et al: Guided tissue regeneration in the treatment of human facial recession: a twelve-case report, *J Periodontol* 63:554, 1992.

18 Restorative Plans and Gingival Grafting

Walter B. Hall

Upon determining that a tooth that is predisposed to recession by lack of adequate attached gingiva has restorative needs or is going to be used as an abutment, the dentist must decide whether grafting to increase the band of attached gingiva is indicated. The patient who elects not to proceed with a graft, when indicated, must be informed of the potential problems.

A If the predisposed tooth requires restoration, the type of restoration and its locale are most important. If the restoration is a Class V but is to be supragingival, there is no need to graft. If the Class V restoration is to be close to the gingival margin (GM) or subgingival, consider a graft. If the restoration is to be of any other class, grafting need not be considered.

B If the predisposed tooth requires a crown and the crown margins are to be supragingival, there is no need to graft; however, if the crown margin is to be placed at the GM or subgingivally, grafting is indicated because the diamond bur will cut soft tissue and tooth structure when carried subgingivally and will produce recession as a consequence of the soft-tissue curettage. If the entire crown of the tooth is to be visible and recession would expose a chamfer, the patient must be aware that not grafting is likely to result in a visible gold margin apical to the porcelain facing. Grafting beforehand is strongly encouraged because the *successful covering of such an exposed chamfer surgically after crown placement is exceedingly unlikely.*

C If the predisposed tooth is to become an abutment for a fixed bridge, consider grafting whether or not a subgingival margin will be placed in the area of inadequate attached gingiva because cleaning either under the pontic or between it and the tooth is likely to produce recession. If a three-quarter crown design is to be used, grafting should be considered but is not as essential as when a full-crown restoration is to be placed.

D If the predisposed tooth will serve as an abutment for a rest-proximal plate-I (RPI) bar-type removable partial denture, a graft should be placed sufficiently large enough that the entire I-bar will be over the gingiva. If this is not done, the patient who removes the partial denture by placing a fingernail under the apical end of the I-bar is likely to cause wounding and to induce recession (Fig. 18-1). A graft usually cannot be placed under an existing I-bar because the space is inadequate for a graft of sufficient thickness to be placed; therefore a new partial denture would have to be constructed following grafting.

E If the predisposed tooth is to be used as an abutment for an overdenture, much the same situation applies. If recession occurs (which is likely when a full denture is placed in the

area), the denture could be relieved and a graft placed, or the denture could be left out while the graft heals. In either case the graft is likely to be moved about and to fail. Instead, a large flange of acrylic must be cut away, the graft placed, and the overdenture rebased once healing is completed. The more advisable course would be to graft on any predisposed tooth before beginning the overdenture treatment. If a graft is to be placed for restorative reasons, the type to be used would involve considering the options among free gingival grafts, pedicle grafts, or connective tissue grafts (see Chapter 15).

References

American Academy of Periodontology: *World workshop in clinical periodontics,* VII-16, Chicago, 1989, American Academy of Periodontology.

Genco EJ, Goldman HM, Cohen DW: *Contemporary periodontics,* St Louis, 1990, Mosby, p 621.

Hall WB: Periodontal preparation of the mouth for restoration, *Dent Clin North Am* 24:195, 1980.

Hall WB: *Pure mucogingival problems,* Berlin, 1984, Quintessence Publishing, p 41.

Maynard JG, Wilson RD: Physiologic dimensions of the periodontium significant to the restorative dentist, *J Periodontol* 50:170, 1979.

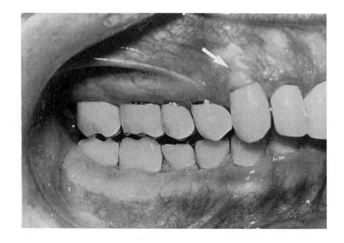

Fig. 18-1 Recession of 3 mm has occurred on the canine, which had inadequate attached gingiva, following crown placement.

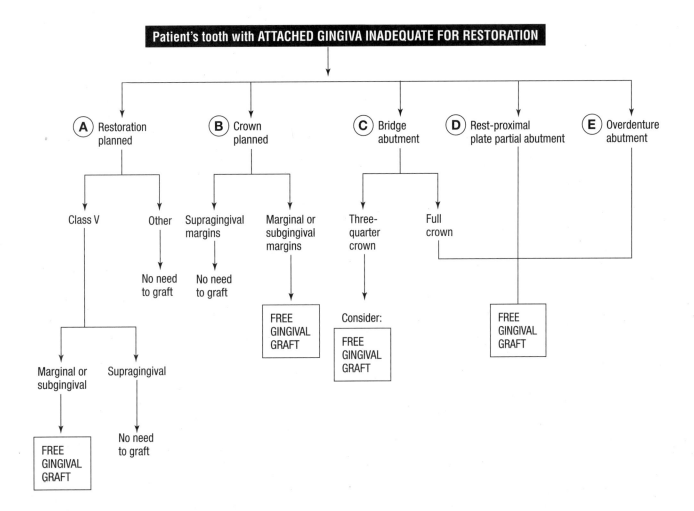

Patient's tooth with ATTACHED GINGIVA INADEQUATE FOR RESTORATION

(A) Restoration planned

Class V
- Marginal or subgingival → FREE GINGIVAL GRAFT
- Supragingival → No need to graft

Other → No need to graft

(B) Crown planned
- Supragingival margins → No need to graft
- Marginal or subgingival margins → FREE GINGIVAL GRAFT

(C) Bridge abutment
- Three-quarter crown → Consider: FREE GINGIVAL GRAFT
- Full crown

(D) Rest-proximal plate partial abutment → FREE GINGIVAL GRAFT

(E) Overdenture abutment

19 Free Gingival Graft

Walter B. Hall

The free gingival graft is perhaps the most predictable of periodontal surgical procedures. The indications for its use have been described (see Chapter 15).

The relative ease of mastering this technique and the mystique of plastic surgical procedures have led to more widespread use of the procedure than some clinicians believe is merited. This surgical procedure, nevertheless, has many important uses: to prevent or control loss of attachment (LOA) resulting from recession, to prevent or control esthetic problems, and to permit restorative or orthodontic treatment without iatrogenic root exposure (LOA). When a patient has a problem of minimal attached gingiva, with or without recession, and the dentist and patient agree that treatment is indicated, a series of decisions in proceeding with this surgery will be needed.

A Whether root coverage is a goal or not will determine how the receptor site is prepared. When root exposure has not occurred, the technique is performed one way. When root exposure has occurred, root coverage may become the goal if esthetic or restorative indications exist. Either a connective tissue graft (see Chapter 20) or guided tissue regeneration (see Chapter 17) are better means of successfully covering exposed roots, but some minimal recession can be managed with a free gingival graft. Most often these indications are present in maxillary anterior and maxillary premolar areas. Often some teeth will need more attached gingiva, whereas an adjacent one may require root coverage. Modify the surgical procedure to meet these individual needs.

B When root coverage is to be attempted, remove all sulcus epithelium and skim the superficial epithelium and connective tissue from adjacent papillae to the level of the cementoenamel junction (CEJ). More apically, separate the alveolar mucosa from the gingiva by an incision immediately coronal to the CEJ and reflect apically to expose a 5- to 6-mm bed. Should the root coverage fail, an adequate band of attached gingiva will have been created to minimize the likelihood of further recession.

C When root coverage is not a goal, prepare the receptor bed with an incision slightly coronal to the mucogingival junction. Expose a bed 5 to 6 mm in height by reflecting the alveolar mucosa with a periosteal elevator. Make a perio-

steal fenestration at the apical extent of the bed to ensure that the graft will not be mobile.

D A combination approach may be indicated when only an occasional tooth with a segment to be grafted requires root coverage.

E When root coverage is to be performed, reduce the prominent root with a back-action chisel so that hemorrhage will not pool peripherally. Reduce the root to keep the dentin free of bacteria or endotoxin. The reduced dimension of the root will make new attachment more likely to occur.

F Once the graft is taken, if root coverage is the goal, suture the graft, stretched tightly between the deepitheliated papillae, with interrupted or single-sling sutures. When root coverage will not be attempted, use single, interrupted sutures in the area of each papilla to stabilize the graft.

G Once the graft is placed, apply pressure with wet gauze for 3 to 4 minutes, place a Stomahesive bandage covering the graft, and provide postoperative instructions on ways to avoid disturbing the graft.

References

Carranza FA, Jr, Newman MG: *Clinical periodontology*, ed 8, Philadelphia, 1996, WB Saunders, p 653.

Hall WB: *Pure mucogingival problems*, Berlin, 1984, Quintessence Publishing, p 127.

Hall WB, Lundergan W: Free gingival grafts-current indications and technique, *Dent Clin North Am* 37(2):227, 1993.

Hall WB, Sutter M, Williams C, Lundergan WD: Aktueller Stand der Anwendung Freier Gingiva Transplantate, *Phillip Journal* 12(10):457, 1995.

Matter J: Creeping attachment of free gingival grafts: a five-year follow-up study, *J Periodontol* 51:681, 1981.

Miller PD: Root coverage using free soft-tissue autograft following citric acid application, Part I: technique, *Int J Periodont Restor Dent* 2:65, 1982.

Rateitschak KH, Rateitschak EM, Wolf HF, Hassell JM: *Color atlas of periodontology*, Stuttgart, 1985, Georg Thieme Verlag, p 230.

Schluger S, Yuodelis R, Page RC, Johnson RH: *Periodontal diseases*, ed 2, Philadelphia, 1990, Lea & Febiger, p 567.

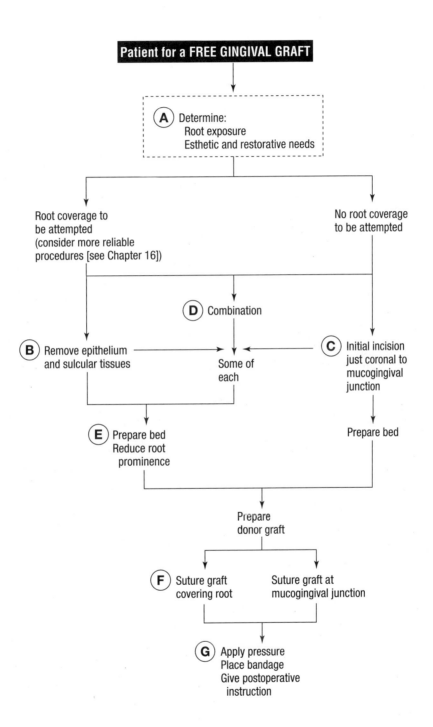

Patient for a FREE GINGIVAL GRAFT

A Determine:
Root exposure
Esthetic and restorative needs

Root coverage to
be attempted
(consider more reliable
procedures [see Chapter 16])

No root coverage
to be attempted

D Combination

B Remove epithelium
and sulcular tissues

Some of
each

C Initial incision
just coronal to
mucogingival
junction

E Prepare bed
Reduce root
prominence

Prepare bed

Prepare
donor graft

F Suture graft
covering root

Suture graft at
mucogingival junction

G Apply pressure
Place bandage
Give postoperative
instruction

20 Connective Tissue Graft

Walter B. Hall

The subepithelial connective tissue graft for root coverage where recession has occurred was described by the Langers in 1985. It has become one of the most predictable approaches to root coverage where facial or lingual recession has occurred. If the donor tissue is obtained from the anterior palate, where the submucosa is fatty, new attachment *may* be obtained because epithelium will not grow to cover fatty tissue until it is replaced with fibrous connective tissue.

The connective tissue graft has been used for regeneration in Class II furca involvements, following this assumption, as described by Han (1992).

A When a patient has a single tooth with facial (or lingual) root exposure on several adjacent teeth with such recession, two approaches to predictable root coverage are available: the connective tissue graft and guided tissue regeneration (GTR). Because the connective tissue graft uses the patient's own tissue and therefore is much less expensive (though more difficult to do), it should be considered first. An adequate donor site of fatty connective tissue must be present. Its presence can be evaluated by repetitive, gentle finger pressure to the area of the rugae and sagittally to it. If the area feels spongy, the submucosa probably is fatty and usable for a connective tissue graft.

B Next, a connective tissue graft requires the lifting of a superficial flap that is 1- or 2-mm thick at its thinnest point. If the rugae are gross (e.g., 3 or 4 mm or more in height), raising a flap of adequate thickness and still leaving tissue for a fatty subepithelial connective tissue graft may not be possible. If the rugae are too substantial, a connective tissue graft should not be attempted. GTR using a membrane should be used.

C Finally, if interdental papillae are receded or involved with pocketing and full root coverage is the goal, the connective tissue graft is not the most promising choice (see Chapter 13). Miller (1985) has shown that root coverage by means of grafting is limited by the height of the interdental papillae and alveolar crests adjacent to the exposed root or roots. The same limitation does *not* apply to GTR by means of a membrane. Regeneration of interproximal tissues with new attachment has been achievable, predictably, since 1989 when the first interproximal membranes for GTR became available. When interproximal height can be gained to increase coverage of exposed roots, GTR by means of a membrane is the technique of choice whether facial or lingual surfaces with or without furcal involvements are present in the area to be treated.

References

Carranza FA, Newman MG: *Clinical periodontology,* ed 8, Philadelphia, 1996, WB Saunders, p 664.

Cole R, Crigger M, Bogle G et al: Connective tissue regeneration to periodontally diseased teeth: a histologic study, *J Periodontol Res* 15:1, 1980.

Hall WB, Sutter M, Williams C, Lundergan WP: Aktueller stand der anwendung freir gingiva transplante, *Phillip Journal* 10:457, 1995.

Han TJ: Connective tissue membrane: treating grade II furcation involvements, *J Calif Dent Assoc* 20:47, 1992.

Langer B, Cologna LJ: Subepithelial graft to correct ridge concavities, *J Prosthet Dent* 44:363, 1980.

Langer B, Langer L: Subepithelial connective tissue graft technique for root coverage, *J Periodontol* 56:715, 1985.

Miller PD: A classification of marginal tissue recession, *Int J Periodont Rest Dent* 2:8, 1985.

Nordland WP: Periodontal plastic surgery; esthetic gingival regeneration, *J Calif Dent Assoc* 17:11, 1989.

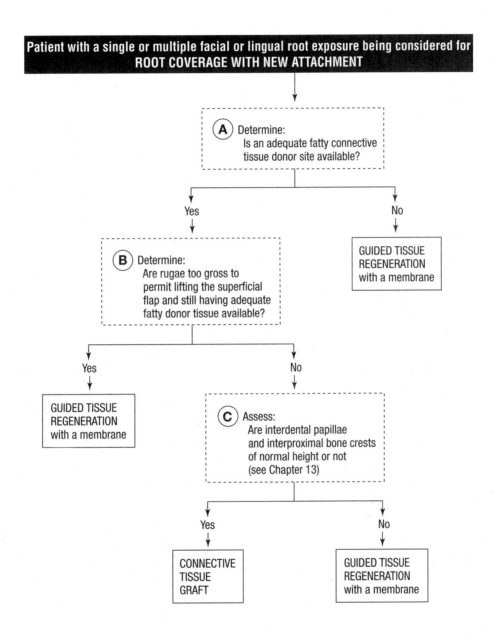

Patient with a single or multiple facial or lingual root exposure being considered for ROOT COVERAGE WITH NEW ATTACHMENT

(A) Determine:
Is an adequate fatty connective tissue donor site available?

Yes

No

(B) Determine:
Are rugae too gross to permit lifting the superficial flap and still having adequate fatty donor tissue available?

GUIDED TISSUE REGENERATION with a membrane

Yes

No

GUIDED TISSUE REGENERATION with a membrane

(C) Assess:
Are interdental papillae and interproximal bone crests of normal height or not (see Chapter 13)

Yes

No

CONNECTIVE TISSUE GRAFT

GUIDED TISSUE REGENERATION with a membrane

21 Guided Tissue Regeneration Strategy to Maximize Esthetics: Selection of the Surgical Approach and the Type of Barrier Membrane

Pierpaolo Cortellini, Giovan Paolo Pini-Prato, Maurizio Tonetti

Objectives of guided tissue regeneration (GTR) in esthetically sensitive sites are: (1) complete resolution of the periodontal defect and (2) preservation of soft tissues.

The selection of the proper regenerative strategy is aimed at overcoming frequent drawbacks of GTR treatment like the uncompleted filling of the bony defect and a soft tissue dehiscence that can result in impaired esthetics.

Deep intrabony defects will benefit most by GTR therapy. The anatomic prerequisites for uneventful procedures are the presence of an adequate band of attached gingiva and the absence of frena in the area of treatment. GTR treatment should be initiated following completion of the initial therapy phase.

A The surgical procedure is selected considering the width of the interdental space (it can be either wide or narrow) and

the correlated thickness of the interdental tissues. The interdental space is considered wide when the interdental tissues exceed 2 mm mesiodistally. If the interdental tissues are less than 2 mm, the interdental space is classified as narrow.

B If the interdental space is wide, the surgical procedure of choice is the modified papilla preservation technique (MPPT) (Cortellini et al, 1995b). In this technique the interdental papilla is horizontally dissected at its base on the buccal side and elevated with the palatal full thickness flap. After completion of membrane positioning the papilla is repositioned through the interdental space to cover the barrier and passively sutured to the buccal flap to obtain primary closure (Fig. 21-1). If the interdental space is narrow, the simplified papilla preservation technique (SPPT) (Cortellini et al)

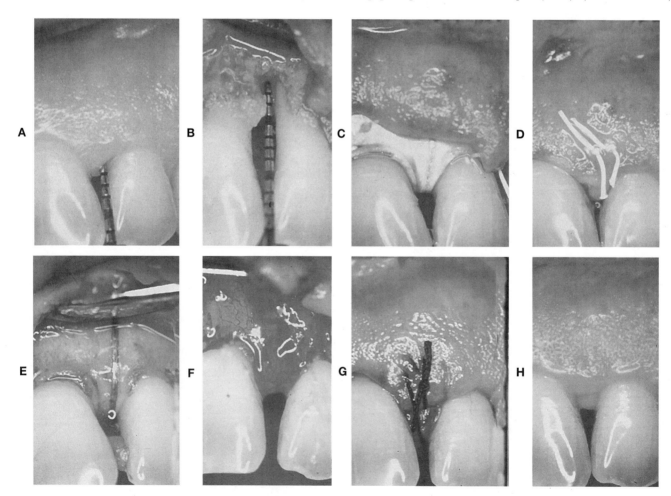

Fig. 21-1 **A,** Preoperative view of a deep defect on the lateral incisor. **B,** The osseous defect has one-walled to three-walled components. **C,** A titanium reinforced e-PTFE interproximal membrane in place. **D,** The modified papilla preservation-designed flap sutured over the membrane. **E,** The membrane exposed 6 weeks after surgery. **F,** Regeneration tissue exposed after membrane removal. **G,** The sutured flaps covering the regeneration tissue. **H,** The healed result.

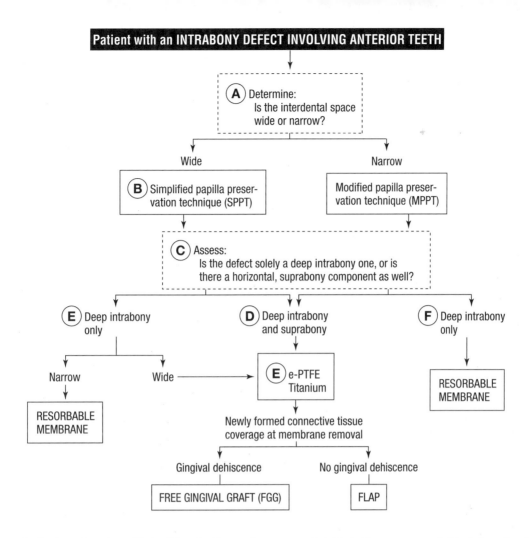

Patient with an INTRABONY DEFECT INVOLVING ANTERIOR TEETH

(A) Determine:
Is the interdental space wide or narrow?

Wide → (B) Simplified papilla preservation technique (SPPT)

Narrow → Modified papilla preservation technique (MPPT)

(C) Assess:
Is the defect solely a deep intrabony one, or is there a horizontal, suprabony component as well?

(E) Deep intrabony only — Narrow → RESORBABLE MEMBRANE — Wide →

(D) Deep intrabony and suprabony → (E) e-PTFE Titanium

(F) Deep intrabony only → RESORBABLE MEMBRANE

Newly formed connective tissue coverage at membrane removal

Gingival dehiscence → FREE GINGIVAL GRAFT (FGG)

No gingival dehiscence → FLAP

should be used. The interdental papilla is obliquely dissected to augment the connective tissue surface for the subsequent primary closure of the flap over the barrier membrane.

C The bony defect associated with the periodontal pocket can be a pure intrabony defect with the residual interproximal bone crest close to the cementoenamel junction (CEJ), or it can have a horizontal component on top of the intrabony component. In the latter case the interproximal bone crest is located at a distance from the CEJ. The recognition of these two different types of osseous defects is relevant for the selection of the barrier membrane.

D An e-PTFE titanium reinforced membrane is selected whenever a horizontal component to the defect is present or when the intrabony defect is wide (Cortellini et al, 1995c). In such cases the self supporting membrane can be positioned and maintained near the CEJ and will not collapse into the wide defect after flap closure.

E When a nonresorbable e-PTFE titanium membrane is used, its removal is planned at approximately 6 weeks. At that time the tissue covering the membrane still can be preserved or, conversely, be dehiscent. In the first instance the regenerated tissue (NFCT) can be properly covered by repositioning the flap. When a gingival dehiscence is present, NFCT coverage is difficult. A proper protection of the regenerated tissue can be achieved with a saddle-shaped free gingival graft (FGG) positioned in the interdental space (Cortellini et al, 1995a).

F A resorbable barrier membrane is preferred whenever a narrow, solely intrabony defect is to be treated (Cortellini

et al, 1996). The anatomy of this defect should allow positioning of the membrane near the CEJ and should prevent its collapse into the defect.

When a resorbable membrane is used, a possible dehiscence of the flap cannot be treated in an early healing phase. An anatomic correction of the consequent soft tissue deficiency should be postponed after completion of the healing until 9 to 12 months after the regenerative procedures.

References

Cortellini P, Pini-Prato G, Tonetti M: Interproximal free gingival grafts after membrane removal in GTR treatment of infrabony defects: a controlled clinical trial indicating improved outcomes, *J Periodontol* 66:488, 1995a.

Cortellini P, Pini-Prato G, Tonetti M: The modified papilla preservation technique: a new surgical approach for interproximal regenerative procedures, *J Periodontol* 66:261, 1995b.

Cortellini P, Pini-Prato G, Tonetti M: Periodontal regeneration of human infrabony defects with titanium reinforced membranes: a controlled clinical trial, *J Periodontol* 66:797, 1995c.

Cortellini P, Pini-Prato G, Tonetti M: The modified papilla preservation technique with bioresorbable barrier membranes in the treatment of intrabony defects: case reports, *Int J Periodon Restor Dent* 16:547, 1996.

Cortellini P, Pini-Prato G, Tonetti M: The simplified papilla preservation flap: a new surgical approach for the management of soft tissues in regenerative procedures, *Int J Periodontol Rest Dent* 1998 (in press).

Tonetti M, Pini-Prato G, Cortellini P: Periodontal regeneration of human infrabony defects, IV: determinants of the healing response, *J Periodontol* 64:934, 1993.

22 Guided Tissue Regeneration Versus Mucogingival Osseous Surgery

Walter B. Hall

Conceptually, guided tissue regeneration (GTR) is always preferable to mucogingival osseous surgery because successful GTR adds to existing support of the tooth while mucogingival osseous surgery usually requires the sacrifice of additional supporting tissue to eliminate pockets and to create a more easily maintainable architecture around the tooth (see Chapter 23). The first decision therefore involves the assessment of the tooth as a GTR candidate.

A GTR may be attempted whenever significant attachment loss has occurred on a tooth; however, extremely periodontally involved teeth or ones with additional problems (e.g., untreatable endodontic problems, unrestorable crowns, deep vertical root cracks) may have to be extracted. Non-strategic teeth do not merit GTR in many cases, especially if less complicated or less expensive alternatives are available.

If many or most of the patient's remaining teeth have extensive loss of attachment (LOA), extraction or maintenance with a hopeless prognosis may be the necessary choice.

B If GTR is a feasible approach, the severity of the problem must be considered. While more severe problems merit GTR, minimal problems (e.g., teeth with LOA of 5 mm or less) may be treated satisfactorily with pocket elimination–mucogingival osseous surgery.

C In the anterior segments of the mouth, even teeth with less than 5 mm of lost attachment may merit GTR rather than mucogingival osseous surgery to improve the esthetic result. Therefore esthetic requirements should be considered to determine whether the patient's esthetic demands would be satisfied better by using GTR.

References

Carranza FA, Newman MG: *Clinical periodontology,* ed 8, Philadelphia, 1996, WB Saunders, p 615.

Genco RJ, Goldman HM, Cohen DW: *Contemporary periodontics,* St Louis, 1990, Mosby, pp 564, 585.

Knowles JW: Results of periodontal treatment related to pocket depth and attachment level: eight years, *J Periodontol* 50:225, 1979.

Pihlstrom BJ, McHugh RB, Oliphant TH, Ortiz-Campos C: Comparison of surgical and non-surgical treatment of periodontal disease, *J Clin Periodontol* 10:524, 1983.

Schluger S, Yuodelis R, Page RC, Johnson RH: *Periodontal diseases,* ed 2, Philadelphia, 1989, Lea & Febiger, p 332.

Smith DH, Ammons WF, Van Belle G: A longitudinal study of periodontal status comparing osseous recontouring with flap curettage: 1—Results after 6 months, *J Periodontol* 51:367, 1980.

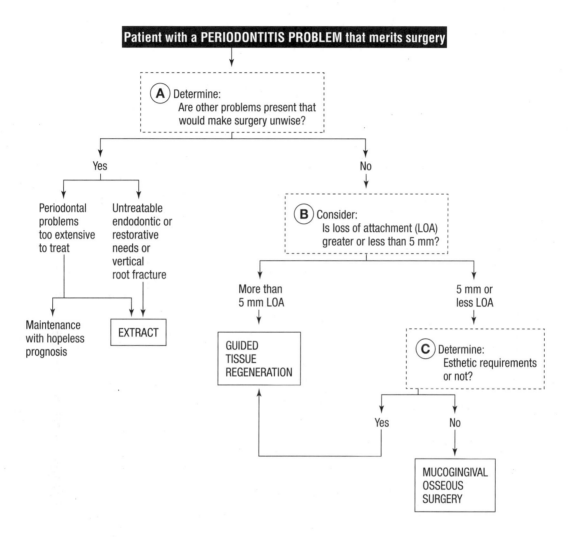

Patient with a PERIODONTITIS PROBLEM that merits surgery

(A) Determine:
Are other problems present that would make surgery unwise?

Yes

No

Periodontal problems too extensive to treat

Untreatable endodontic or restorative needs or vertical root fracture

Maintenance with hopeless prognosis

EXTRACT

(B) Consider:
Is loss of attachment (LOA) greater or less than 5 mm?

More than 5 mm LOA

5 mm or less LOA

GUIDED TISSUE REGENERATION

(C) Determine:
Esthetic requirements or not?

Yes

No

MUCOGINGIVAL OSSEOUS SURGERY

23 Selection of Mucogingival-Osseous Surgical Approaches: Resection or Regeneration

Walter B. Hall

Many patients with complex dental problems require mucogingival-osseous surgery. Most have been affected by adult periodontitis and have a number of teeth with pocket depth, bone loss, and loss of attachment. The character of the bone loss present determines the type of mucogingival-osseous surgery indicated.

A The dentist must first decide whether the problem is one of horizontal bone loss only, vertical loss only, or a mixed problem (some teeth with horizontal and some with vertical bone loss). If the patient has only horizontal bone loss, the severity of loss and the number of severely involved teeth are the factors that determine the treatment plan. If many teeth are severely affected, mucogingival-osseous surgery is contraindicated. The teeth should either be extracted or given a hopeless prognosis and maintained. The restorative plan is determined by which if any teeth could be used. If the horizontal bone loss is not severe or generalized, pocket elimination surgery with osteoplasty to create the most readily maintainable contours is best.

B If vertical bone loss is involved, the types of osseous defects present determine the type of surgery indicated. One-walled defects that are shallow should be managed with pocket elimination surgery and osseous resection (ostectomy and osteoplasty). If a one-walled defect is moderate to deep, the value of the individual tooth to the overall treatment plan should be considered. If the tooth is of little value, extraction is the best approach. If the tooth is critical to the overall treatment plan, guided tissue regeneration (GTR) with or without concomitant or second-stage osseous resection should be used.

C For two-walled defects the surgical approach depends on whether the defects are craters (defects between adjacent teeth where facial and lingual cortical plates remain) or the less common type affecting only one tooth (either a facial or a lingual cortical plate and a wall against the adjacent tooth remain). If a crater is present and is a shallow defect, pocket elimination surgery with osseous resection is best. If the crater is moderate to deep, GTR should be used. If the two-walled defect affects only a single tooth, its value to the overall treatment plan determines whether GTR or extraction is best (Figs. 23-1 and 23-2).

D For three-walled defects the depth and horizontal width from root to osseous crest are the factors that determine the surgical approach. A narrow defect (less than 1 mm horizontally from root to osseous crest) is amenable to a "Prichard fill" technique wherein total débridement is followed by bone fill and new attachment on a predictable basis. If the defect is wide (more than 1 mm horizontally from root to osseous crest) and moderate to deep, GTR is a predictable means of gaining new attachment. If the defect is wide and shallow, pocket elimination with osseous resection is best.

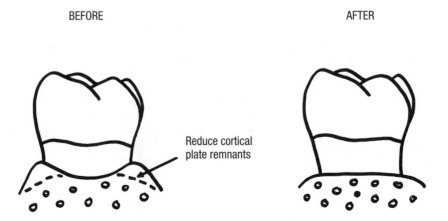

BEFORE　　　　　　　　　　　　AFTER

Reduce cortical plate remnants

Fig. 23-1　A shallow, two-walled infrabony "crater" is treated by osseous resection.

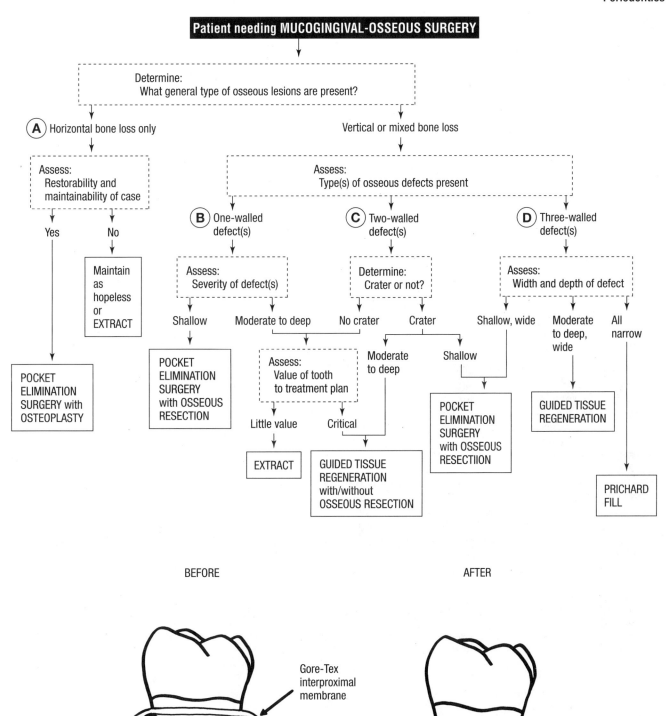

Patient needing MUCOGINGIVAL-OSSEOUS SURGERY

Determine:
What general type of osseous lesions are present?

A Horizontal bone loss only

Vertical or mixed bone loss

Assess:
Restorability and maintainability of case

Assess:
Type(s) of osseous defects present

Yes | No

B One-walled defect(s)

C Two-walled defect(s)

D Three-walled defect(s)

Maintain as hopeless or EXTRACT

Assess:
Severity of defect(s)

Determine:
Crater or not?

Assess:
Width and depth of defect

Shallow | Moderate to deep

No crater | Crater

Shallow, wide | Moderate to deep, wide | All narrow

POCKET ELIMINATION SURGERY with OSTEOPLASTY

POCKET ELIMINATION SURGERY with OSSEOUS RESECTION

Assess:
Value of tooth to treatment plan

Moderate to deep

Shallow

POCKET ELIMINATION SURGERY with OSSEOUS RESECTIION

GUIDED TISSUE REGENERATION

Little value | Critical

EXTRACT

GUIDED TISSUE REGENERATION with/without OSSEOUS RESECTION

PRICHARD FILL

BEFORE

AFTER

Gore-Tex interproximal membrane

Fig. 23-2 A deep, two-walled infrabony "crater" is treated by tissue regeneration.

References

Carranza FA: *Clinical periodontology*, ed 7, Philadelphia, 1990, WB Saunders, p 792.

Genco RJ, Goldman HM, Cohen DW: *Contemporary periodontics*, St Louis, 1990, Mosby, pp 564, 585.

Knowles JW: Results of periodontal treatment related to pocket depth and attachment level: eight years, *J Periodontol* 50:225, 1979.

Pihlstrom BJ, McHugh RB, Oliphant TH, Ortiz-Campos C: Comparison of surgical and non-surgical treatment of periodontal disease, *J Clin Periodontol* 10:524, 1983.

Schluger S, Yuodelis R, Page RC, Johnson RH: *Periodontal diseases*, ed 2, Philadelphia, 1989, Lea & Febiger, p 332.

Smith DH, Ammons WF, Van Belle G: A longitudinal study of periodontal status comparing osseous recontouring with flap curettage: 1—results after 6 months, *J Periodontol* 51:367, 1980.

24 Guided Tissue Regeneration Versus Osseous Fill

Steven A. Tsurudome

The goal of guided tissue regeneration (GTR) is to regenerate lost periodontal structures. The lost periodontal structures include the alveolar bone, periodontal ligament, and cementum. The two most commonly used materials for GTR today are barrier membranes and graft materials.

A When a periodontal patient is evaluated for a GTR procedure, the radiographs must first be evaluated to assess the type of bone loss. Patients with a horizontal type of bone loss are usually not amenable to GTR procedures, while patients with vertical or intrabony type of bone loss are possible candidates for GTR procedures.

B If the patient has a vertical or intrabony radiographic defect, the clinician should consider a preliminary treatment plan that may consist of several different GTR technique options; however, the definitive treatment option should be made at the time of surgery when the surgical site is reflected, débrided, and the intrabony defect exposed for direct visual inspection. The overall defect depth, width, and the number of associated bony walls will ultimately dictate the type of regenerative technique used by the clinician.

C If the intrabony defect is narrow and deep with only one osseous wall, then the combination technique of a "bone graft and absorbable barrier membrane" is recommended for creation and maintenance of the critical space for regeneration. The use of barrier membranes alone may cause the membrane to collapse into the defect and obliterate this critical space. Currently, absorbable membranes are the preferred membranes over the nonabsorbable types because of the necessity of a secondary surgery for removal of nonresorbable membranes. This second procedure represents additional trauma to the patient and the newly regenerated tissues. Thus most GTR procedures around natural teeth should benefit from using resorbable membranes.

D If the intrabony defect is narrow and deep with two or three walls, then the "membrane alone" technique may be considered. The two or three walls in narrow-deep osseous defects should provide adequate space maintenance and wound stabilization for predictable regeneration without the additional use of a bone graft. Absorbable barrier membranes alone have shown consistent ability to promote periodontal regeneration because the unique epithelial exclusion afforded by the barrier membranes effectively inhibits the proliferation of the junctional epithelium into the periodontal defect. Upon visual inspection of the intrabony defect, if the membrane alone does not provide adequate space maintenance, then the clinician always has the option of the combination "bone graft and absorbable barrier membrane" technique, as described for the narrow, deep, one-walled intrabony defects.

E If the intrabony defect is narrow and shallow with only one wall, the benefits of GTR become minimal because the potential gain in regenerated periodontium in shallow defects is inconsequential. Considering the cost and inherent risks involved in GTR surgery, osseous resective surgery should be the treatment of choice because of its greater predictability in shallow, wide defect cases.

F If the intrabony defect is narrow and shallow with two or three walls, then a bone graft alone may be considered because the defect size is sufficient to accommodate the small quantity of autogenous bone usually harvested from the oral cavity. In addition, if bone grafts such as demineralized freeze-dried bone allografts (DFDBA) are used, the predictability of the regenerative techniques caused by their possible release of bone-inducing proteins (known as bone morphogenic proteins [BMPs], as well as maintaining the critical space for regeneration, can be helpful. The inorganic alloplastic graft materials, in contrast, may not be recommended because studies have shown encapsulation with little bone fill and periodontal regeneration; thus they serve as space fillers only. In addition, barrier membranes are not recommended for shallow defects because the risks and benefits may not warrant their use. The cost of the membrane plus the inherent increased risk of complications may outweigh the potential benefit of only a slight gain in regenerated periodontium.

G If the intrabony defect is wide and deep with only one wall, the prognosis for the tooth decreases dramatically. The clinician must consider the possibility of extraction in these cases.

H If the intrabony defect is wide and deep with two or three walls, the prognosis is only slightly better than that for a wide and deep defect with only one wall. Extraction again is a possible option, but if the tooth is strategically important, the clinician may consider the use of a titanium reinforced membrane with or without the use of a bone graft to maintain the space and to stabilize the wound for possible regeneration to occur. However, the clinician must be aware that the predictability for regeneration of a wide and deep osseous defect is not great.

I, J If the intrabony defect is wide and shallow with either one, two, or three walls, the recommended procedure is osseous resection. The rationale is similar to the recommendations given earlier for narrow shallow intrabony defects.

In conclusion, the unique epithelial exclusion and wound stabilization afforded by the barrier membranes and the enhanced osteogenic, space maintaining, and wound stabilizing potential afforded by bone grafts (allogenic or autogenic) should increase the potential of regeneration; thus it is logical and prudent to combine the two techniques whenever possible to increase the predictability of regeneration of the periodontium destroyed by periodontal disease and to ultimately improve the clinical outcome.

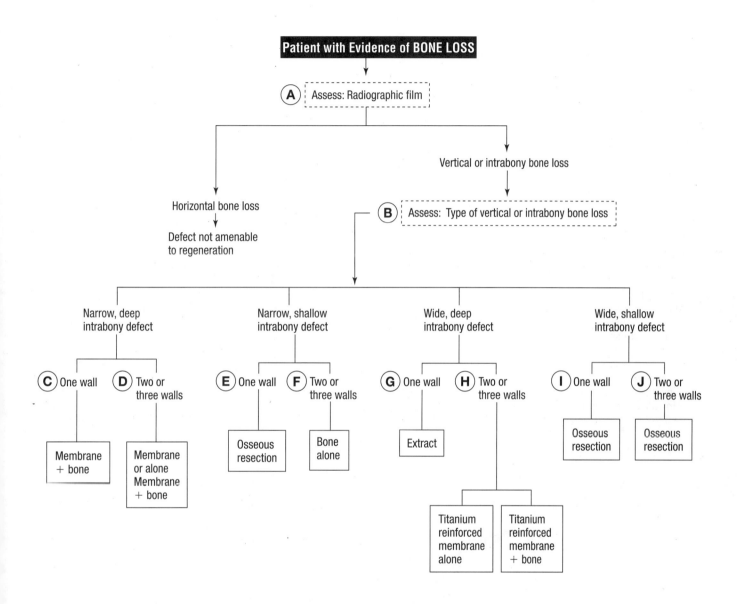

Patient with Evidence of BONE LOSS

(A) Assess: Radiographic film

Horizontal bone loss

Defect not amenable
to regeneration

Vertical or intrabony bone loss

(B) Assess: Type of vertical or intrabony bone loss

Narrow, deep
intrabony defect

(C) One wall   (D) Two or
three walls

Membrane
+ bone

Membrane
or alone
Membrane
+ bone

Narrow, shallow
intrabony defect

(E) One wall   (F) Two or
three walls

Osseous
resection

Bone
alone

Wide, deep
intrabony defect

(G) One wall   (H) Two or
three walls

Extract

Titanium
reinforced
membrane
alone

Titanium
reinforced
membrane
+ bone

Wide, shallow
intrabony defect

(I) One wall   (J) Two or
three walls

Osseous
resection

Osseous
resection

References

The American Academy of Periodontology: *Proceedings of the world workshop in clinical periodontics,* Princeton, August, 1987, The American Academy of Periodontology, p VI 2.

Annals of Periodontology: *1996 world workshop in periodontics,* Lansdowne, November, 1996, The American Academy of Periodontology, p 626.

Genco R, Goldman H, Cohen DW: *Contemporary periodontics,* St Louis, 1990, Mosby, p 585.

Wilson T, Kornman K: *Fundamentals of periodontics,* Chicago, 1996, Quintessence Publishing, p 405.

25 Furcation Involvements

Walter B. Hall

The type and severity of furcation involvements on molar teeth represent a critical concern in treatment planning, particularly when surgery is being considered. Furcation involvements are categorized as follows: Class I, incipient; Class II, definite; or Class III, through and through (Fig. 25-1).

Each furcation should be explored with a pig-tailed type of explorer or "furca finder." Insert the instrument into the furca and move it laterally and coronally to determine whether the instrument can slip out. The type of furcation involvement is recorded on the chart, and the options for its treatment are then considered.

A An incipient (Class I) furca exists when the instrument slips out of the furca when moved anteriorly, posteriorly, or coronally or in proximal furcas when moved facially, lingually, and coronally. It is recorded with the symbol "∧" placed appropriately on the tooth diagram. Such furcas are unlikely to influence the treatment plan but should be documented. If the incipient involvement is a deep one that does not produce a definite catch because adjacent roots are fused, guided tissue regeneration (GTR) (see Chapter 26) should be considered.

B A definite (Class II) furca exists when a definite catch prevents removal of the furca finder coronally or laterally but definitely stops before going "through and through" to another furca opening. It is recorded with the symbol "Δ"

placed in the appropriate furca on the tooth diagram. The severity of the involvement horizontally determines the best treatment option. If the furca finder can be advanced less than 3 mm horizontally into the defect, osseous resection and pocket elimination represent a good treatment option. If the furca finder can be advanced 3 mm or more into the defect, GTR is a predictable approach for regaining lost attachment and creating a maintainable situation. Often the horizontal measurement is recorded in millimeters apical to the symbol of the chart.

C A through and through (Class III) furca exists when the furca finder is inserted and appears to connect directly with one or more other furcas. It is recorded by placing the symbol "▲" in each of the appropriate furca areas on the tooth diagram; therefore more the one "▲" symbol must be used on a tooth to document a Class III situation. If a tooth with a Class III furca is not critical to the overall treatment plan, it should be extracted. If its retention does not jeopardize the overall treatment plan, it may be maintained. GTR has become a predictable treatment for such teeth only recently. If the tooth is a critical one and its retention can be achieved by hemisection or root amputation in a maintainable and useful manner, such an approach, although expensive, often can significantly improve the overall treatment plan for a complex case.

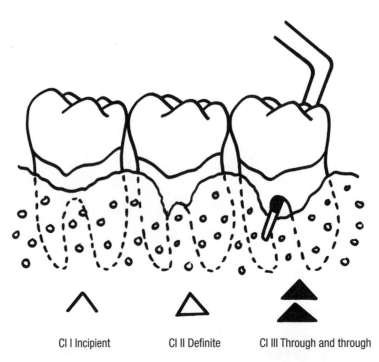

| CI I Incipient | CI II Definite | CI III Through and through |

Fig. 25-1 Classes of symbols and appearance of furcation involvements.

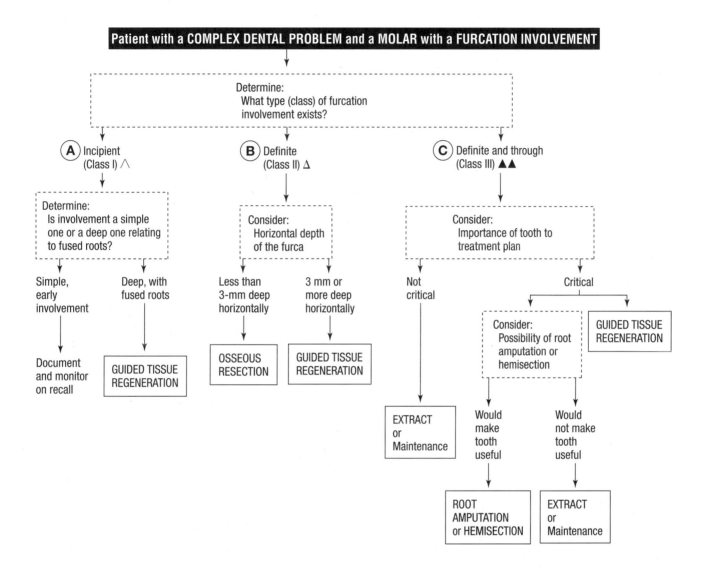

Patient with a COMPLEX DENTAL PROBLEM and a MOLAR with a FURCATION INVOLVEMENT

Determine:
What type (class) of furcation involvement exists?

A Incipient (Class I) ∧

B Definite (Class II) Δ

C Definite and through (Class III) ▲▲

Determine:
Is involvement a simple one or a deep one relating to fused roots?

Consider:
Horizontal depth of the furca

Consider:
Importance of tooth to treatment plan

Simple, early involvement

Deep, with fused roots

Less than 3-mm deep horizontally

3 mm or more deep horizontally

Not critical

Critical

Document and monitor on recall

GUIDED TISSUE REGENERATION

OSSEOUS RESECTION

GUIDED TISSUE REGENERATION

Consider:
Possibility of root amputation or hemisection

GUIDED TISSUE REGENERATION

EXTRACT or Maintenance

Would make tooth useful

Would not make tooth useful

ROOT AMPUTATION or HEMISECTION

EXTRACT or Maintenance

References

Carranza FA, Newman MG: *Clinical periodontology,* ed 8, Philadelphia, 1996, WB Saunders, p 640.

Easley JF, Drennan GA: Morphological classification of the furca, *J Can Dent Assoc* 35:12, 1969.

Genco RJ, Goldman HM, Cohen DW: *Contemporary periodontics,* St Louis, 1990, Mosby, pp 344, 354.

Grant DA, Stern JB, Listgarten MA: *Periodontics,* ed 6, St Louis, 1988 Mosby, p 921.

Heins PJ, Carter SR: Furca involvement: a classification of bony deformities, *Periodontics* 6:84, 1968.

Schluger S, Yuodelis R, Page RC, Johnson RH: *Periodontal diseases,* ed 2, Philadelphia, 1990, Lea & Febiger, p 545.

Tarnow D, Fletcher P: Classification of the vertical component of furcation involvement, *J Periodontol* 55:283, 1984.

26 Evaluation of Furcation Status of Molars Before Surgery

Walter B. Hall

When initial therapy evaluation is performed several weeks or more following root planing and any other aspects of initial treatment, the status of furcation involvements of molar teeth becomes an important consideration in deciding whether surgery would be beneficial to the patient. If furcations are readily accessible for plaque removal and root planing, maintenance by regular root planing several times a year is a reasonable option for controlling progress of inflammatory periodontal disease. If the furcations are not accessible for plaque removal and root planing, surgery may make them accessible, thus improving the prognosis for the tooth. An individual molar should be treated on the basis of the worst furcation involvement present (Fig. 26-1).

A The type of furcation involvement must be assessed in deciding upon treatment options. If the furcations are not involved, maintenance by root planing alone usually is a good option. The status of adjacent teeth and pocket depths on the individual molar may make surgery a desirable option in some cases, even when furcations are not involved. Class I (incipient) and Class II (definite) involvements (see Chapter 25) require considerable decision making. Class III ("through and through") involvements are discussed in Chapter 25. Mandibular molars have two furcations that must be evaluated in deciding upon further therapy at the time of initial therapy evaluation; whereas, maxillary molars have three furcations to be evaluated.

B If the worst involvement is incipient (Class I), maintenance with regular root planing several times a year may suffice. If the roots are fused, a Class I furcation may be all that is present to the apex of the tooth; therefore pocket depth and type of osseous defect present become critical factors. If pocket depth is slight, the tooth may be maintained; however if it is extensive, guided tissue regeneration (GTR) may be possible with the expectation of regenerating lost attachment. Most defects associated with fused roots will have three osseous walls, making them good candidates for GTR. Should the roots be tortuous and the defect not accessible to instrumentation surgically, extract the tooth or maintain it with a hopeless prognosis.

C If the molar has a Class II (definite) involvement, access for plaque removal and root planing is a most important consideration in deciding upon the possible value of surgery. Because maxillary molars have proximal furcations, access is a greater problem in that arch than in the mandibular one. If access is good, maintenance with regular root planing several times a year may be sufficient. The status of adjacent teeth however may make including molars with Class II furcations in surgery a desirable option, even though they are accessible for maintenance. If the access is not good, so that adequate plaque removal and root planing are difficult or impossible to accomplish, loss of attachment and type of osseous defect present become the chief factors in deciding upon treatment. If the defect is less than 3 mm straight in, mucogingival-osseous surgery with an apically positioned flap approach will make the area accessible for instrumentation and plaque removal. If the defect is 3 mm or more straight in, a three-walled osseous defect usually will be present on facial or lingual furcas, whereas proximal ones may be two- or three-walled. All are good candidates for GTR. If only one root is severely involved, root amputation or hemisection may be better options (see Chapter 72).

D Class III "through and through" furcas are amenable to predictable GTR now. The decision-making process for treating them is presented in Chapter 30.

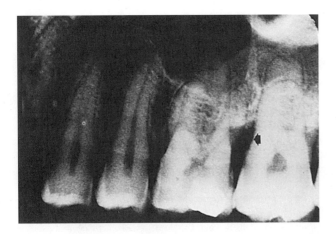

Fig. 26-1 A distal furcation involvement on the first molar with apparent second molar root proximity.

References

Carranza, Jr, FA, Newman MG: *Clinical periodontology*, ed 8, Philadelphia, 1996, WB Saunders, p 640.

Genco RJ, Goldman HM, Cohen DW: *Contemporary periodontics*, St Louis, 1990, Mosby, p 344.

Hemp SE, Nyman S, Lindhe J: Treatment of multi-rooted teeth: results after 5 years, *J Clin Periodontol* 2:126, 1975.

Lindhe J: *Textbook of clinical periodontology*, ed 2, Copenhagen, 1989, Munksgaard, p 515.

Schluger S, Yuodelis R, Page RC, Johnson RH: *Periodontal diseases*, ed 2, Philadelphia, 1990, Lea & Febiger, p 541.

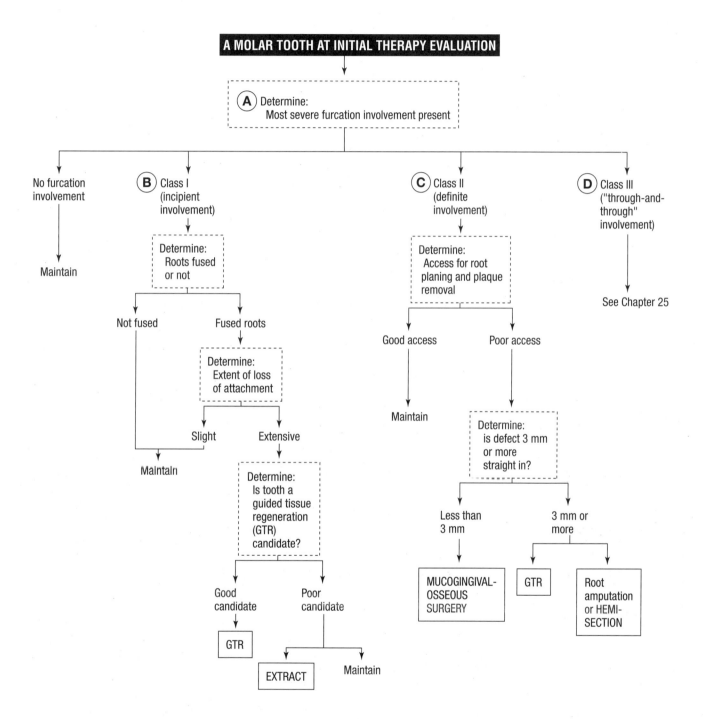

A MOLAR TOOTH AT INITIAL THERAPY EVALUATION

A Determine:
Most severe furcation involvement present

No furcation involvement

Maintain

B Class I (incipient involvement)

Determine:
Roots fused or not

Not fused

Fused roots

Determine:
Extent of loss of attachment

Slight

Extensive

Maintain

Determine:
Is tooth a guided tissue regeneration (GTR) candidate?

Good candidate

Poor candidate

GTR

EXTRACT

Maintain

C Class II (definite involvement)

Determine:
Access for root planing and plaque removal

Good access

Poor access

Maintain

Determine:
is defect 3 mm or more straight in?

Less than 3 mm

3 mm or more

MUCOGINGIVAL-OSSEOUS SURGERY

GTR

Root amputation or HEMI-SECTION

D Class III ("through-and-through" involvement)

See Chapter 25

27 Guided Tissue Regeneration for Treatment of Vertical Osseous Defects

Burton E. Becker, William Becker

The biologic principles of guided tissue regeneration (GTR) are based upon epithelial exclusion and connective tissue exclusion. If the epithelium can be delayed from contacting the root surface long enough for the clot to organize, new cementum, periodontal ligament, and bone may have the potential to regenerate. The use of membranes to exclude the epithelium has been shown to achieve this clinically and histologically.

A GTR has been shown to be the most successful treatment for the deep vertical defect. The deep defect is detected best by probing depths greater than 5 mm, attachment loss greater than 5 mm, and radiographic evidence of a vertical defect. The Teflon barrier excludes epithelial cells and flap connective tissues. GTR creates a space for the clot to form and protects the clot during the early phases of wound healing. Teflon membranes made of e-PTFE (Gore-Tex) and resorbable membranes have been used as barriers for GTR.

B A shallow defect is described as having pocket depths less than 5 mm, attachment loss less than 5 mm, and radiographic evidence of a small vertical defect. This type of defect can be treated with flap débridement or apically positioned flaps with or without osseous resection.

C When osseous defects that are greater than 5 mm in depth are exposed, the number of osseous walls that remain determine the treatment options. A deep, one-walled defect may require extraction or be amenable to maintenance (even with a poor prognosis) after mucogingival-osseous surgery. GTR may be attempted but is not totally predictable.

D Two- or three-walled defects that have pocket depths deeper than 5 mm and attachment loss greater than 5 mm can be treated with several modalities of therapy. This type of defect can be treated with flap débridement, GTR, or GTR in combination with either freeze-dried bone or synthetic grafting materials. GTR has been shown to achieve greater pocket reduction and greater gain of attachment than flap débridement alone, but there is no evidence to suggest that GTR with grafting creates any significant increase in attachment. Synthetic materials act as fillers. Although decreased probing depths have been demonstrated with their use, little or no attachment gain has been shown. Defects that have pocket depths greater than 5 mm, attachment loss greater than 5 mm, and upon entry, two- or three-walled vertical defects deeper than 5 mm in conjunction with a Class II furcation have several options for therapy. Flap débridement may be used; however, this type of defect responds well to GTR. Grafting materials may be used with GTR, but there is no evidence that allogenic or allographic grafting significantly improves the result. The presence of a deep Class II furcation makes this an ideal type of defect to treat with GTR.

E Most defects that have pocket depths greater than 5 mm and attachment loss greater than 5 mm may be treated with GTR. These defects, which usually are found to wrap around the lingual or palatal aspects of teeth, use the barrier to keep the space in the defect open for the clot to form. The deep, three-walled intrabony defect is the ideal type of defect for treatment with GTR. This type of defect has been shown to heal with new bone after thorough débridement. GTR has been shown to provide a predictable reduction in pocket depth and pain and to result in significant new attachment.

F The presence of a Class II furca may alter the likelihood of success with GTR. Class II furcas, however, do not have as good a prognosis for successful GTR, therefore maintenance or extraction should be considered.

References

Becker W, Becker B, Berg L et al: Clinical and volumetric analysis of three-walled intrabony defects following open flap débridement, *J Periodontol* 57:277, 1986.

Becker W, Becker B, Berg L et al: Root isolation for new attachment, *J Periodontol* 58:819, 1987.

Becker W, Becker B, Berg L et al: New attachment after treatment with root isolation procedures: report for treated Class III and Class II furcations and vertical defects, *Int J Periodont Restor Dent* 3(3):9, 1988.

Cortellini P et al: Periodontal regeneration of human intrabony defects, V: effect on oral hygiene and long term stability, *J Clin Periodontol* 21:606, 1994.

Gottlow J, Nyman S, Karring I et al: New attachment formation in human periodontium by guided tissue regeneration, *J Periodontol* 57:727, 1986.

Melcher HH: On the repair potential of periodontol tissues, *J Periodontol* 47:256, 1976.

Schallhorn RG, McClain PR: Combined osseous composite grafting, root conditioning and guided tissue regeneration, *Int J Periodontol Restor Dent* 8(4):9, 1988.

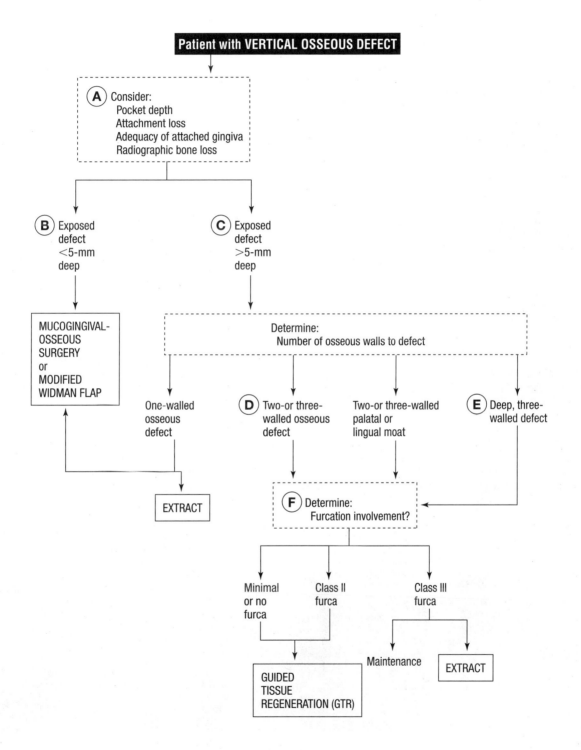

Patient with VERTICAL OSSEOUS DEFECT

A Consider:
Pocket depth
Attachment loss
Adequacy of attached gingiva
Radiographic bone loss

B Exposed defect <5-mm deep

C Exposed defect >5-mm deep

MUCOGINGIVAL-OSSEOUS SURGERY or MODIFIED WIDMAN FLAP

Determine:
Number of osseous walls to defect

One-walled osseous defect

D Two-or three-walled osseous defect

Two-or three-walled palatal or lingual moat

E Deep, three-walled defect

EXTRACT

F Determine:
Furcation involvement?

Minimal or no furca

Class II furca

Class III furca

Maintenance

EXTRACT

GUIDED TISSUE REGENERATION (GTR)

28 Management of a Three-Walled Osseous Defect on an Abutment Tooth

Walter B. Hall

A three-walled osseous defect on an abutment tooth offers significant opportunities for treatment that can "make or break" a treatment plan in a complex case. The opportunities for regaining lost attachment have improved impressively with the development of guided tissue regeneration (GTR). Implants offer opportunities that were not predictable 5 to 10 years ago. The dentist has an obligation to discuss these possibilities with the patient and to select a treatment that best meets the patient's individual objectives and means.

A The severity of the three-walled defect (Fig. 28-1) affects which options offer the most predictable results for the patient. A shallow three-walled defect (1 to 2 mm in depth) often is best managed with pocket elimination mucogingival-osseous surgery when the defect can be eliminated without affecting the use of the tooth as an abutment or with respect to esthetic demands while improving access for plaque removal and recall root planing. If esthetics would be compromised, the defect is shallow, or surgery can or should be avoided for health or personal reasons, maintenance care may suffice.

B If the defect is 3 mm or greater in depth but is narrow (1 mm or less measured horizontally from root to crest of bone), it is amenable to osseous fill with new attachment by the Prichard method in which complete débridement of the narrow defect results in the formation of new bone and creation of a new connective tissue attachment filling the defect.

C If the defect is 3 mm or more in depth and is wider than 1 mm from root to osseous crest measured horizontally, a Prichard approach would only result in filling in the narrower, deeper portion with a residual defect remaining.

GTR using a Gore-Tex barrier (see Chapters 21 and 29) predictably results in a new attachment regenerating from the ligament, often with significant new bone formation (Fig. 28-2). Neither the extremity of the depth of the defect nor the presence of a furcation involvement (as long as it is not through and through [Class III]), makes this approach less predictable. A potential abutment thus involved had little chance of being usable before the development of GTR. Now this approach is the treatment of choice if the tooth is a critical one. If it is not a critical abutment, it could be extracted. If GTR fails, an implant may be considered. Because GTR is a more predictable procedure than a single tooth implant and is far less expensive, it should be used before considering an implant.

References

Bowers GM, Schallhorn RG, Mellonig JR: Histologic evaluation of new attachment in human intrabony defects: a literature review, *J Periodontol* 53:509, 1982.

Carranza FA: *Clinical periodontology*, ed 7, Philadelphia, 1990, WB Saunders, p 836.

Caton J, Nyman S, Zander H: Histometric evaluation of periodontal surgery. II. Connective tissue attachment levels after four regenerative procedures, *J Clin Periodontol* 7:224, 1980.

Prichard JF: The infrabony technique as a predictable procedure, *J Periodontol* 28:202, 1957.

Prichard JF: A technique for treating intrabony pockets based on alveolar process morphology, *Dent Clin North Am* 3:85, 1960.

Schallhorn RG, Hiatt WH: Human allografts of iliac cancellous bone and marrow in periodontal osseous defects. II. Clinical observations, *J Periodontol* 43:67, 1972.

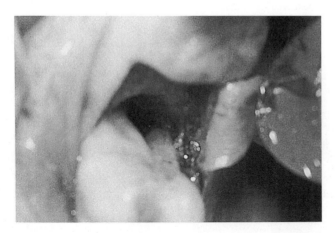

Fig. 28-1 A deep, wide three-walled osseous defect on a critical abutment tooth exposed for guided tissue regeneration.

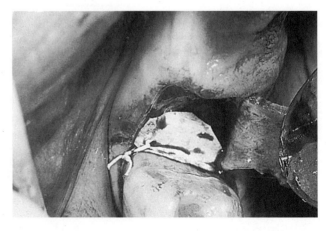

Fig. 28-2 A Gore-Tex membrane has been sutured and covers the débrided defect.

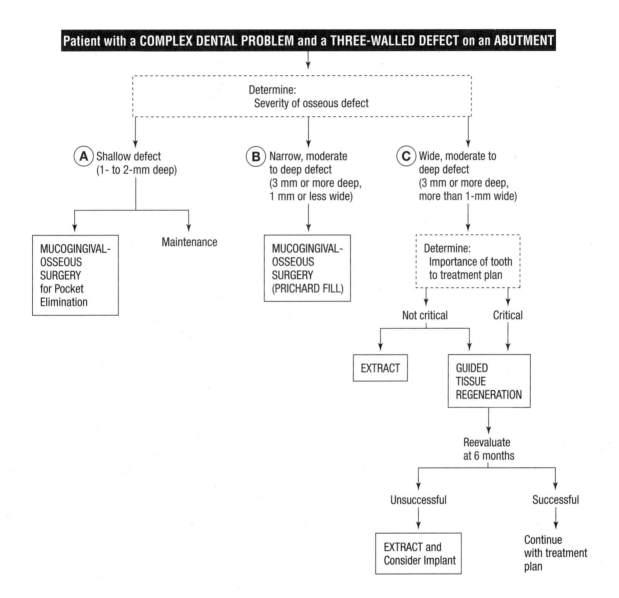

Patient with a COMPLEX DENTAL PROBLEM and a THREE-WALLED DEFECT on an ABUTMENT

Determine:
Severity of osseous defect

A Shallow defect
(1- to 2-mm deep)

B Narrow, moderate
to deep defect
(3 mm or more deep,
1 mm or less wide)

C Wide, moderate to
deep defect
(3 mm or more deep,
more than 1-mm wide)

MUCOGINGIVAL-
OSSEOUS
SURGERY
for Pocket
Elimination

Maintenance

MUCOGINGIVAL-
OSSEOUS
SURGERY
(PRICHARD FILL)

Determine:
Importance of tooth
to treatment plan

Not critical

Critical

EXTRACT

GUIDED
TISSUE
REGENERATION

Reevaluate
at 6 months

Unsuccessful

Successful

EXTRACT and
Consider Implant

Continue
with treatment
plan

29 Guided Tissue Regeneration in Three-Walled Osseous Defects

Alberto Sicilia, Jon Zabelegui

Of all the bone defects created by periodontal disease, the three-walled defect has the highest predictability of successful regeneration. A three-walled defect is delimited by three bony walls: buccal, mesial or distal, and lingual. The fourth wall is always the surface of the root of the tooth. Radiographic examination and periodontal probing help to diagnose a three-walled defect; two different osseous levels at the same site—one parallel to the pattern of bone level and the other aiming toward the apex of the root—suggest a three-walled defect. Probings on a possible three-walled defect are shallow at the line angles and deep in the interproximal area under the contact.

A If the defect is shallow (1- or 2-mm deep) and wide, possible approaches include an apically positioned flap with osseous recontouring of the architecture or an open flap débridement.

B If the defect is deep and wide with deep surrounding vestibular depth, perform guided tissue regeneration (GTR). Choose the wraparound configuration that best covers the defect, overlapping 2 to 3 mm over the osseous walls. An autograft or allograft of autogenous bone is sometimes used. Denudation with secondary intention healing may be useful with narrow defects.

C If the defect is deep with shallow surrounding vestibular depth, perform GTR. Choose the wraparound configuration that best covers the defect, overlapping 2 to 3 mm over the osseous walls. An autograft or allograft of autogenous bone may be used so that the gingival tissue does not push the GTR membrane into the defect (which would not allow enough space for the regenerative tissue to form). Denudation with secondary intention healing is a less satisfactory alternative. Extraction of the tooth may be necessary if the restorative plan is extensive and the prognosis of the tooth cannot be improved by other treatment methods. Extraction may be necessary if the three-walled defect totally surrounds the four surfaces of the tooth and trauma from occlusion cannot be controlled.

The most critical factor in obtaining maximum results with GTR is the availability of good access for root débridement. Collapse of the periodontal membrane used into the defect must be avoided by properly managing the sutures and surrounding (hard and soft) tissues-to-membrane relationships. The flap should be elevated so that no tension occurs at the time of closure; either vertical releasing incisions or extending two teeth aside of the treated area is recommended for this purpose.

References

Becker W, Becker B, Berg L, Sansom O: Clinical and volumetric analysis of three-walled intrabony defects following open flap débridement, *J Periodontol* 57:277, 1986.

Becker W, Becker B, Berg L et al: New attachment after treatment with root isolation procedures: report for treated Class III and Class II furcations and vertical defects, *Int J Periodont Restorat Dent* 8(3):9, 1988.

Carranza FA, Newman MG: *Clinical periodontology*, ed 8, Philadelphia, 1996, WB Saunders, p 626.

Gottlow J, Nyman S, Karring T, Wennstrom J: New attachment formation in human periodontium by guided tissue regeneration, *J Periodontol* 57:727, 1986.

Schallhorn RC, McClain PR: Combined osseous composite grafting, root conditioning and guided tissue regeneration, *Int J Periodontol Restor Dent* 8(4):9, 1988.

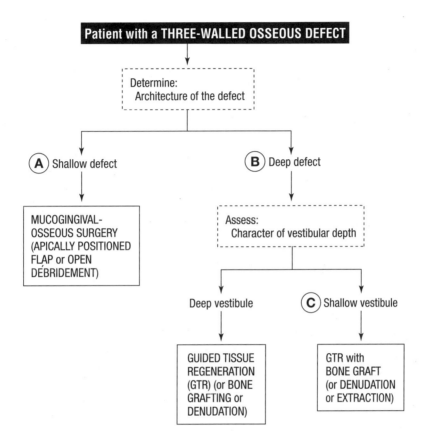

Patient with a THREE-WALLED OSSEOUS DEFECT

Determine:
Architecture of the defect

A Shallow defect

B Deep defect

MUCOGINGIVAL-
OSSEOUS SURGERY
(APICALLY POSITIONED
FLAP or OPEN
DEBRIDEMENT)

Assess:
Character of vestibular depth

Deep vestibule

C Shallow vestibule

GUIDED TISSUE
REGENERATION
(GTR) (or BONE
GRAFTING or
DENUDATION)

GTR with
BONE GRAFT
(or DENUDATION
or EXTRACTION)

30 Guided Tissue Regeneration or Alternatives for Treating Furcation Involvements

Alberto Sicilia, Jon Zabelegui

One of the most common difficulties encountered in treating periodontal disease is the presence of a furcation involvement. The ultimate goal of periodontal therapy is the regeneration of the periodontium to a state of health and function. Historically, with furcation involvement, treatment and prognosis have been difficult. Results with conventional therapy are unpredictable, but guided tissue regeneration (GTR) in some furcations consistently has been reported to be predictable if certain characteristics are found.

A A furcation involvement exists when attachment exposes the furcation to probing. Depending on how much attachment has been lost, it can be classified as Class I, II, or III. Furcation involvements are a periodontal hazard because they are difficult to clean even by professional means. Class I furcations are those where the tip of the probe does not catch within the furcation. This situation is easy to control; mild modification of the contour (odontoplasty) of the crown with a cylindrical finishing bur allows the tooth to be cleaned.

B When the probe catches in the furcation when moved coronally or in either lateral direction, a Class II or Class III furcation involvement is present. If an instrument goes into one furcation and comes out of another, a through-and-through or Class III furcation involvement is present; if it cannot do so, a definite or Class II furcation involvement is present.

C With Class II or III furcation involvement, a decision whether GTR or resective surgery should be performed is based on the apical depth of the furca involvement in relation to the bone levels between the involved molar and adjacent teeth. This may be assessed radiographically and by probing.

D If the furcation pocket depth is deep to that of the crestal bone between the involved tooth and its adjacent neighbors, GTR should be considered; however, if root proximity (see Chapter 32) limits access for débridement (e.g., there is only a narrow opening), resective surgery is a better option unless the roots are fused.

In some GTR situations, bone grafting to fill out a space into which regeneration tissue can grow (and prevent collapse of the membrane into the defect) may be helpful, or a coronal placement of the flap may be useful.

E If the furcation pocket depth is more shallow than the level of the crestal bone between the involved tooth and its adjacent neighbors, options include resective surgery (see Chapter 23), hemisection or root amputation, (see Chapter 72), or extraction (see Chapter 3).

References

Anderegg OR, Martin SJ, Gray JL et al: Clinical evaluation of the use of decalcified freeze-dried bone allograft with guided tissue regeneration in the treatment of molar furcation invasions, *J Periodontol* 62:264, 1991.

Becker W, Becker B, Berg L et al: New attachment after treatment with root isolation procedures: report for treated Class III and Class II furcations and vertical osseous defects, *Int J Periodontol Restor Dent* 3(3):9, 1988.

Carranza FA, Newman MG: *Clinical periodontology,* cd 8, Philadelphia, 1996, WB Saunders, p 626.

Gottlow J, Nyman S, Karring T, Wennstrom J: New attachment formation in human periodontium by guided tissue regeneration, *J Periodontol* 57:727, 1986.

Pontoriero R, Lindhe J, Nyman S et al: Guided tissue regeneration in degree II furcation involved mandibular teeth, *J Clin Periodontol* 15:247, 1988.

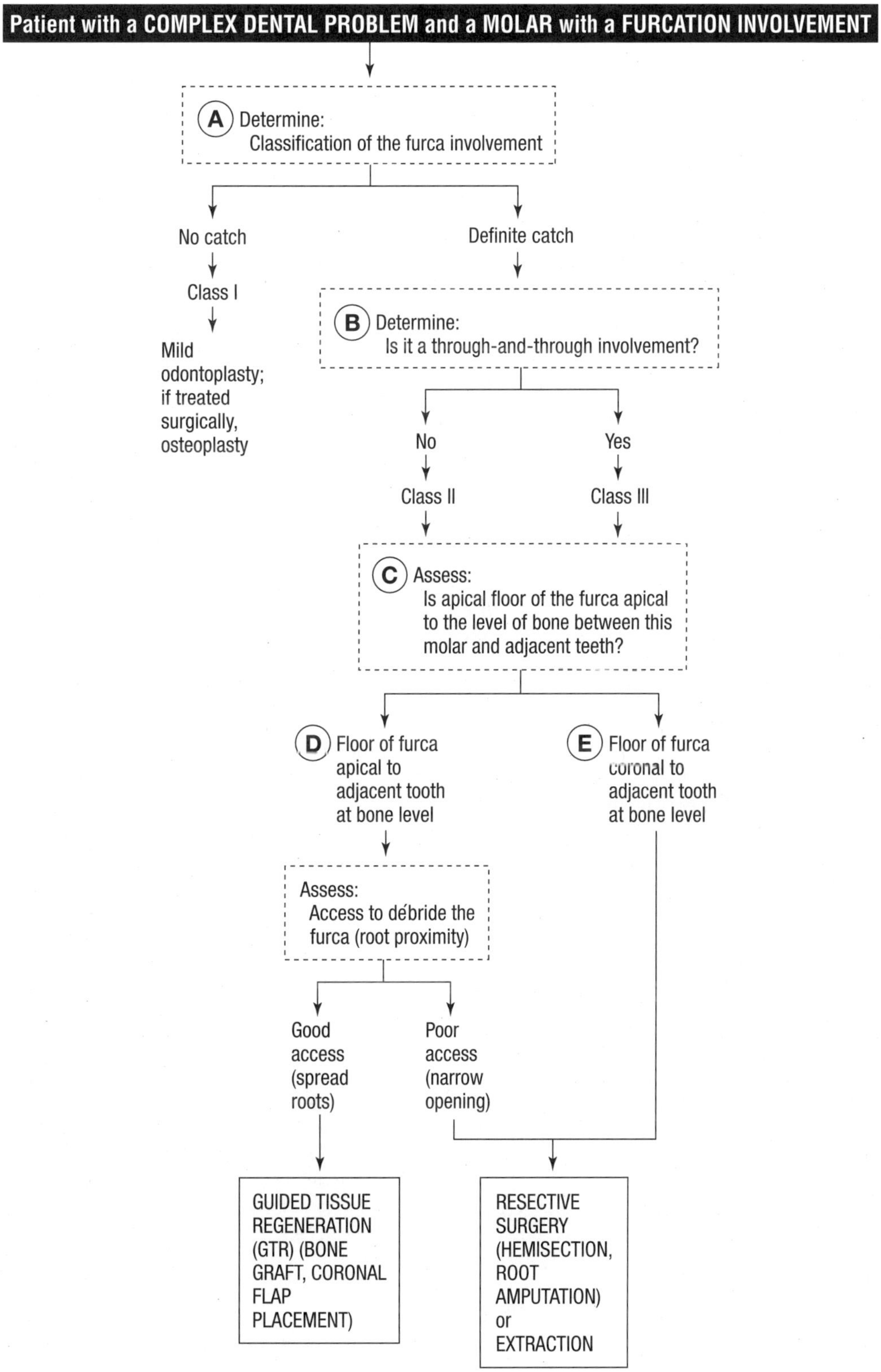

Patient with a COMPLEX DENTAL PROBLEM and a MOLAR with a FURCATION INVOLVEMENT

A Determine:
Classification of the furca involvement

No catch

Class I

Mild odontoplasty; if treated surgically, osteoplasty

Definite catch

B Determine:
Is it a through-and-through involvement?

No

Class II

Yes

Class III

C Assess:
Is apical floor of the furca apical to the level of bone between this molar and adjacent teeth?

D Floor of furca apical to adjacent tooth at bone level

E Floor of furca coronal to adjacent tooth at bone level

Assess:
Access to débride the furca (root proximity)

Good access (spread roots)

Poor access (narrow opening)

GUIDED TISSUE REGENERATION (GTR) (BONE GRAFT, CORONAL FLAP PLACEMENT)

RESECTIVE SURGERY (HEMISECTION, ROOT AMPUTATION) or EXTRACTION

31 Guided Tissue Regeneration in Two-Walled Osseous Defects

Alberto Sicilia, Jon Zabelegui, Francisco Enrile

Before studying the possible indication for a guided tissue regeneration (GTR) technique, the general condition of the patient should be evaluated. Characteristics of the patient such as systemic diseases, healing capacity, smoking habits, psychologic aspects, and manual ability (which can affect treatment and plaque control) must be taken into consideration.

A After this evaluation, the focus is on dental examination. First, the size of the intraosseous component of the defect (small, moderate, or large) must be determined. In the shallow defects (< 2 mm) regeneration is difficult to achieve or very little regeneration can be obtained. The cost-benefit relationship when compared with other kinds of treatment is unfavorable; GTR is not recommended.

B In moderate (2-4 mm) and deep defects (: 4 mm) the prognosis of the adjacent tooth or teeth must be evaluated, and if hopeless (see Chapter 3) the case is unfavorable for GTR on the middle tooth.

C If the tooth is treatable, analyze the local conditions. Positive findings include: (1) an adequate separation (: 2 mm) that exists between the roots of the adjacent teeth; (2) the anatomy of the affected dental surface allows a good adaptation of the membrane and closure of the defect; (3) a good quantity of healthy periodontium remains close to the defect (such as occurs in narrow and deep defects); and (4) a thick periodontium and adequate vestibule, which facilitate viability and stability of the flap that covers the membrane remains. When one or more negative conditions appear, the case will be considered as unfavorable for GTR.

D If local conditions are positive, evaluate the anatomy of the defect. If this permits the natural creation of space, a favorable situation exists. Evaluate the convenience of performing GTR in a conventional way with an expanded polytetrafluoroethylene membrane (ePTFE) or whether the use of a resorbable one[1] would be more efficacious (Fig. 31-1).

E If the morphology of the defect does not allow the natural creation of space, the case will not be as favorable. However, if the rest of the local conditions mentioned earlier are favorable, GTR can be attempted using procedures to maintain the space below the barrier, which in terms of predictability according to actual studies could be: (1) titanium reinforced membranes (TR), (2) TR membranes plus bone graft (BG), (3) ePTFE membranes plus BG, or (4) resorbable membrane plus BG.

---

[1]Short-term scientific data exists to support the use of membranes made from pure Lactide and glycolide polymers (Reslolut)or a physical blend of Poly-D, L-Lactide, and Poly-L-Lactide softened with Acetyl-μ-butyl citrate (Guidor).

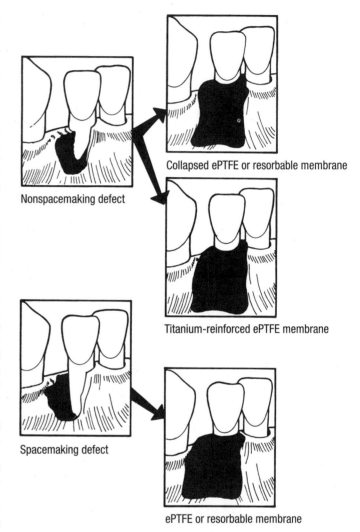

Collapsed ePTFE or resorbable membrane

Nonspacemaking defect

Titanium-reinforced ePTFE membrane

Spacemaking defect

ePTFE or resorbable membrane

Fig. 31-1 Selection of membranes for spacemaking and nonspacemaking defects.

References

Becker W, Becker BE: Treatment of mandibular 3-wall intrabony defects by flap debridement and expanded polytetrafluoroethylene barrier membranes. Long-term evaluation of 32 treated patients, *J Periodontol* 64:1138, 1993.

Cortellini P, Pini-Prato G, Tonetti MS: Periodontal regeneration of human infrabony defects with titanium reinforced membranes: a controlled clinical trial, *J Periodontol* 66:797, 1995.

Cortellini P, Pini-Prato G, Tonnetti MS: Periodontal regeneration of human intrabony defects with bioresorbable membranes: a controlled clinical trial, *J Periodontol* 67:217, 1996.

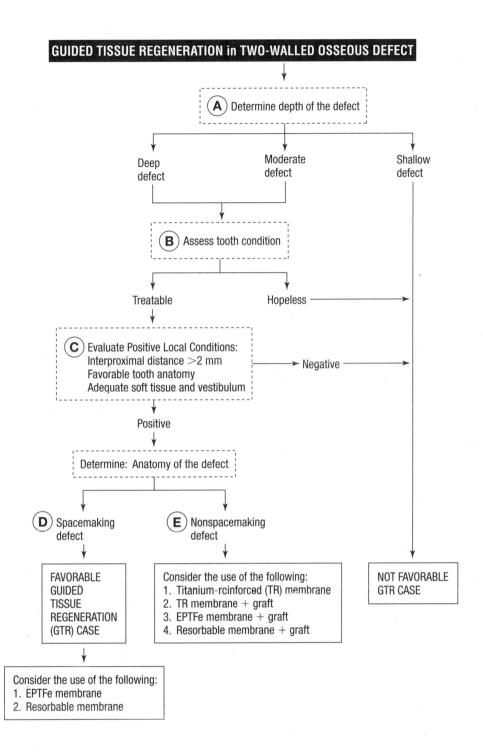

GUIDED TISSUE REGENERATION in TWO-WALLED OSSEOUS DEFECT

A Determine depth of the defect

Deep defect Moderate defect Shallow defect

B Assess tooth condition

Treatable Hopeless

C Evaluate Positive Local Conditions:
Interproximal distance >2 mm
Favorable tooth anatomy
Adequate soft tissue and vestibulum

Negative

Positive

Determine: Anatomy of the defect

D Spacemaking defect

E Nonspacemaking defect

FAVORABLE GUIDED TISSUE REGENERATION (GTR) CASE

Consider the use of the following:
1. Titanium-reinforced (TR) membrane
2. TR membrane + graft
3. EPTFe membrane + graft
4. Resorbable membrane + graft

NOT FAVORABLE GTR CASE

Consider the use of the following:
1. EPTFe membrane
2. Resorbable membrane

Laurell L, Falk H, Johard G, Gottlow J: Clinical use of a bioresorbable matrix barrier in guided tissue regeneration therapy: case series, *J Periodontol* 65:967, 1994.

McClain PK, Shallhorn RG: Long-term assessment of combined osseous composite grafting, root conditioning, and guided tissue regeneration, *Int J Periodont Rest Dent* 13:9, 1993.

Sanz M, Zabelegui I, Villa A, Sicilia A: Guided tissue regeneration in human class II furcation and interproximal infrabony defects after using a bioabsorbable membrane barrier, *Int J Periodont Rest Dent* (in press).

Tonetti MS, Pini-Prato G, Cortellini P: Factors affecting the healing response of intrabony defects following guided tissue regeneration and access flap surgery, *J Clin Periodontol* 23:548, 1996.

32 Maxillary Molars with Root Proximity and Periodontal Problems

Walter B. Hall

Maxillary molar teeth with periodontal problems complicated by root proximity (roots so close together that plaque removal and root planing cannot be accomplished because plaque removal devices and curettes cannot be manipulated in the available space) are a common treatment planning puzzle. A surgical procedure that eliminates pocketing but leaves an area in which plaque removal by the patient and root planing by the therapist cannot effectively be performed is not a wise choice for therapy. Extraction or root amputation on one or both of the molars can create a sound, maintainable, functional unit but one that involves extensive treatment including endodontics or prosthodontics as well as periodontal treatment. Such treatment is expensive and must be within the patient's means. Guided tissue regeneration (GTR) is not feasible if root proximity negates the possibility of thorough débridement of the periodontal defect; however, if the area can be thoroughly débrided, GTR could be an effective and comparatively inexpensive approach. See Fig. 32-1.

A If the defect between the two molars can be thoroughly débrided with a curette or new thin ultrasonic tip following flap displacement, GTR is the best option.

B If GTR is not feasible, the endodontic status of the two molars should be determined next. If no pulpal problem exists, a determination should be made whether root canal therapy and a root amputation can be done. If so, the restorability of the teeth and their value to the overall treatment plan should be assessed. If restoration is feasible and useful and the periodontal problem can be resolved by root amputation on either or both of the molars (and the patient consents to and can afford this approach), endodontics followed by root amputation and periodontal surgical therapy should be performed and the teeth restored appropriately. If root canal therapy or root amputation cannot be done (e.g., root tips are fused) or if the restorative and periodontal problems cannot be resolved by root amputation, either or both of the molars may have to be extracted and the problem resolved prosthodontically or with implants.

C If either or both of the molars also have endodontic problems, the possibility of performing a successful root canal therapy should be evaluated first. If they can be treated, the sequence of decision making would be the same as in *B:* (1) Can a root amputation be done? (2) Can the periodontal problem be resolved and the teeth restored to usefulness in the overall treatment plan? (3) Can the patient accept and afford this approach?

If the answer to each question is positive, proceed with endodontics, root amputation and periodontal surgery, and restoration. If the answer to any of the questions is negative, extraction of one or both molars and a prosthodontic or implant solution should be considered.

D If one or both of the molars have existing endodontics, the adequacy of the existing endodontics (including "cracked tooth" signs or symptoms) should be evaluated first. If the endodontics is satisfactory and no vertical root fractures can be detected, the sequence of decision making would be the same as in *C.* If the answer to each question is positive and no endodontic treatment is needed, root amputation and elimination of the periodontal defects should be performed and followed by appropriate restoration. If the answer to each question is positive and the existing endodontics is unsatisfactory, but it can be redone successfully or the problem is around the root to be amputated, necessary endodontic retreatment followed by root amputation and periodontal surgery and restoration should be planned. If any answers are negative, extraction and a prosthodontic or implant alternative should be used.

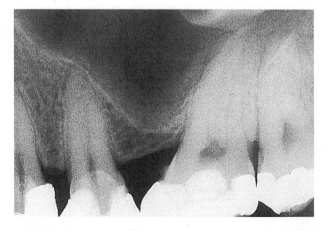

Fig. 32-1 Root proximity between second and third molars appears to jeopardize access to successfully treat or maintain the distal furcation involvement on the second molar.

References

Carranza FA, Newman MG: *Clinical periodontology,* ed 8, Philadelphia, 1996, WB Saunders, p 538.

Genco RJ, Goldman HM, Cohen DW: *Contemporary periodontics,* St Louis, 1990, Mosby, pp 582, 589.

Hall WB: Periodontal preparation of the mouth for restoration, *Dent Clin North Am* 24:197, 1980.

Hall WB: Removal of third molars: a periodontal viewpoint. In McDonald RE, Hurt WC, Gilmore HW, Middleton RH, editors: *Current therapy in dentistry,* St Louis, 1980, Mosby, p 228.

Schluger S, Yuodelis R, Page RC, Johnson RH: *Periodontal diseases,* ed 2, Philadelphia, 1990, Lea & Febiger, pp 102, 343, 511.

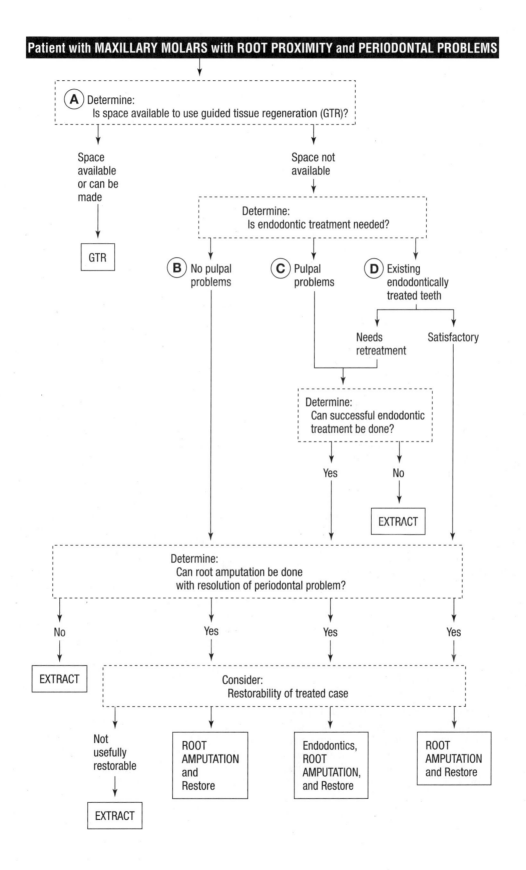

Patient with MAXILLARY MOLARS with ROOT PROXIMITY and PERIODONTAL PROBLEMS

(A) Determine:
Is space available to use guided tissue regeneration (GTR)?

Space available or can be made

GTR

Space not available

Determine:
Is endodontic treatment needed?

(B) No pulpal problems

(C) Pulpal problems

(D) Existing endodontically treated teeth

Needs retreatment

Satisfactory

Determine:
Can successful endodontic treatment be done?

Yes

No

EXTRACT

Determine:
Can root amputation be done with resolution of periodontal problem?

No

Yes

Yes

Yes

EXTRACT

Consider:
Restorability of treated case

Not usefully restorable

ROOT AMPUTATION and Restore

Endodontics, ROOT AMPUTATION, and Restore

ROOT AMPUTATION and Restore

EXTRACT

33 Guided Tissue Regeneration Versus Implants

William P. Lundergan

Rapid progress in the field of implantology and the development of guided tissue regeneration (GTR) were among the many advances in the 1980s. In the 1990s the dentist must consider these treatment alternatives when confronted with a periodontally compromised tooth. Should the tooth be treated using GTR or should it be extracted and replaced with an implant? Choosing between these two procedures or an alternative therapy requires careful consideration.

A The nature of the periodontal bony defect is important when assessing the prospects for success with GTR. The procedure is less successful in treating areas of horizontal bone loss because of the difficulty of maintaining a space in which regeneration can occur. New membrane designs, however, have facilitated regeneration in these areas. GTR is most predictable in treating two- and three-walled vertical defects and Class II furcation involvements. (Mandibular molar furcations are more predictable than maxillary molar furcations.) Success in treating one-walled vertical defects and Class III furcation involvements is less predictable. Consider implant therapy if GTR procedures are unlikely to be successful.

B The anatomy of the tooth in question must be evaluated when considering GTR. Root concavities and furcation involvement can complicate the procedure because complete adaptation of the membrane to the tooth is critical. If the membrane is poorly adapted, epithelial cells are able to migrate apically along the root surface and prevent regeneration. Thus when treating a tooth with furcation involvement, a long root trunk is preferred to a short root trunk as the chances of successfully adapting the membrane are enhanced. The clinician must also consider the potential postsurgical maintenance problems created by root concavities, grooves, and furcation exposure. Root morphology and length should also be evaluated. If the tooth is eventually to serve as an abutment, will the periodontal support be adequate even if GTR is successful? All these factors must be considered.

C Before performing GTR the ultimate restorability of the tooth should be evaluated. If the tooth is fractured, perforated, or internally-externally resorbed, can these complicating factors be satisfactorily resolved? If the tooth requires endodontic therapy, what are the prospects for successful treatment? If the roots are severely dilacerated or the canals calcified, the chance for success may not be good. The position of the tooth in the arch should also be considered from the standpoints of strategic location and maintainability. If the tooth is not in a favorable position, is orthodontic therapy indicated, and what are the prospects for success? If esthetic concerns are involved, can the tooth be restored with an acceptable esthetic result? Finally, the decision must consider the overall treatment plan for the patient. Is GTR compatible with the overall treatment plan, or would extraction be more appropriate?

D GTR procedures may be contraindicated for patients with heart valve defects, prosthetic devices, uncontrolled diabetes, or compromised immune conditions. Any factor that contraindicates periodontal surgery also contraindicates GTR; in such cases, an alternative therapy should be considered.

E The dentist must consider several factors when planning the surgical placement of an implant. Anatomic considerations include the type of bone present, available vertical bone height, buccolingual width of the alveolar ridge, maxillary sinus location, mandibular nerve location, and surgical access. Some potentially limiting anatomic factors can be corrected using advanced surgical techniques (e.g., sinus lift, mandibular nerve repositioning procedure) but not without increased cost and risk of complications. Alveolar ridge deficiencies may be corrected using ridge augmentation procedures (i.e., bone grafting or GTR). Medical contraindications for the surgical placement of implants might include recent myocardial infarction, poorly controlled diabetes, immunosuppression, head and neck radiation therapy, risk for endocarditis, dependency on alcohol and drugs, and mental health status. The dentist must also consider patient acceptance of the overall surgical and prosthetic treatment plan including factors such as time, cost, and risk. Any single factor may make implant therapy inappropriate and require consideration of an alternative treatment plan.

F The dentist must evaluate several prosthetic considerations when considering a dental implant: temporomandibular joint status, maxillary-mandibular ridge relationship, available interarch distance, the existence of parafunctional habits, the occlusal relationship of the remaining teeth, the patient's oral hygiene and motivation, and the patient's esthetic requirements. Any single factor may make implant therapy inappropriate and require consideration of an alternative treatment plan.

References

Bahat O: Surgical planning, *J Calif Dent Assoc* 20(5):31, 1992.

Carranza FA, Newman MG: *Clinical periodontology*, Philadelphia, 1996, WB Saunders, pp 626, 688.

Patient with a COMPLEX DENTAL PROBLEM INVOLVING a TOOTH REQUIRING GUIDED TISSUE REGENERATION or an IMPLANT

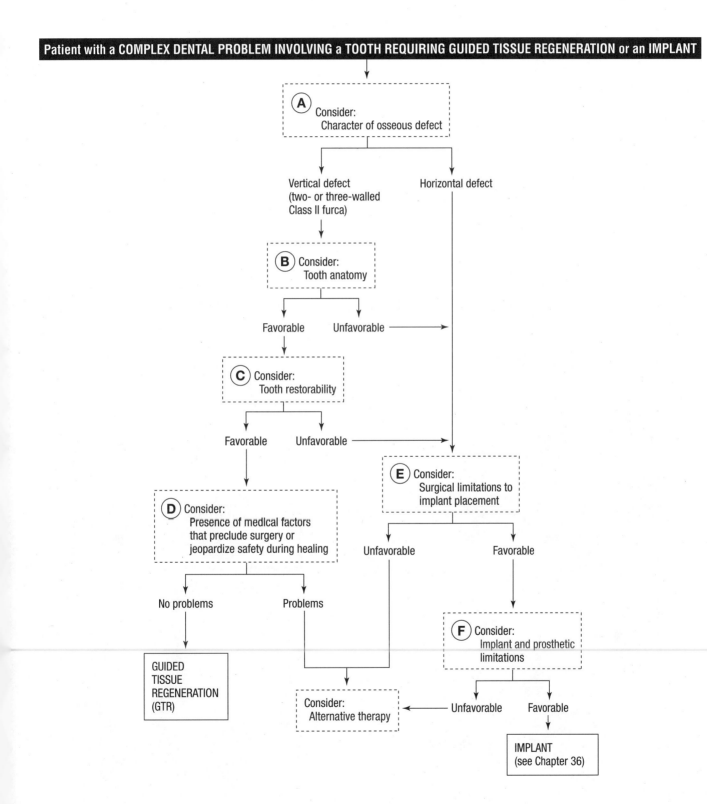

Guided Tissue Regeneration in Osseous Dehiscences

Alberto Sicilia, Jon Zabelegui, Pedro Buitrago

Having verified the suitability of the patient for a regenerative periodontal treatment from a general point of view (see Chapter 22) and established the diagnosis of an osseous dehiscence by the usual methods (see Chapter 15), the dentist should approach the treatment in the following way.

A In the shallow dehiscences (< 3 mm) regeneration is difficult to achieve or scant regeneration can be obtained. If the cost-benefit relationship when compared with other kinds of treatment is unfavorable, GTR is not recommended.

B In moderate (3-5 mm) and deep (> 6 mm) dehiscences, determine the prognosis of the affected tooth or teeth, and if hopeless (see Chapter 3), do not attempt GTR.

C If the tooth is treatable, evaluate the adequacy of the vestibulum and attached gingiva. If they are adequate, GTR is indicated because it would be easier to keep the membrane covered during the treatment, preventing gingival recession and contamination of the barrier, which might endanger regeneration. If desirable conditions do not exist, evaluate the need for mucogingival surgical procedures, with or without membranes, as alternatives.

D The anatomy of the osseous dehiscence and the root prominence must be such as to permit adaptation of the membrane ideally to the cementum-enamel junction of the tool, completely covering the defect and creating a space beneath the membrane.

E If the root is not prominent and the form of the osseous defect makes it easier to create space, a favorable case exists (Fig. 34-1). Use GTR with an e-PTFE or resorbable membrane.[1] Narrow dehiscences with thick bony walls make it easier to achieve these objectives because a greater quantity of adjacent donor cells exists near the surface in which regeneration should take place.

---

[1]Short-term scientific data exists to support the use of membranes made from pure Lactide and glycolide polymers (Resololut), polyglycolactic acid (Vicryl) or a physical blend of Poly-D, L-Lactide, and Poly-L-Lactide softened with Acetyl-μ-butyl citrate (Guidor).

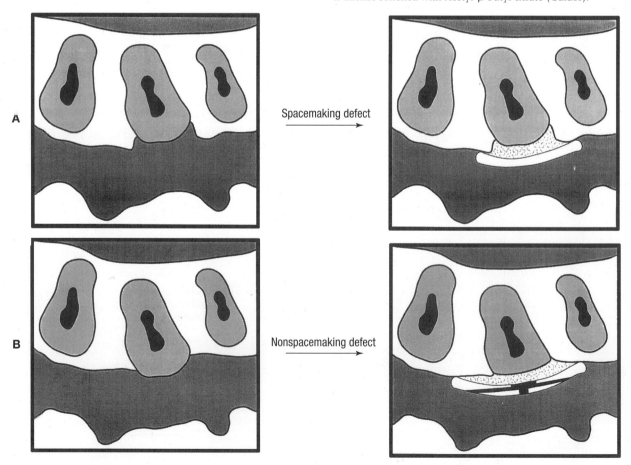

Fig. 34-1 **A**, Spacemaking defect. **B**, Nonspacemaking defect using titanium-supported membrane.

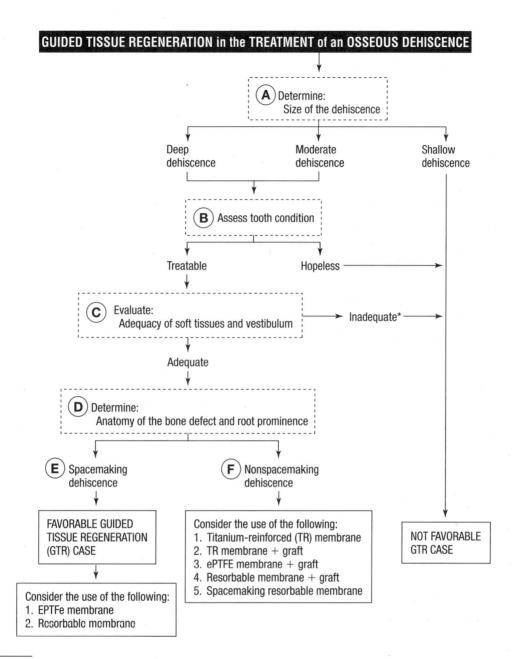

GUIDED TISSUE REGENERATION in the TREATMENT of an OSSEOUS DEHISCENCE

A Determine: Size of the dehiscence

- Deep dehiscence
- Moderate dehiscence
- Shallow dehiscence

B Assess tooth condition

- Treatable
- Hopeless

C Evaluate: Adequacy of soft tissues and vestibulum → Inadequate*

- Adequate

D Determine: Anatomy of the bone defect and root prominence

E Spacemaking dehiscence

FAVORABLE GUIDED TISSUE REGENERATION (GTR) CASE

Consider the use of the following:
1. EPTFe membrane
2. Resorbable membrane

F Nonspacemaking dehiscence

Consider the use of the following:
1. Titanium-reinforced (TR) membrane
2. TR membrane + graft
3. ePTFE membrane + graft
4. Resorbable membrane + graft
5. Spacemaking resorbable membrane

NOT FAVORABLE GTR CASE

*Consider mucogingival procedures, with or without membranes.

F If the osseous defect and the morphology of the root do not allow creation of a space, a space can be created using: (1) titanium reinforced membranes (TR) alone or accompanying osseous grafts (OG), (2) ePTFE membranes with OG, (3) resorbable space-creating membranes (Guidor), or (4) resorbable membranes with OG.

References

Cortellini P, Clauser C, Pini-Prato GP: Histological assessment of new attachment following the treatment of a buccal recession by means of a guided tissue regeneration procedure, *J Periodontol* 64:387, 1993.

Echeveria JJ, Manzanares C: Guided tissue regeneration in severe periodontal defects in anterior teeth: case reports, *J Periodontol* 66:295, 1995.

Pini-Prato G, Clauser C, Magnani C, Cortellini P: Resorbable membranes in the treatment of human buccal recession: a nine-case report, *Int J Periodontol Rest Dent* 15(3):259, 1995.

Rachlin G, Koubi J, Dejou J, Franquin JC: The use of a resorbable membrane in mucogingival surgery: case series, *J Periodontol* 67:621, 1996.

Roccuzzo M, Lungo M, Corrente G, Gandolfo S: Comparative study of a bioresorbable and non-resorbable membrane in the treatment of human buccal gingival recessions, *J Periodontol* 67:7, 1996.

Tinti C, Vincenzi G, Cortellini P, Pini-Prato GP, Clauser C: Guided tissue regeneration in the treatment of human facial recession: a twelve case report, *J Periodontol* 63:554, 1992.

Tinti C, Vincenzi G, Cocchetto R: Guided tissue regeneration in mucogingival surgery, *J Periodontol* 64:1184, 1993.

35 Third Molar Extraction and Guided Tissue Regeneration

Daniel Etienne, Mithri Davarpanah

Guided tissue regeneration (GTR) is an accepted way for treating deep intrabony defects. The principle is based on numerous animal and clinical studies in which barrier membranes were used to isolate periodontal defects from gingival epithelium and gingival connective tissues, allowing cells from the periodontal ligament to repopulate the detached root surface. To date, the majority of studies relating to GTR have used expanded polytetrafluoroethylene (e-PTFE) barrier membranes, which are considered "the gold standard."

The hoped-for outcome of removing impacted third molars is to do so without injury of the adjacent tooth. Improper surgical technique can cause postoperative pain and may result in intrabony defects adjacent to second molars. Partially impacted third molars are frequently accompanied by periodontal breakdown of the adjacent tooth. In a retrospective study, Kugelberg et al reported that, 2 years after impacted third-molar surgery, 43.3% of the cases showed probing depths more than 7 mm, and 32.1% showed intrabony defects greater than 4 mm on the distal surface of the adjacent second molar. Of patients older than 26 years of age, 44% demonstrated intrabony defects distal to second molars that were greater than 4 mm. Of patients younger than 25 years of age, 4% developed defects greater than 4 mm.

GTR is an accepted method for treating advanced periodontal defects. Pecora et al (1993) have evaluated the possibilities of using GTR procedures to prevent and treat periodontal lesions after third-molar extractions (the use of e-PTFE membranes to regenerate tissue lost as a result of periodontal diseases has been well documented).

In this study, periodontal healing of 20 vertical intrabony defects located distal to the second molar was monitored for 7 years after impacted third-molar surgery. Data showed that all defects healed with a combination of a recession and a decrease in probing depths. In the test group the mean decrease in probing depths was 5.7 mm, compared with 4 mm in the control group. There was a mean gain of probing attachment level of 4.3 mm for the test group, compared with 1.9 mm for the control group. The use of e-PTFE membrane significantly enhanced the gain of attachment level in the test sites compared with the control sites (p < .01); however, both treatment modalities resulted in a significant reduction in pocket depth.

The proper diagnosis of an intrabony defect on the distal surface of the second molar is important for successful treatment during third-molar surgery. The preoperative anatomic relationship with the second molar is also a critical factor.

Age is a main contributing factor. Subjects 25 years of age or younger exhibit less postoperative intrabony pockets. The extent of the intrabony defect on distal of the second molar is also a critical parameter. Dental plaque affects the wound healing of older patients.

A The Kugelberg's "Risk Index M3" is an index predicting the risk for periodontal defects. A value of 1 is no risk, 2 is low risk, 3 is moderate risk, and 4 and above is high risk. An index of 0 is correlated with an estimated defect of 2 mm; an index of 2 is correlated with an intrabony defect of 3 to 4 mm.

B For patients who have a Kugelberg's Risk Index M3 less than 2 (patients with no periodontal involvement on the adjacent second molar, patients whose asymptomatic third molars are being removed for orthodontic reasons, or patients with 3 mm or less infrabony defects on the adjacent second molar), membrane therapy is not necessary.

C For patients with a Kugelberg's Risk Index M3 greater than 2, with deep pockets and narrow, deep infrabony defects on the adjacent second molar, the possibility of closing the flaps completely over the third molar extraction socket or not determines whether a resorbable or a nonresorbable membrane should be used. If full coverage of the membrane is possible, a resorbable membrane should be used for GTR. In all other instances a nonresorbable membrane is necessary.

D For patients with a Kugelberg's Risk Index M3, those with deep pockets and deep, wide infrabony defects, a nonresorbable membrane with titanium reinforcement is used to avoid membrane collapse.

The use of reinforced membranes is well established for wide intrabony defects or guided bone regeneration around implants. The blood clot is well protected from membrane collapse when using a titanium reinforced membrane, but the outcome and the advantage for comparison with conventional e-PTFE membranes has to be validated for third molar surgery and wide spaces.

Treatment modalities will evolve with resorbable membranes (Resolut, Guidor). These membranes, made of polymers, are well-integrated within the soft tissue, but they collapse in wide defects. If an optimal bone level is expected, e-PTFE membranes will be better.

GTR is an appropriate way of treating periodontal diseases associated with horizontally impacted third molars.

References

Kugelberg C: Third molar surgery: oral and maxillofacial surgery and infections, *Curr Opin Dentistry* 2:9, 1992.

Pecora G, Celletti R, Davarpanah M, Convani U, Etienne D: The effects of guided tissue regeneration on healing after impacted mandibular third-molar surgery: 1 year results, *Int J Periodont Rest Dent* 13:397, 1993.

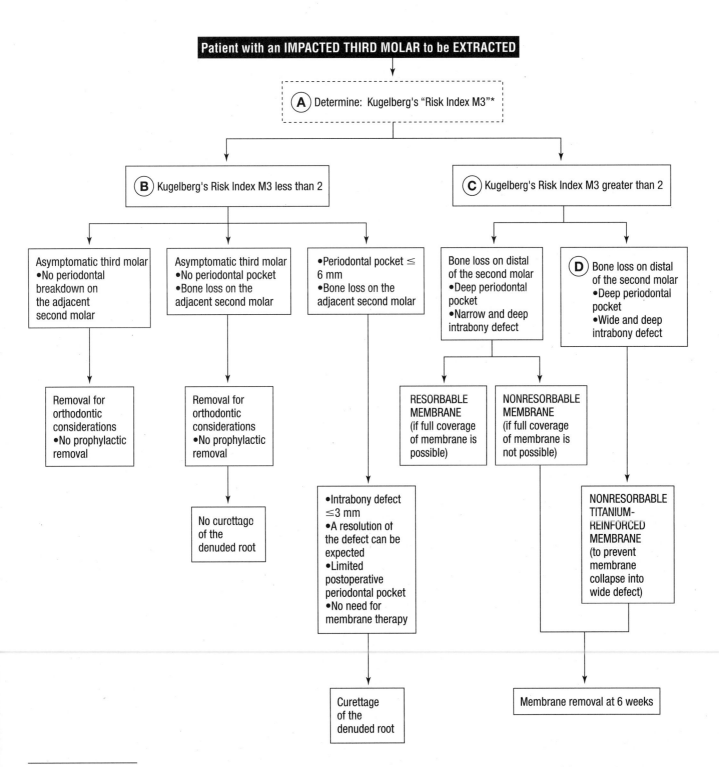

Patient with an IMPACTED THIRD MOLAR to be EXTRACTED

(A) Determine: Kugelberg's "Risk Index M3"*

(B) Kugelberg's Risk Index M3 less than 2

(C) Kugelberg's Risk Index M3 greater than 2

Asymptomatic third molar
•No periodontal breakdown on the adjacent second molar

Asymptomatic third molar
•No periodontal pocket
•Bone loss on the adjacent second molar

•Periodontal pocket ≤ 6 mm
•Bone loss on the adjacent second molar

Bone loss on distal of the second molar
•Deep periodontal pocket
•Narrow and deep intrabony defect

(D) Bone loss on distal of the second molar
•Deep periodontal pocket
•Wide and deep intrabony defect

Removal for orthodontic considerations
•No prophylactic removal

Removal for orthodontic considerations
•No prophylactic removal

RESORBABLE MEMBRANE
(if full coverage of membrane is possible)

NONRESORBABLE MEMBRANE
(if full coverage of membrane is not possible)

No curettage of the denuded root

•Intrabony defect ≤3 mm
•A resolution of the defect can be expected
•Limited postoperative periodontal pocket
•No need for membrane therapy

NONRESORBABLE TITANIUM-REINFORCED MEMBRANE
(to prevent membrane collapse into wide defect)

Curettage of the denuded root

Membrane removal at 6 weeks

*Kugelberg's Risk Index M3. Each of the following criteria has a value of 1: on distal of second molar: (1) plaque, (2) pocket depth greater than 6 mm, (3) intrabony defect greater than 3 mm, (4) root resorption; third molar, (5) sagittal inclination < 50°, (6) third molar widened follicles < 2.5 mm, (7) large contact area between third and second molar, (8) smoker.

36 Basic Considerations in Selecting a Patient for Implants

E. Robert Stultz, Jr., William Grippo

When a patient is considering an implant approach to the edentulous or partially dentulous status, information may be sought from a general dentist or a specialist. In each case a series of decisions is made to determine whether the patient is a reasonable candidate for implant therapy. The initial decisions involve medical and psychologic qualification for implant therapy. Once these considerations are met successfully, the dental indications and contraindications can be evaluated.

A A medical evaluation is made from a questionnaire, a patient interview, and any medical consultations necessitated by the patient's health history. Conditions that make surgery dangerous or adversely affect healing must be considered. Examples of absolute contraindications are recurrent myocardial infarction, acquired immunodeficiency syndrome (AIDS), debilitating or transmissible hepatitis, pregnancy, granulocytopenia, poorly controlled diabetes, and drug or alcohol dependency. Other conditions (e.g., prolonged corticosteroid use, blood dyscrasias, collagen diseases, malignancies, heavy smoking) make implant a questionable alternative. If any significant medical contraindication exists and cannot be resolved promptly, implants are not indicated, and alternative approaches are required.

B If no medical contraindications are detected, the psychologic status of the patient and the reasonableness of expectations are evaluated. If the patient is psychologically unstable or the expectations of implant therapy are unrealistic, alternative approaches should be considered.

C If the patient is psychologically well adjusted and does not expect "miracles" in esthetics or functional benefits of an implant approach, the consequences of the totally edentulous or partially dentulous status should be considered next. The status of teeth to be retained are a complicating factor in this decision process. Position of these teeth, their periodontal status, and their restorability must be considered.

D To determine whether adequate support exists for implants, the quantity of bone available at implant sites must be evaluated. If the height or width of the recipient ridge areas is inadequate or if the trajectory is unsatisfactory, an implant may not be feasible. Bony undercuts also present problems, as does the position of anatomic features such as the mental foramen. These factors can be examined with simple dental radiographs, Panorex films, tomographic or cephalometric film, or computerized tomography scan imaging. If the ridge is inadequate for any reason, an implant is inappropriate, and alternatives should be considered.

E If bone "quantity" is satisfactory, bone "quality" should be considered next. The most ideal alveolar bone is the dense cortical bone of the mandibular anterior ridge; the least desirable is the thin cortical, loose trabecular bone typically found in the maxillary posterior region. Bone quality may be classified as follows:
- Class I: Dense cortical bone
- Class II: Dense cortical bone with dense trabecular bone
- Class III: Moderate cortical and trabecular bone
- Class IV: Thin cortical bone with poor trabecular bone

Patients with Class I or II bone are good candidates for osseointegrated implants. Those with Class III or IV bone require bone augmentation before osseointegrated implants or a subperiosteal approach.

References

Branemark PI, Zarb G, Albrectson T: *Tissue integrated prosthesis: osseointegration in clinical dentistry,* Chicago, 1985, Quintessence Publishing, p 1.

Golec TS: Implants, what and when, *Calif Dent Assoc J* 15:49, 1987.

Jensen O: Site classification for the osseointegrated implant, *J Prosthet Dent* 61:228, 1989.

Misch C, Judy K: Classification of partially edentulous arches for implant dentistry, *Int J Oral Implant* 12:688, 1986.

Stambaugh R: Surgical management of the complicated periodontal-prosthesis patient, *Calif Dent Assoc J* 17:31, 1989.

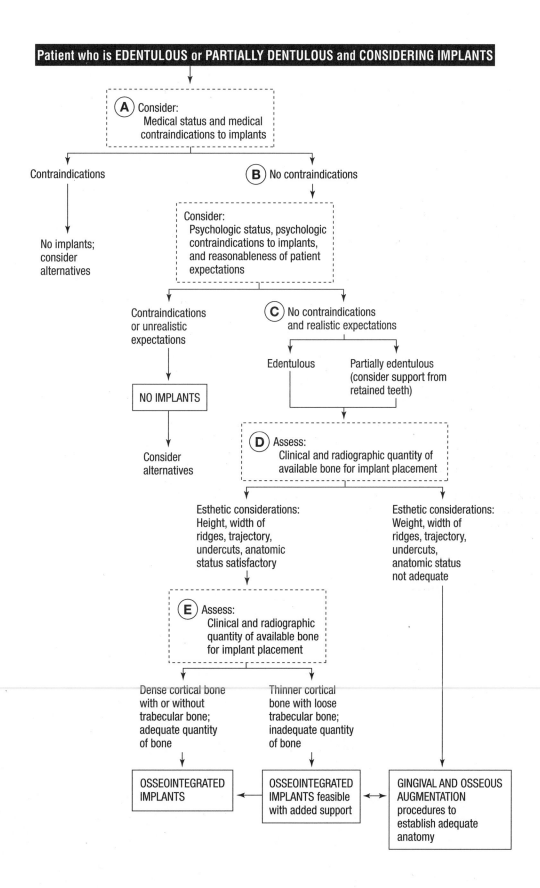

37 Selection of Implant Modalities for Partially Dentulous Patients

E. Robert Stultz, Jr., William Grippo

Once the basic factors that determine the eligibility of a patient for implant therapy have been met (see Chapter 36), the periodontal status of teeth to be retained must be determined.

A If the remaining teeth are healthy periodontally, an implant approach to implant therapy for the partially dentulous patient becomes feasible.

B If significant periodontal problems are detected (e.g., deep pockets, furcation involvement, poor crown-to-root ratio), the likelihood of treatment making affected teeth useful in the overall treatment plan must be assessed. The ability of the patient to perform adequate plaque control can be evaluated during the periodontal treatment phase. If the periodontal problems are refractory (i.e., response is poor) or good plaque control is not demonstrated, implants are not likely to be helpful, and alternatives should be explored.

C If the periodontal problems appear resolvable, their efficacy must be established following treatment. Unsuccessful cases should not receive implant therapy; implant therapy is feasible in successful cases.

D The available bone support is considered next. If alveolar bone height is greater than 10 mm, its width greater than 6 mm, and the trajectory less than 25 degrees, endosseous cylinder implants are the best approach.

E If the available bone height is less than 10 mm, the width only 4 to 6 mm, or the trajectory greater than 25 degrees, endosseous blade implants are indicated.

F If inadequate bone height or width is present for endosseous root from implants, the following various procedures may be used to create an adequate ridge: (1) membrane-assisted hard tissue grafts, (2) monocortical onlay grafts from the chin or ascending ramus, (3) ridge expansion techniques, and (4) sinus elevation procedures in the maxilla.

If these procedures succeed, the adequacy of the available bone can be reassessed. In some cases guided bone augmentation can be used at the time of placement of the cylinder implant into an extraction socket.

G In selected cases where the alveolar ridge is deficient in height but adequate in width (> 6 mm), a subperiosteal implant may be the treatment of choice. I find this choice most useful in the posterior mandible where monocortical onlay grafting or nerve lateralization is not recommended.

References

Branemark PI, Zarb G, Albrectson T: *Tissue integrated prosthesis: osseointegration in clinical dentistry,* Chicago, 1985, Quintessence Publishing, p 1.

Golec TS: Implants, what and when, *Calif Dent Assoc J* 15:49, 1987.

Jensen O: Site classification for the osseointegrated implant, *J Prosthet Dent* 61:228, 1989.

Meffert RM, Block MS, Kent JN: What is osseointegration? *Int J Periodontol Restor Dent* 11:135, 1987.

Misch C, Judy K: Classification of partially edentulous arches for implant dentistry, *Int J Periodontol Restor Dent* 12:688, 1986.

Smiler DG: Evaluation and treatment planning, *Calif Dent Assoc J* 15:35, 1987.

EVALUATING PERIODONTAL STATUS of PATIENT WHO MEETS BASIC CRITERIA for IMPLANT THERAPY

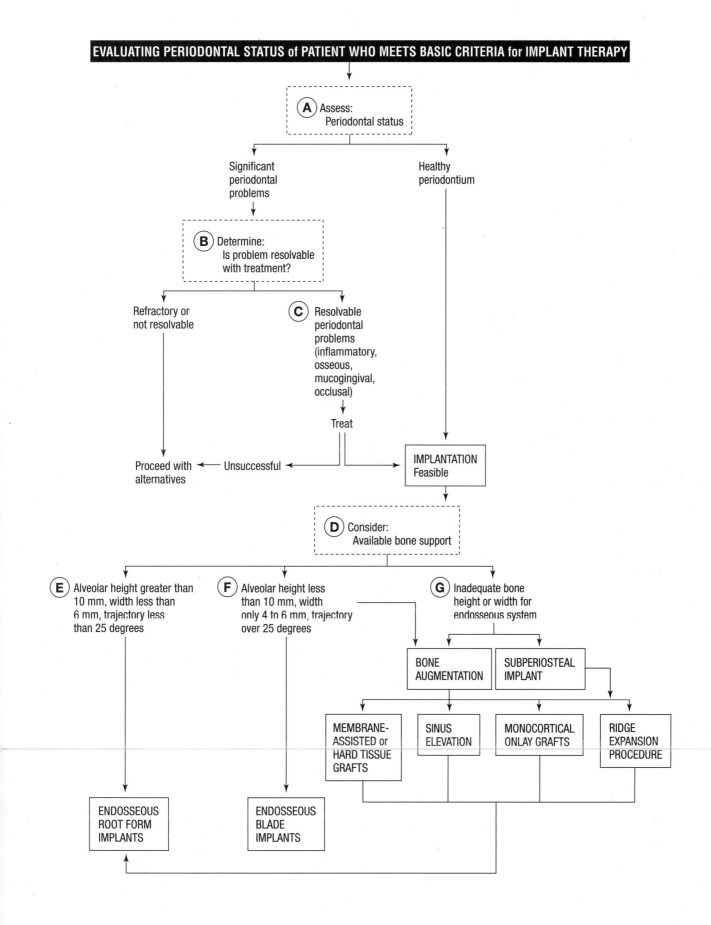

38 Osseointegrated Implants for the Partially Edentulous Maxilla

Joan Pi Urgell

When evaluating the distally edentulous maxilla, the following important factors for the long-term prognosis of the implant-supported restoration should be considered:

- Quantity of bone, limited by the floor of the sinus
- Quality of bone decreases in the posterior maxilla
- Available space intermaxillary
- Major occlusal forces

A The method of choice to evaluate both quantity and quality of bone is the computerized tomography scanner, available with a wide range of software.

B If the remaining alveolar crest is more than 8 mm below the floor of the sinus, assess the quality of that bone.

C If it is good quality bone, consider the width of the ridge. If there is more than 6 mm of width, place wide fixtures, one per missing tooth. If there is 5 to 6 mm of width, use regular fixtures. If there is less than 4-mm width, the fixtures should be placed simultaneously with guided bone regeneration (GBR).

D When less than 8 mm of bone is present below the sinus floor, determine if it has been caused by vertical resorption or an enlargement of the sinus.

E In the case of vertical resorption the treatment of choice is to rebuild the maxilla. When less than 4 mm is needed to place the fixtures simultaneously with a reinforced membrane, bone chips may be used to augment the residual ridge height. If more than 4 mm is needed, graft the remaining ridge using an onlay graft, and secure the graft with mini screws. Place the fixtures after 6 to 8 months.

F If the lack of residual bone is caused by enlargement of the sinus, evaluate the possibility of placing a fixture in the pterygomaxillary fissurae.

G If there is enough bone anterior to the sinus and a fixture could be placed in the pterygomaxillary fissurae, the treatment of choice will be two fixtures in the premolar area and one in the pterygomaxillary region.

H If there is no possibility of placing fixtures anterior to the sinus and in the pterygomaxillary fissurae because of a large pneumatized sinus, evaluate the residual ridge below the floor of the sinus again. If 3 to 8 mm of residual ridge remains, the treatment of choice is a lateral antrectomy. Raise the Schneiderian membrane, graft with autologous bone, and place the fixtures simultaneously. When less than 3 mm of residual ridge remains, treatment should be to graft the sinus with autologous bone (block or particulate). After 6 to 8 months, the fixtures may be placed.

References

Dahlin C, Andersson L, Linde A: Bone augmentation at fenestrated implants by an osteopromotive membrane technique: a controlled clinical study, *Clin Oral Implants Res* 2:159, 1991.

Hochwald DA, Davis HW: Bone grafting in the maxillary sinus floor. In Worthington P, Branemark PI, editors: *Advanced osseointegration surgery,* Chicago, 1992, Quintessence Publishing.

Jemt T, Lekholm U, Adell R: Osseointegrated implants in the treatment of partially edentulous patients: a preliminary study on 876 consecutively placed fixtures, *Int J Oral Maxillofac Implants* 4:211, 1989.

Langer B: Solutions for specific bone situations: use of wide diameter implants, *Int J Oral Maxillofac Implants* 9:19, 1994.

Palmer RM et al: Healing of implant dehiscence defects with and without expanded polytetrafluoroethylene membranes: a controlled clinical and histological study, *Clin Oral Implants Res* 5:98, 1994.

Simion M, Baldoni M, Zaffe D: Jawbone enlargement using immediate implant placement associated with a split-crest technique and guided tissue regeneration, *Int J Periodont Res Dent* 12:463, 1992.

Tatum H, Jr: Maxillary sinus and implant reconstruction, *Dent Clin North Am* 30:107, 1986.

Tulasne JF: Implant treatment of missing posterior dentition. In Albrectson T, Zarb G, editors: *The Branemark osseointegrated implant,* Chicago, 1989, Quintessence Publishing.

Tulasne JF: Osseointegrated fixtures in the pterygoid region. In Worthington P, Branemark PI: *Advanced osseointegration surgery,* Chicago, 1992, Quintessence Publishing.

Van Steenberghe D, Lekholm U, Bolender C: The applicability of osseointegrated oral implants in the rehabilitation of partial edentulism: a prospective multicenter study of 558 fixtures, *Int J Oral Maxillofac Implants* 5:272, 1990.

Patient Considering Osseointegrated Implants for the DISTAL PARTIALLY EDENTULOUS MAXILLA

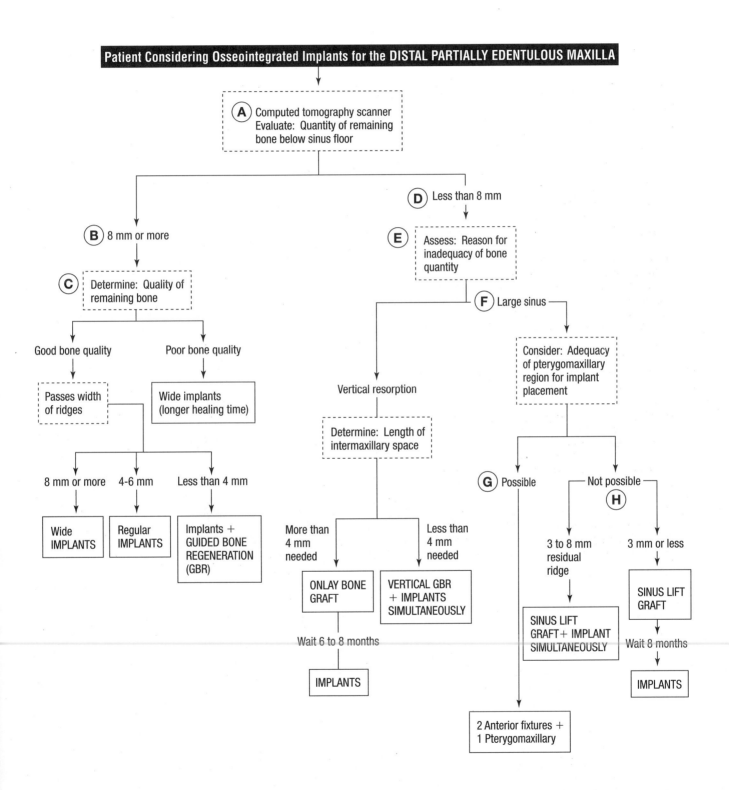

(A) Computed tomography scanner
Evaluate: Quantity of remaining bone below sinus floor

(B) 8 mm or more

(D) Less than 8 mm

(C) Determine: Quality of remaining bone

(E) Assess: Reason for inadequacy of bone quantity

(F) Large sinus

Good bone quality

Poor bone quality

Passes width of ridges

Wide implants (longer healing time)

Consider: Adequacy of pterygomaxillary region for implant placement

Vertical resorption

Determine: Length of intermaxillary space

8 mm or more

4-6 mm

Less than 4 mm

(G) Possible

Not possible

(H)

Wide IMPLANTS

Regular IMPLANTS

Implants + GUIDED BONE REGENERATION (GBR)

More than 4 mm needed

Less than 4 mm needed

3 to 8 mm residual ridge

3 mm or less

ONLAY BONE GRAFT

VERTICAL GBR + IMPLANTS SIMULTANEOUSLY

SINUS LIFT GRAFT + IMPLANT SIMULTANEOUSLY

SINUS LIFT GRAFT

Wait 6 to 8 months

Wait 8 months

IMPLANTS

IMPLANTS

2 Anterior fixtures + 1 Pterygomaxillary

39 Osseointegrated Implants for the Partially Edentulous Mandible

Joan Pi Urgell

A The partially edentulous posterior mandible has an important anatomic structure that affects the possibility of implant placement and the necessity for some reconstructive surgery— its inferior alveolar nerve and vascular component. Assess the distance between the neurovascular bundle of dental nerve and the top of the remaining residual ridge with a computerized tomography (CT) scanner.

B When there is more than 8 mm of residual ridge, assess the presence and adequacy of posterior abutment(s). If there is a posterior tooth that needs to be restored and it is not a long span, a conventional fixed bridge is the treatment of choice. If any remaining teeth are sound, one implant per tooth may be placed as a self-retained bridge.

C In a free-end saddle situation, assess the width of the residual ridge. A ridge width of 8 mm or more will allow installation of wide fixtures, which are most favorable in posterior areas. Conventional implants of 4 to 6 mm are used. If the ridge has less than 4 mm of width, the fixtures are installed and guided bone regeneration (GBR) is performed simultaneously using bone chips as a spacemaker.

D If there is less than 8 mm of bone height between the crest of the ridge and the dental nerve, determine the presence of remaining distal teeth for a conventional fixed bridge. If the situation is a free-end saddle, evaluate the intermaxillary space for a favorable crown-to-root ratio. If less than 4 mm is needed to increase the height of the ridge for an optimal crown-to-root dimension, simultaneous fixture placement and GBR with a titanium reinforced membrane and bone chips are used.

E If more than 4 mm of vertical augmentation is needed, assess the amount of residual ridge above the dental nerve. When there is 4 mm or more of bone above the neurovascular canal, simultaneously install the fixtures with an onlay bone graft (usually taken from the chin). If less than 4 mm of bone is present above the dental nerve, decide whether to perform an onlay graft secured with miniscrews and delayed fixture placement for a self-retained bridge, or consider nerve lateralization and fixture placement without augmenting the ridge.

References

Astrand P: Onlay bone grafts to the mandible. In Worthington P, Branemark PI: *Advanced osseointegration surgery*, Chicago, 1992, Quintessence Publishing.

Dahlin C, Andersson L, Linde A: Bone augmentation at fenestrated implants by an osteopromotive membrane technique: a controlled clinical study, *Clin Oral Implants Res* 2:159, 1991.

Jemt T, Lekholm U, Adell R: Osseointegrated implants in the treatment of partially edentulous patients: a preliminary study on 876 consecutively placed fixtures, *Int J Oral Maxillofac Implants* 4:211, 1989.

Langer B: Solutions for specific bone situations: use of wide diameter implant, *Int J Oral Maxillofac Implants* 9:19, 1994.

Palmer RM et al: Healing of implant dehiscence defects with and without expanded polytetrafluoroethylene membranes: a controlled clinical and histological study, *Clin Oral Implants Res* 5:98, 1994.

Rosenquist B: Implant placement in combination with nerve transpositioning: experiences with the first 100 cases, *Int J Oral Maxillofac Implants* 9:522, 1994.

Simion M, Dahlin C, Trisi P, Piatelli A: Qualitative and quantitative comparative study on different filling materials used in bone regeneration, *Int J Periodontal Rest Dent* 14:199, 1994.

Tinti C, Parma S, Polizze G: Vertical ridge augmentation. What is the limit? *Int J Periodontal Rest Dent* 16:221, 1996.

Van Steenberghe D, Lekholm U, Bolender C: The applicability of osseointegrated oral implants in the rehabilitation of partial edentulism: a prospective multicenter study of 558 fixtures, *Int J Oral Maxillofac Implants* 5:272, 1990.

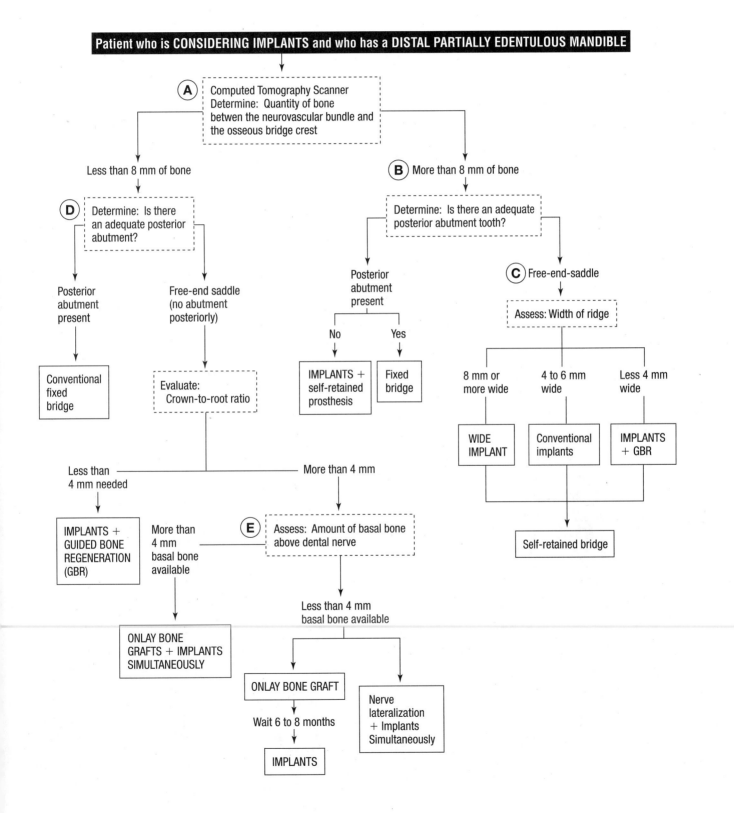

Patient who is CONSIDERING IMPLANTS and who has a DISTAL PARTIALLY EDENTULOUS MANDIBLE

(A) Computed Tomography Scanner
Determine: Quantity of bone betwen the neurovascular bundle and the osseous bridge crest

Less than 8 mm of bone

(B) More than 8 mm of bone

(D) Determine: Is there an adequate posterior abutment?

Determine: Is there an adequate posterior abutment tooth?

Posterior abutment present

Free-end saddle (no abutment posteriorly)

Posterior abutment present

(C) Free-end-saddle

Conventional fixed bridge

Evaluate: Crown-to-root ratio

No

Yes

Assess: Width of ridge

IMPLANTS + self-retained prosthesis

Fixed bridge

8 mm or more wide

4 to 6 mm wide

Less 4 mm wide

WIDE IMPLANT

Conventional implants

IMPLANTS + GBR

Less than 4 mm needed

More than 4 mm

Self-retained bridge

IMPLANTS + GUIDED BONE REGENERATION (GBR)

More than 4 mm basal bone available

(E) Assess: Amount of basal bone above dental nerve

ONLAY BONE GRAFTS + IMPLANTS SIMULTANEOUSLY

Less than 4 mm basal bone available

ONLAY BONE GRAFT

Nerve lateralization + Implants Simultaneously

Wait 6 to 8 months

IMPLANTS

40 Guided Bone Augmentation for Osseointegrated Implants

William Becker, Burton E. Becker

The principles of guided tissue regeneration (GTR) that have been used for periodontal regeneration can be used for root form dental implants as well. The tissues involved in the healing of an extraction socket are flap connective tissue and bone. Membrane barriers may be used to exclude flap connective tissue from collapsing into an extraction socket that has received an immediately placed implant, thus allowing the necessary cells for bone formation access to the area. The barrier creates a space and protects the clot during the early healing phase, creating an environment for potential bone formation around the portion of the implant that is not fully encompassed by bone (Fig. 40-1). A specially designed ePTFE membrane (Gore-Tex) is used for this purpose. The oval-shaped material has an inner portion that is totally occlusive and a peripheral portion that allows for the ingrowth of connective tissue fibrils. The use of guided bone augmentation (GBA) with osseointegrated implants has been shown to be successful on a predictable basis.

A Successful use of GBA for implants placed into extraction sockets requires careful case selection. Teeth that have advanced untreatable periodontitis, recurrent endodontic lesions, or fractures that are not exposable by crown lengthening are ideal candidates for extraction accompanied by immediate implant placement. To obtain maximum implant stability, there should be a minimum of 3 to 5 mm of bone apical to the root tip. Implants placed into thin edentulous ridges may result in fenestrations. These defects can be treated with GBA.

B When the site is exposed surgically, the type of defect and site that are present are evaluated, and the stability of an implant potentially or after placement is assessed. If a stable implant cannot be placed, alternative restorative plans should be proposed.

C Fenestration defects that result from placing the implant close to the facial surface of the implant can be treated with GBA. The implant must be completely stable. If the fenestration exposes only one or two threads, no barrier is necessary. When a large fenestration is present, exposing three or more threads of the implant, a barrier should be placed over the defect for GBA.

D When an implant has been placed into an extraction socket, an intraalveolar defect may exist. When implants are placed into extremely narrow sockets, as those present on mandibular anterior teeth, or into extremely wide bone and leave no exposure of the implant in the adjacent socket, no GTR is necessary. Defects that are less than 3-mm deep and do not expose more than three threads may have a barrier placed. GBA should be considered when defects are greater than 3-mm deep and expose more than three threads.

E An implant that is placed into an extraction socket that is missing one or more bony walls may be treated with GBA. If two walls cannot be stabilized, the implant should be removed immediately. Many times, one or two bony walls are partially missing, and the implant is stable. This is the ideal defect in which to use GBA.

F When any of the aforementioned defects occur in conjunction with a narrow ridge, GBA may be used to attempt to augment the width of the ridge.

When barriers are used for implant augmentation, complete flap closure over the barrier should be obtained before removal; the barrier occasionally becomes exposed. If a small area becomes exposed before 30 days, the area may be cleaned by the patient with chlorhexidine swabs. If the barrier has a large exposed area and inflammation is present, it should be removed immediately. Ideally, the barrier should remain completely covered until its removal at 4 to 6 weeks after placement.

Allogenic bone and alloplasts used under membranes act as fillers and do not contribute to osseointegration. Autologous bone is the best graft material for implant or ridge augmentation.

Fig. 40-1 An implant with exposed body knurling covered with a membrane for guided bone augmentation.

References

Becker W, Becker BE, Prichard J et al: Root isolation for new attachment procedures: a surgical and suturing method: three case reports, *J Periodontol* 58:819, 1987.

Becker W, Becker BE, Ochsenbein O et al: Bone formation at dehisced dental implant sites treated with implant augmentation material: a pilot study in dogs, *Int J Periodontal Restor Dent* 9:333, 1989.

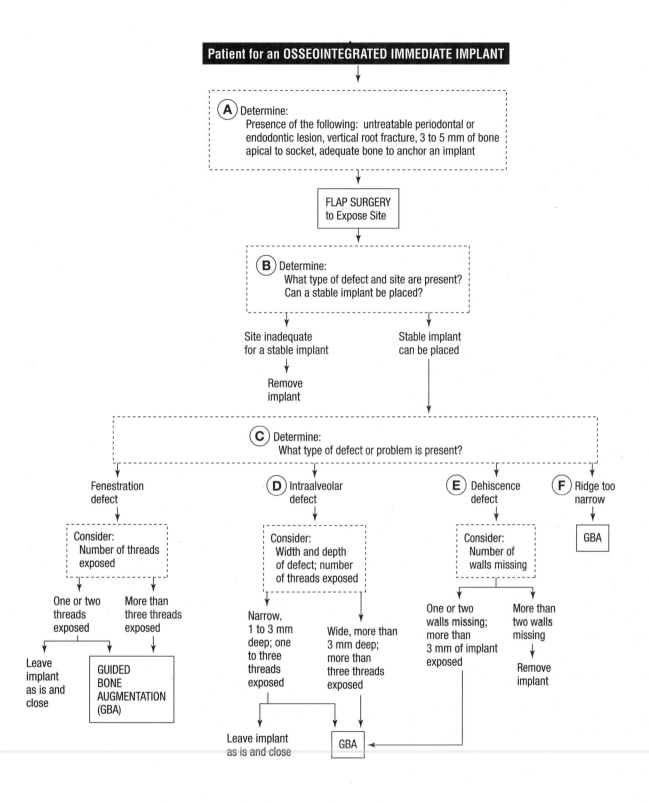

Patient for an OSSEOINTEGRATED IMMEDIATE IMPLANT

A Determine:
Presence of the following: untreatable periodontal or endodontic lesion, vertical root fracture, 3 to 5 mm of bone apical to socket, adequate bone to anchor an implant

FLAP SURGERY to Expose Site

B Determine:
What type of defect and site are present?
Can a stable implant be placed?

Site inadequate for a stable implant → Remove implant

Stable implant can be placed

C Determine:
What type of defect or problem is present?

Fenestration defect
Consider: Number of threads exposed
- One or two threads exposed → Leave implant as is and close
- More than three threads exposed → GUIDED BONE AUGMENTATION (GBA)

D Intraalveolar defect
Consider: Width and depth of defect; number of threads exposed
- Narrow, 1 to 3 mm deep; one to three threads exposed → Leave implant as is and close
- Wide, more than 3 mm deep; more than three threads exposed → GBA

E Dehiscence defect
Consider: Number of walls missing
- One or two walls missing; more than 3 mm of implant exposed → GBA
- More than two walls missing → Remove implant

F Ridge too narrow → GBA

Dahlin C, Sennerby L, Lekholm U et al: Generation of new bone around titanium implants using a membrane technique: an experimental study in rabbits, *Int J Oral Maxillofac Implants* 4:19, 1989.

Gottlow J, Nyman S, Lindhe J: New attachment formation as a result of controlled tissue regeneration, *J Clin Periodontol* 11:494, 1984.

Lazzara RJ: Immediate implant placement into extraction sites: surgical and restorative advantages, *Int J Periodontal Restor Dent* 9:333, 1989.

Nyman S, Lang NP, Buser D, Bragge U: Bone regeneration adjacent to titanium dental implants using guided tissue regeneration: a report of two cases, *Int J Oral Maxillofac Implants* 5:9, 1990.

41 Soft Tissue Surgery Around Implants

Roberto Barone, Carlo Clauser, Giovan Paolo Pini-Prato

The role of masticatory mucosa around implants is still controversial. There are cases where a band of masticatory mucosa is desirable for esthetic or hygienic reasons. To obtain a significant amount of masticatory mucosa requires surgery. Because the benefit of masticatory mucosa is doubtful or limited, it is important to keep the additional surgery to a minimum. In the case of osseointegrated submerged implants, adequate masticatory mucosa can be obtained in most cases without additional surgical sessions. The nonsubmerged implants pose different problems. The final amount of masticatory mucosa must be obtained before implant installation because the soft tissue closure at installation is critical. Both width and thickness of the masticatory mucosa may be relevant for the esthetics of the final restoration.

A Evaluate the need for masticatory mucosa; screw-type machined implants in totally edentulous patients do not have special requirements for attached gingiva. One animal experiment has shown different behaviors of tissues around plasma-sprayed implants with and without masticatory mucosa during periimplantitis. Masticatory mucosa, however, may be considered clinically useful in partial cases, especially in esthetic areas and to improve hygiene. If no need for masticatory mucosa is apparent, each implant system has its standard protocols for surgery and rehabilitation.

B In the upper arch there is no need for augmentation procedures before installation of the implants because it is possible to increase the bank of buccal masticatory mucosa (using the palatal mucosa) at phase 2 surgery in any case without increasing the number of surgical sessions.

C In the lower arch it may not be possible to create a significant width of masticatory mucosa at phase 2 surgery if the preexistent tissue is too scant. Placing a masticatory tissue graft before implant surgery is necessary. Thus it is possible to evaluate the adequacy of the healed graft and to correct it at phase 2 surgery, if needed.

D The choice of 2 mm of masticatory mucosa as a minimum for the lower arch is related to the difficulty of obtaining an appreciable increase in the width of masticatory mucosa by means of an apically positioned flap.

E Installation of implants is carried out as usual according to the standard protocol. Before suturing the flaps, the distance between bone margin (on the buccal aspect of the implant) and mucogingival junction is measured. A periodontal probe is aligned horizontally with the mucogingival junction of the adjacent teeth at the releasing incisions. A second periodontal probe measures the vertical distance between the first probe mucogingival junction to the buccal bone margin at the emergence of the implant. In that way an estimate is obtained of the width of the masticatory mucosa that is expected to be attached to bone upon completion of the implant therapy. This measurement is recorded and serves as a basis to plan the second stage surgery, when it would be difficult to locate the head of the implant exactly before incising. If the expected width of keratinized gingiva is judged inadequate at implant installation, the flap design at phase 2 will be modified to increase the width of masticatory mucosa. A threshold of 3 mm was chosen arbitrarily to have a safety margin against flap shrinkage and measurement errors. The adequacy of this threshold value has been validated in a clinical study.

F The thickness of the keratinized tissue on the buccal side of the implants also may have a critical role in obtaining and maintaining an esthetic appearance. It may be important in preventing recession; therefore augmentation of the buccal tissue thickness to facilitate the fabrication of the fixed prosthesis and to improve aesthetics is indicated. This problem is more common in the upper arch.

G The apically positioned flap is designed to increase the width of the masticatory mucosa. The horizontal incision is made slightly on the palatal-lingual side of the crest to exploit all the masticatory mucosa that lies directly over the cover screw. A full-thickness flap is elevated over the implant while the periosteum is left in place on the buccal side. The vertical releasing incisions are extended into the vestibule. At the end of the operation the flap is moved apically to leave the abutment uncovered and anchored to the periosteum.

H In the roll technique a flap is elevated from the palate. The palatal portion of the flap is deepithelialized and inserted between the buccal side of the bone crest and the buccal portion of the flap to increase the thickness of the buccal masticatory mucosa. The flap is secured at the original level (repositioned) or apically.

I Gingivectomy is a means of removal of masticatory mucosa covering the implant via a circular incision over the head of the implant. A circular blade usually is used. The gingivectomy approach is indicated in presence of a wide, flat crest with thick tissues where no gingival inadequacy would be produced by the procedure.

J The repositioned flap is indicated when the alveolar crest is narrow. A horizontal linear incision is made on the crest to locate and uncover the cover screws. The margins of the wound are elevated without releasing incisions. After the abutment connection the flaps are adapted with single sutures without dislocation and with little or no trimming of the tissues.

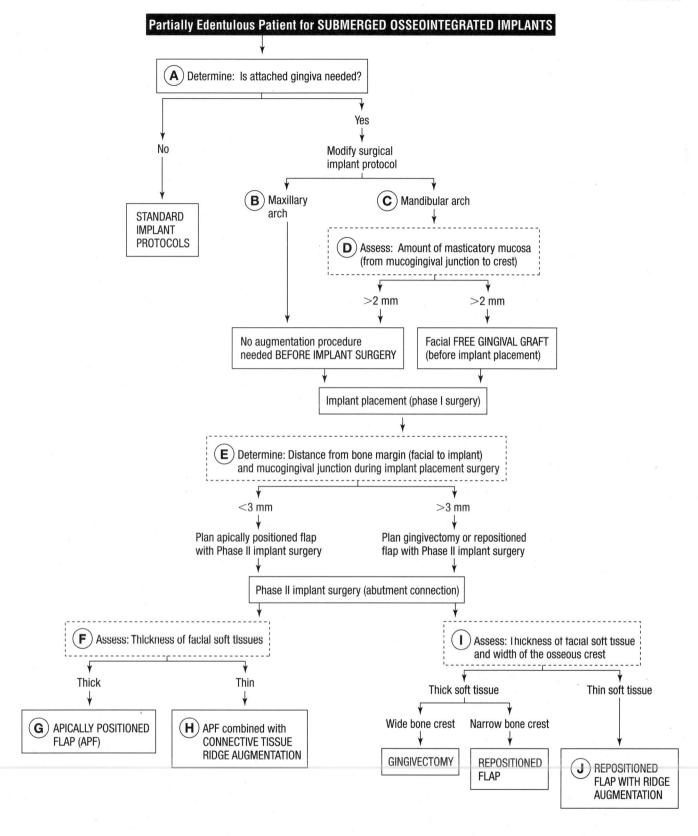

Partially Edentulous Patient for SUBMERGED OSSEOINTEGRATED IMPLANTS

A. Determine: Is attached gingiva needed?

No → STANDARD IMPLANT PROTOCOLS

Yes → Modify surgical implant protocol

B. Maxillary arch

C. Mandibular arch

D. Assess: Amount of masticatory mucosa (from mucogingival junction to crest)

>2 mm → No augmentation procedure needed BEFORE IMPLANT SURGERY

>2 mm → Facial FREE GINGIVAL GRAFT (before implant placement)

Implant placement (phase I surgery)

E. Determine: Distance from bone margin (facial to implant) and mucogingival junction during implant placement surgery

<3 mm → Plan apically positioned flap with Phase II implant surgery

>3 mm → Plan gingivectomy or repositioned flap with Phase II implant surgery

Phase II implant surgery (abutment connection)

F. Assess: Thickness of facial soft tissues

Thick → G. APICALLY POSITIONED FLAP (APF)

Thin → H. APF combined with CONNECTIVE TISSUE RIDGE AUGMENTATION

I. Assess: Thickness of facial soft tissue and width of the osseous crest

Thick soft tissue
Wide bone crest → GINGIVECTOMY
Narrow bone crest → REPOSITIONED FLAP

Thin soft tissue → J. REPOSITIONED FLAP WITH RIDGE AUGMENTATION

References

Barone R, Clauser C, Grassi R, Merli M: *Rationale for soft tissue treatment around implants,* Paris, Clinical communication at Europerio 1, May 12-15, 1994.

Sharf DR, Tarnow DP: Modified roll technique for localized alveolar ridge augmentation, *Int J Periodontics Rest Dent* 12:415, 1992.

Warrer K, Buser D, Lang N, Karring T: Plaque induced peri-implantitis in the presence or absence of keratinized mucosa: an experimental study in monkeys, *Clin Oral Implants Res* 6:131, 1995.

Wennstrom JL, Bengazi F, Lekholm U: The influence of the masticatory mucosa on the peri-implant soft tissue condition, *Clin Oral Implants Res* 5:1, 1994.

42 Periimplantitis: Etiology of the Ailing, Failing, or Failed Dental Implant

Mark Zablotsky, John Kwan

The discipline of implant dentistry has gained clinical acceptance owing to long-term studies that suggest high success and survival rates in both partially and completely edentulous applications; however, in a small percentage of cases, implant failure and morbidity have been reported. Implant failure caused by surgically overheating bone has been minimized with the advent of slow-speed, high-torque internally, and often externally, irrigated drilling systems. After integration (either bio- or osseointegration), the major cause of implant failure is thought to be a result of biomechanical (i.e., overload, heavy lateral interferences, lack of a passive prosthesis fit, etc.) or infectious (plaque-induced) etiology.

Complications can be eliminated or minimized if clinicians plan treatment adequately. Mounted study models with diagnostic waxups or tooth setups are mandatory to evaluate ridge relationships, occlusal schemes, and restorative goals. When taken with adequate radiographs and clinical examination, the implant team (restoring dentist, surgeon, and laboratory technician) can adequately plan for the location, number, and trajectory of implants to ensure the most healthy, esthetic, and functional prosthesis. Often, additional implants may be proposed to satisfy the implant team and patient requirements (i.e., fixed versus removable prostheses). The final restoration should be one that is esthetic, adequately engineered (enough implants of sufficient length in sufficient quality and quantity of supporting bone), and accessible for the patient for adequate home care. When evaluating the ailing or failing implant, often one or more of the aforementioned criteria have not been met.

A When referring to a dental implant as ailing, failing, or failed, one really is referring to the status of the periimplantis supporting tissues (unless the implant is fractured). The ailing implant is one that displays progressive bone loss and pocketing but no clinical mobility. The failing implant is one that displays similar features to the ailing implant but is refractory to therapy and continues to progress downhill. This implant is also immobile. The term *ailing* suggests a somewhat more favorable prognosis than the term *failing*.

B A failed implant is one that is fractured, has been totally refractory to all methods of treatment, or demonstrates clinical mobility or circumferential periimplant radiolucency. These implants must be removed immediately because progressive destruction of surrounding osseous tissues may occur.

C The etiology of periimplant disease is often multifactorial. Many times the clinician must do detective work to discover the potential etiology. Meffert has coined the terms the *traditional* and *retrograde* pathways when differentiating bacterial versus biomechanical etiologies.

Although a hemidesmosomal attachment of soft tissues to titanium has been reported, it is doubtful that this histologic phenomenon has clinical relevance around titanium implant abutments. The periimplant seal is thought to originate from a tight adaptation of mucosal tissues around the abutment via an intricate arrangement of circular gingival fibers and a tight junctional epithelium. Because this "attachment" is tenuous at best, it can be extrapolated that a plaque-induced (traditional pathway) periimplant gingivitis may not truly exist and that plaque-induced inflammation of periimplant tissues may directly extend to the underlying supporting osseous tissues.

The periodontal ligament acts as a "shock absorber" around the natural tooth when excessive occlusal or orthodontic forces are present. In the absence of bacterial plaque, occlusal trauma does not cause a loss of attachment to teeth; however, because implants lack a periodontal ligament, force can be transmitted to the implant-bone interface. If significant enough, microfractures of this interface can occur and allow for an ingress of soft tissues and secondary bacterial infection.

In fixed bridgework that does not fit passively and is cemented on natural teeth, orthodontic movement of abutments occurs owing to the presence of the periodontal ligament. In this scenario, little if any damage occurs around abutments because of this orthodontic movement. When this same phenomenon occurs on dental implant abutments (either screw-retained or cemented), one of a few complications can result. The restoration may become loose either as a result of cement failure, screws backing out, or fracture. Abutments can loosen or fracture, or the implant body may fracture or have bone loss because of progressive microfractures at the interface (retrograde pathway); therefore it is imperative that frameworks fit precisely. Lateral interferences or excessive off-axis loading has led to greater stresses on components as well as implant-bone interface and should be minimized. Bruxism can be extremely destructive and should be addressed by modifying occlusal schemes to eliminate lateral contacts in function or parafunction; alternatively, the patient should commit to permanent splint-nightguard treatment before placement of the implant. In some instances, it is possible to plan a removable prosthesis to address this concern.

When evaluating the ailing or failing implant, clinical signs of periimplant problems include increased probing depths, bleeding on probing, suppuration, erythema and flaccidity of tissues, and radiographic bone loss. Pain may be present, but usually it is a late symptom. If plaque is absent with minimally inflamed tissues, one must suspect occlusal etiology. Often this can be confirmed via culture and sensitivity testing. If bacteria associated with gingival health are present (i.e., *Streptococcus* sp. or *Actinomyces* sp.), then an occlusal component is strongly suggested. If, however, periodontal pathogens (i.e., *P. gingivalis, P. intermedius,* etc.) are present, one should have a high suspicion for periimplant infection. This is not to say that there is not also an occlusal component. Inspect restorations for fit. If the restoration is loose, it is always bad. Remove and evaluate each component until the loose or failed component is found. If the implant is loose, it is a failure and should be removed immediately. It will never reintegrate and be functional. Replace-

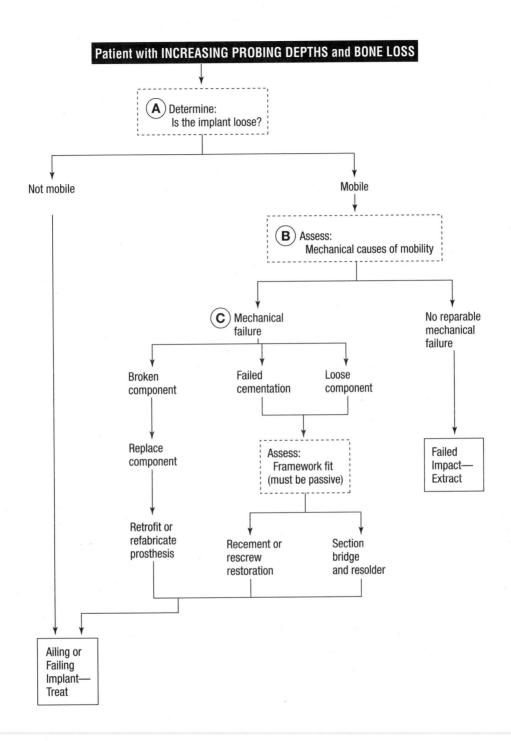

Patient with INCREASING PROBING DEPTHS and BONE LOSS

(A) Determine:
Is the implant loose?

Not mobile

Mobile

(B) Assess:
Mechanical causes of mobility

(C) Mechanical failure

No reparable mechanical failure

Broken component

Failed cementation

Loose component

Replace component

Assess:
Framework fit
(must be passive)

Failed Impact—Extract

Retrofit or refabricate prosthesis

Recement or rescrew restoration

Section bridge and resolder

Ailing or Failing Implant—Treat

ment implants can be placed either at the time of implant removal or within 6 months of implant removal, as various regenerative techniques may be contemplated to maintain alveolar height and width.

References

Meffert R: Periodontitis vs. peri-implanting. The same disease? The same treatment? *Br Rev Oral Biol Med* 7:278, 1996.

Meffert R, Block M, Kent J: What is osseointegration? *Int J Periodontol Restor Dent* 11(2):88, 1987.

Newman M, Fleming T: Periodontal considerations of implants and implant associated microbiota, *J Dent Educ* 52(12):737, 1988.

Rosenberg E, Torosian J, Slots J: Microbial differences in 2 distinct types of failures of osseointegrated implants, *Clin Oral Implant Res* 2(3):135, 1991.

43 Initial Therapy for the Ailing or Failing Dental Implant

Mark Zablotsky, John Kwan

A differential diagnosis should be made as early as possible in the initial stages of implant therapy because information garnered may be critical in the follow-up and maintenance of the ailing or failing implant. If an accurate assessment of the etiology has not been established, then any interceptive therapy may be compromised.

A Effective patient-performed plaque control is mandatory, and the patient must accept this responsibility. The therapist should customize a hygiene regimen for each implant patient. The use of conventional oral hygiene aids (i.e., brush, floss, etc.) can be augmented with any number of instruments (i.e., superfloss, yarn, plastic-coated proxibrushes, electric toothbrushes, etc.). If the patient's oral hygiene is suspect, the addition of a topical application of chemotherapeutics (i.e., chlorhexidine), either by rinsing or applying locally (via dipping brushes, etc.), may be beneficial in maintenance. The restorative dentist must give the patient hygiene access to implant abutments circumferentially.

B Evaluate occlusion, and eliminate centric or lateral prematurities and interferences via occlusal adjustment. Initiate nightguard-splint therapy if parafunctional activity is suspected. Often, the clinician can remove the prosthesis and place healing cuffs on the implants in hopes of getting a positive response by reducing the load if occlusal etiology is suspected. Single implants that are attached to mobile natural teeth may be overloaded as a result of the compression of the tooth and subsequent relative cantilevering of the prosthesis from the implant. If occlusal etiology is suspected in this case, contemplate the attachment of more implants to the existing weakened implant to support the cantilever of periodontally weak teeth. If one suspects bacterial etiology, initial conservative treatment may consist of subgingival irrigation with a blunt-tipped, side-port irrigating needle. Chlorhexidine is probably the irrigant of choice. Local application of tetracycline via monolithic fibers may be an effective adjunct.

C Perform culture and sensitivity testing to guide therapy if systemic antibiotics are contemplated. Consider débridement of hyperplastic periimplant tissues using hand or ultrasonic plastic (if the implant or abutment is going to be touched) instrumentation.

D Ideally, the implant abutment should emerge through attached keratinized mucosa. This will give the patient an ideal mucosa. It will also give the patient an ideal environment to perform home care because moveable alveolar mucosal margins can be irritating and cause difficulty in effecting oral hygiene. Increased failures of implants and morbidity have been associated with areas that are deficient in attached keratinized gingival tissues. Soft-tissue augmentation procedures can be performed either before implant placement, during integration, at uncovering (stage 2), or for repair procedures.

E Consider reevaluation of periimplant tissues 2 to 4 weeks after initial therapy. Probing depths should be reduced, and there should be no bleeding on probing or suppuration. The clinician must decide whether the improvement in clinical indices is a predictable long-term endpoint. One must remember that the success of periodontal therapy depends upon the therapist's ability to remove plaque, calculus, and other bacterial products from radicular surfaces. Because it is not possible or recommended to "root plane" the implant surfaces (because of the detrimental effects of conventional curettes or ultrasonics), one must consider that the titanium abutment or the hydroxylapatite-coated titanium implant surface is contaminated with bacteria and their products (i.e., endotoxin), therefore one must conclude that the implant and periimplant tissues would benefit from surgical intervention.

If the therapist feels that a successful endpoint has been attained, close maintenance with monitoring of clinical, radiographic, and microbiologic parameters is imperative. If prompt recurrence of problems occurs, one must question either the initial diagnosis (incorrect etiology) or the predictability of the more conservative nonsurgical therapy. In this instance the clinician should strive to stabilize or arrest the active disease process (nonsurgically), then reevaluate to determine a clinical endpoint. Commonly, cases that are refractory to nonsurgical therapy do well after surgical intervention because the contaminated implant surface can be addressed more adequately.

References

Gammage D, Bowman A, Meffert R: Clinical management of failing dental implants: four case reports, *J Oral Implants* 15(2):124, 1989.

Kwan J: Implant maintenance, *J Cal Dent Assoc* 19(12):45, 1991.

Kwan J, Zablotsky M: The ailing implant, *J Cal Dent Assoc* 19(12):51, 1991.

Orton G, Steele D, Wolinsky L: The dental professional's role in monitoring and maintenance of tissue-integrated prostheses, *Int J Oral Maxillofac Implants* 4:305, 1989.

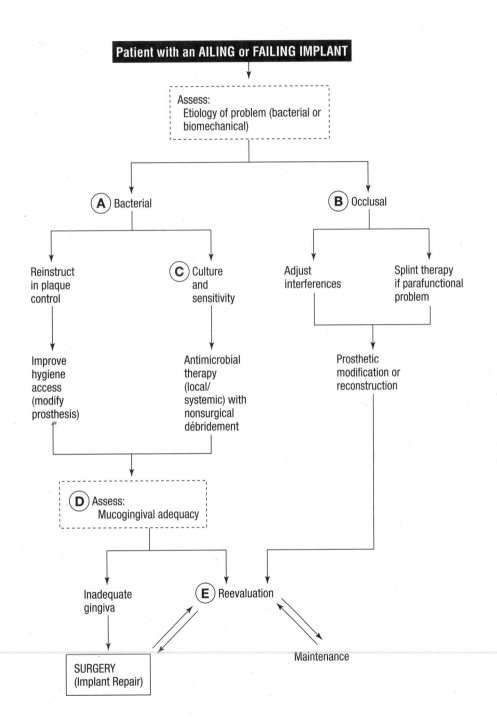

Patient with an AILING or FAILING IMPLANT

Assess:
Etiology of problem (bacterial or biomechanical)

A Bacterial

B Occlusal

Reinstruct in plaque control

C Culture and sensitivity

Adjust interferences

Splint therapy if parafunctional problem

Improve hygiene access (modify prosthesis)

Antimicrobial therapy (local/systemic) with nonsurgical débridement

Prosthetic modification or reconstruction

D Assess: Mucogingival adequacy

Inadequate gingiva

E Reevaluation

Maintenance

SURGERY (Implant Repair)

44 The Surgical Management of Periimplantitis: Implant Repair

Mark Zablotsky, John Kwan

The surgical repair of the ailing or failing implant is dependent on an accurate diagnosis and effective nonsurgical intervention to stabilize or arrest the progression of the active periimplant lesion (Figs. 44-1, 44-2, 44-3).

A It is important to assess the mucogingival status of periimplant tissues before repair surgery. If only mucogingival defects exist around the ailing or failing implant, subsequent osseous repair surgery may not be necessary when soft-tissue augmentation is performed around the ailing or failing implant. If indicated, osseous repair surgery is less technically demanding when dealing with keratinized tissues.

B Modifications of periodontal surgical procedures, either resective or regenerative, have been reported with some success. After making the initial incisions and degranulating the osseous defect (open débridement), one must evaluate the defect before selecting the appropriate surgical modality.

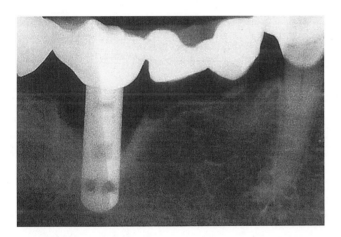

Fig. 44-1 Preoperative radiograph of an "ailing" implant before guided bone augmentation repair.

C Periimplant osseous defects that are predominantly horizontal in nature respond most predictably to resective procedures (i.e., definitive osseous surgery) with or without fixture modification.

D Fixture modification is performed to remove macroscopic or microscopic features that interfere with subsequent plaque control in the supracrestal aspect of the defect. Fixture modification consists of smoothing with a series of rotary instruments in descending grit (i.e., fine diamond, white stone, rubber points) and using copious irrigation because significant heat can be generated by these instruments. For those with concerns of contaminating implant surfaces or periimplant tissues with rotary instruments, some have reported a healthy soft-tissue response against hydroxylapatite-coated or plasma-sprayed titanium implant surfaces. If the patient's oral hygiene is suspect, consider fixture modification for these microscopically rough surfaces.

E Regenerative procedures (bone grafting with or without guided tissue regeneration [GTR]) has been reported for the repair of the ailing or failing implant. Regenerative procedures are most appropriate when the adjacent osseous crest is close to the rim of the implant (i.e., narrow two- or three-walled moat or dehiscence and fenestration defects). When these procedures are contemplated, fixture modification is not recommended.

F Detoxification procedures to treat the infected implant surface are recommended before regenerative modalities. It appears that a 30-second to 1-minute application of a supersaturated solution of citric acid (pH 1) burnished with a cotton pledget may be beneficial in detoxifying the infected hydroxylapatite-coated implant surface. If the coating appears pitted and altered, however it should be

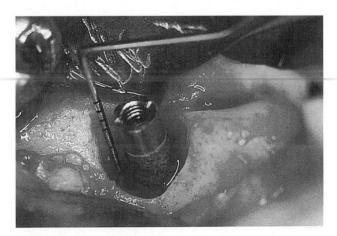

Fig. 44-2 The defect surgically exposed before Gore-Tex membrane placement.

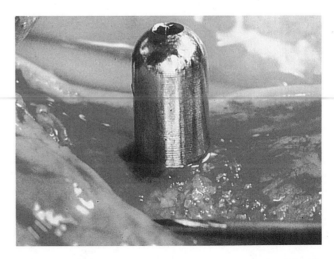

Fig. 44-3 The defect is filled with hard tissue 6 months following guided bone augmentation.

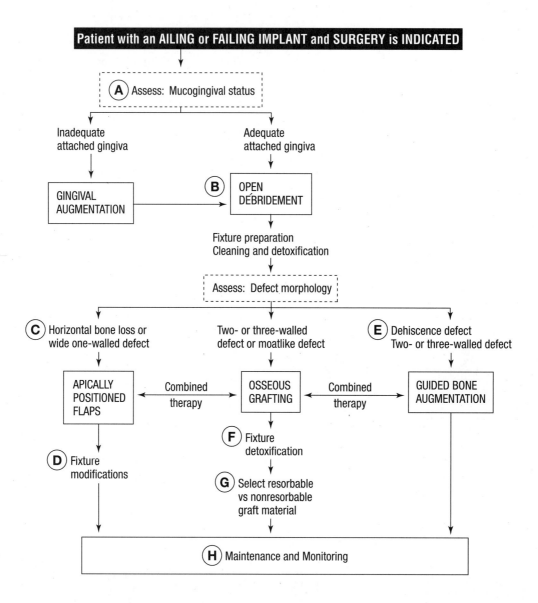

Patient with an AILING or FAILING IMPLANT and SURGERY is INDICATED

A Assess: Mucogingival status

Inadequate attached gingiva

Adequate attached gingiva

GINGIVAL AUGMENTATION

B OPEN DÉBRIDEMENT

Fixture preparation
Cleaning and detoxification

Assess: Defect morphology

C Horizontal bone loss or wide one-walled defect

Two- or three-walled defect or moatlike defect

E Dehiscence defect Two- or three-walled defect

APICALLY POSITIONED FLAPS

Combined therapy

OSSEOUS GRAFTING

Combined therapy

GUIDED BONE AUGMENTATION

D Fixture modifications

F Fixture detoxification

G Select resorbable vs nonresorbable graft material

H Maintenance and Monitoring

removed either with ultrasonic or air and powder abrasives. A short application of an air and powder abrasive detoxifies the titanium implant surface. Extreme caution is recommended if the defect to be treated with the air and powder abrasive is a narrow intrabony defect because pressurized air may enter the marrow spaces and there may be a risk of embolism.

G Choice of bone-grafting materials should be based on the clinician's level of certainty that the site to be grafted is free of bacterial contaminants. If the clinician is certain that the defect is not contaminated, resorbable materials (i.e., autogenous bone, demineralized freeze-dried bone allografts [DFDBA], or resorbable hydroxylapatite, or GTR materials alone) may be considered. If the surface of the implant is suspect, nonresorbable materials (i.e., dense nonresorbable hydroxylapatite) should be considered. Use nonresorbable bone-grafting materials to obturate apical vents and basket holes because osseous regeneration probably will not occur in these anatomically contaminated environments.

Contemplate combined therapies whenever defect combinations include horizontal bone loss and dehiscence or intrabony defects. Postoperative care is much like that for periodontal surgical procedures, with close follow-up and reevaluation before placing the patient back on a supportive maintenance schedule.

H The goals of periimplant surgical and nonsurgical therapies are to reestablish a healthy perimucosal seal and to regenerate a soft- or hard-tissue attachment to the implant and abutment. This requires a definitive diagnosis, comprehensive therapy, and effective maintenance. At this time, no prospective or retrospective studies exist when dealing with the short- or long-term results attained through implant repair procedures; therefore close follow-up for recurrence of disease is warranted. Although the goals of therapy are clear, the clinician must be willing to accept and recognize failure when it occurs. The dental implant that is refractory to all attempts at treatment is a failure and should be removed as soon as this diagnosis is made.

References

Lozada J, James R et al:. Surgical repair of peri-implant defects, *J Oral Implant* 16(1):42, 1990.

Meffert R: How to treat ailing and failing implants, *Implant Dent* 1:25, 1992.

Meffert R: Periodontitis vs. peri-implantitis: the same disease? The same treatment? *Brit Rev Oral Biol Med* 7:278, 1996.

Zablotsky M: The surgical management of osseous defects associated with endosteal hydroxylapatite-coated and titanium dental implants, *Dent Clin North Am* 36(1):117, 1992.

Zablotsky M, Diedrich D, Meffert R, Wittrig E: The ability of various chemotherapeutic agents to detoxify the endotoxin infected HA-coated implant surface, *Int J Oral Maxillofac Implants* 8(2):45, 1991.

Zablotsky M, Diedrich D, Meffert R: The ability of various chemotherapeutic agents to detoxify the endotoxin-contaminated titanium implant surface, *Implant Dent* 1:154, 1997.

45 Approaches to the Distal Ridge Pocket

Walter B. Hall

Deep pockets on the distal surface of the most posterior teeth in either arch present unique options for treatment planning. Such defects are common to distal second molars where impacted or partially erupted third molars have been removed (see Chapter 29). Difficulty in cleaning the distal surfaces of the most posterior teeth make pocket formation there more likely to occur. Heavy function on distal ridges may lead to fibrotic enlargement and pocket deepening. In other situations, where a two-walled defect exists between two teeth and the most posterior tooth is extracted, an osseous defect remains distal to the remaining tooth. Pocket elimination in shallower defects or regenerative procedures (Prichard type, guided tissue regeneration [GTR]) are the treatments of choice. The development of highly predictable GTR procedures has changed treatment planning for more severely involved teeth radically (see Chapter 35). The anatomic complexities of maxillary and mandibular distal ridge areas necessitate some variations in the design of flaps to avoid vascular and nerve injuries.

A When pocket depth is present but no osseous defect is detectable, several surgical approaches to pocket elimination exist. If an adequate band of gingiva is present on the distal line angles of the teeth so that gingival excision will not create a pure mucogingival problem, gingivectomy may be used. When a fatty retromolar pad is involved in the mandibular arch, electrosurgery or laser surgery (which produces a fibrotic scarring in healing) are preferable to a surgical approach. In all other areas of this type the surgical approach is easier and less complicated to perform. If no osseous defect is present but gingivectomy would produce a pure mucogingival problem on a distal line angle of the most posterior tooth, a distal wedge or trap-door approach (Figs. 45-1 and 45-2) will permit pocket elimination without creating pure mucogingival problems.

B If an osseous defect is present distal to the most posterior tooth, gingivectomy or electrosurgery are not appropriate approaches. The type of osseous defect that is present should be determined by probing and radiographic evaluation. If a one- or two-walled noncrater type defect is present, guided tissue regeneration may be appropriate. Pocket elimination by osseous resection and apical positioning of the flap is the treatment of choice for shallow defects. Occasionally, a one-walled or two-walled noncrater type defect distal to the most posterior tooth will be so deep that the tooth should be extracted or maintained with frequent root planing. Should such a tooth have severe furcation problems or severe defects on its other surfaces, it also might be untreatable.

C If a three-walled osseous defect is present distal to the most posterior tooth, the width of the defect from the osseous crest to the root will determine the approach to be used. A narrow, three-walled defect (1 mm or less in width) has a high predictability of success with a bone regeneration approach (see Chapter 27).

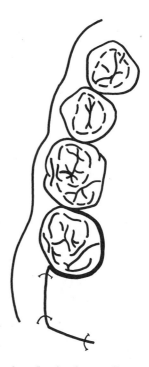

Fig. 45-1 Distal trap-door flap for the maxillary arch when a narrow, three-walled defect is present on the most posterior tooth.

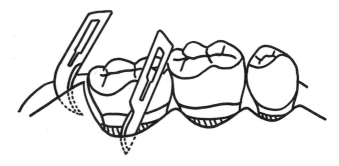

Fig. 45-2 Distal "three-cornered tear" type of trap-door flap used in the mandibular arch when a narrow, three-walled defect is present on the most posterior tooth.

D If the defect is wider than 1 mm from root to osseous crest measured horizontally, the vertical depth of the three-walled defect will determine the surgical approach. If the defect is relatively shallow (1-3 mm), at lease some of its apical portion will be a narrow defect (1 mm or less from root to osseous crest measured horizontally). In such cases osseous resection may be used to eliminate the wider, coronal portion and a Prichard-type regenerative approach can be used to gain back lost attachment in the deeper portion (see Chapter 28). The trap-door flap design should be used so that the suture used to close the flap does not lie over the defect to be filled.

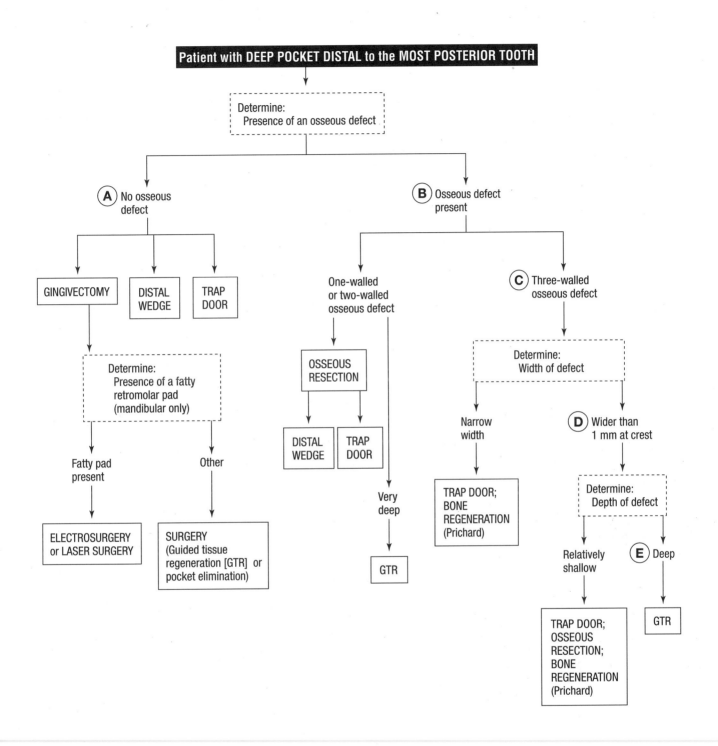

References

Braden BE: Deep distal pockets adjacent to terminal teeth, *Dent Clin North Am* 113:161, 1969.

Carranza, Jr, FA: *Glickman's clinical periodontology,* ed 7, Philadelphia, 1990, WB Saunders, p 821.

Genco RJ, Goldman HM, Cohen DW: *Contemporary periodontics,* St Louis, 1990, Mosby, p 563.

Robinson RE: The distal wedge operation, *Periodontics* 4:256, 1966.

Schluger S, Yuodelis R, Page RC, Johnson RH: *Periodontal diseases,* ed 2, Philadelphia, 1990, Lea & Febiger, p 493.

E If a three-walled defect is deep (more than 3 mm measured vertically) and wide (more than 1 mm from root to bone crest measured horizontally), GTR is a highly predictable approach unless the tooth has a Class III (through and through) furcation involvement, a vertical crack making it untreatable (see Chapter 5) or severe defects on other surfaces that make it hopeless. In hopeless cases extraction or maintenance would be the options. When GTR is used, the distal wedge flap design is preferred because the position of the suture is not a factor and the distal wedge holds the barrier in position better.

46 Timing of Restoration Following Periodontal Surgery

Walter B. Hall

The timing of restorations following periodontal surgery depends upon what types of treatment have been done, both presurgically and surgically. A patient who has been splinted presurgically, generally speaking, can wait a longer time before deciding upon permanent restorations than one who has not been splinted. If procedures that have a lower predictability of success have been used surgically (i.e., guided tissue regeneration [GTR], new attachment), a longer time should be allowed before making a decision upon the restorative plan than if a more definitive approach were used.

A When temporary splinting or provisional splinting has been used before periodontal surgery, the teeth involved usually are so loose that the dentist has decided that splinting is necessary for comfort and function during the surgical period. Provisional splinting is done for periods up to 2 years in cases that will ultimately require extensive reconstruction and in which some of the teeth have a guarded prognosis. Temporary splinting often is extracoronal (such as a nightguard or wire and composite splint); in these cases restorative decisions can be made 3 months or more after the last surgery, unless a new attachment or bone regeneration approach was used, in which case a 6-month wait would be indicated. If intracoronal temporary splinting or provisional splinting was used, a minimal waiting period of 6 months after surgery is necessary before reevaluation. If the provisionally splinted case is an extensive one, a waiting period up to 2 years after surgery may be indicated before reevaluation and permanent restoration.

B If a patient who has had mucogingival-osseous surgery and has not required splinting and has had pocket elimination surgery (apically positioned flap with osseous recontouring or gingivectomy), reevaluation before restoration can be performed as early as 1 month after the last surgery. Healing following such surgery usually is clinically completed this soon; however, if there are any significantly compromised teeth, the reevaluation should be delayed until 3 to 6 months after surgery so that a more reliable prognosis can be made.

C If a new attachment procedure or a GTR procedure has been used, reevaluation before restoration should not be performed sooner than 6 months after the last surgery. Restoration should be delayed in these cases until the long-term prognoses for these teeth are clearly established. With new attachment and osseous regeneration approaches, extensive and expensive restorations should not be placed unless the teeth have a reasonable prognosis 6 months after surgery.

References

Carranza, Jr, FA, Newman MG: *Clinical periodontology*, ed 8, Philadelphia, 1996, WB Saunders, p 710.

Donaldson D: Gingival recession associated with temporary crowns, *J Periodontol* 44:691, 1973.

Nyman S, Lindhe J: A longitudinal study of combined periodontal and prosthetic treatment of patients with advanced periodontal disease, *J Periodontol* 50:163, 1979.

Schluger S, Yuodelis R, Page RC, Johnson RH: *Periodontal diseases*, ed 2, Philadelphia, 1990, Lea & Febiger, p 612.

Seibert JS, Cohen DW: Periodontal considerations in preparation for fixed and removable prosthodontics, *Dent Clin North Am* 31:529, 1987.

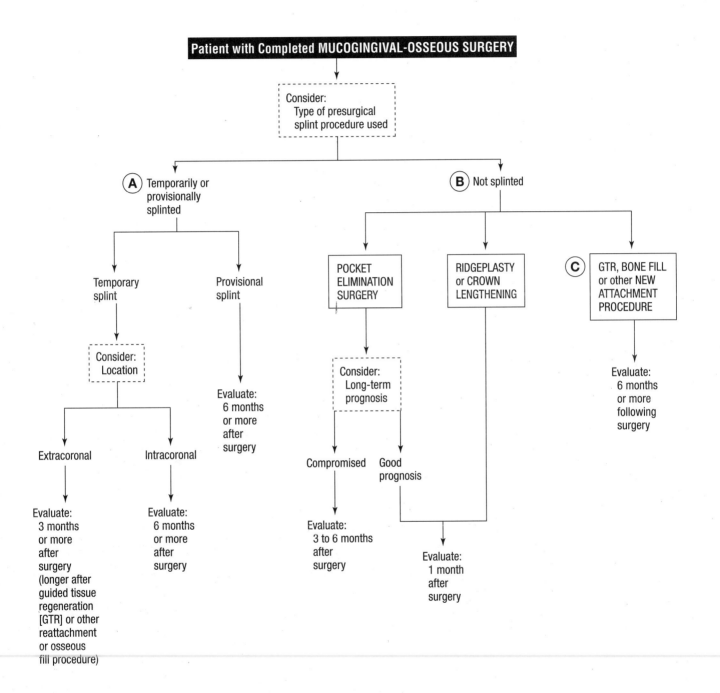

Patient with Completed MUCOGINGIVAL-OSSEOUS SURGERY

Consider:
Type of presurgical
splint procedure used

(A) Temporarily or provisionally splinted

(B) Not splinted

Temporary splint

Provisional splint

Consider:
Location

Evaluate:
6 months
or more
after
surgery

Extracoronal

Intracoronal

Evaluate:
3 months
or more
after
surgery
(longer after
guided tissue
regeneration
[GTR] or other
reattachment
or osseous
fill procedure)

Evaluate:
6 months
or more
after
surgery

POCKET
ELIMINATION
SURGERY

RIDGEPLASTY
or CROWN
LENGTHENING

(C) GTR, BONE FILL
or other NEW
ATTACHMENT
PROCEDURE

Consider:
Long-term
prognosis

Evaluate:
6 months
or more
following
surgery

Compromised

Good
prognosis

Evaluate:
3 to 6 months
after
surgery

Evaluate:
1 month
after
surgery

47 Behavioral Approach to Recall Visits

Walter B. Hall

The timing of recall visits for periodontal patients can be planned in several ways. Some dentists, citing long-term studies of periodontal treatment based on a uniform recall interval, recall all patients at 3-month intervals. They believe that they can predict success rates of various forms of treatment more accurately on this basis; however, the problem with this approach is the patient's response. For years many dentists recalled patients twice a year because studies indicated that between visits caries would not develop so rapidly as to endanger many teeth. In "behavioral" terms, however, many patients "learned" that they had to return to the dentist every 6 months whether they needed it or not (i.e., whether they had made a good effort at oral hygiene or not). Patients understood this message long before dentists did, and oral hygiene and the incidence of caries improved little during that era. An approach that uses the long-term study concepts in a more behaviorally sound way is to "reward" patients depending on the adequacy of their home care efforts between visits; if a patient is doing well (based on assessments of plaque, inflammation, and pocket depth), the time before the next recall is extended, offering a direct reward for individual efforts and reinforcing desirable behavior. With a large group of patients the average recall time is likely to be 3 months; however, no individual patient is likely to be recalled regularly at 3-month intervals.

The greatest advantage of the behavioral approach to recall visit timing is that patients are given an immediate reinforcing reward for good or poor effort. The patients can see either that their efforts have paid off or that lack of effort has brought appropriate consequences.

In the fixed interval (every 3 months) approach, only praise or scolding are available to the dentist. The more tangible rewards of less cost (in time, money, and discomfort) is much more likely to prove successful. Additionally, the dentist can demonstrate how the treatment was altered in response to patient behavior between visits, and patients must take responsibility for their progress and its costs.

A When an individual patient's first recall visit is to be scheduled, information on which to base the recall interval is not clearly defined. The patient may have remaining areas of compromise, such as individual teeth for which definitive treatment was impossible (because these teeth already had lost too much attachment) or for which selection of a less definitive treatment was made for financial reasons. Some patients are compromised by the status of their health. Others may be compromised by less than ideal restorative work or tooth alignment. If the patient has areas of compromise, they should be annotated and the recall interval decreased. If a compromised patient has shown little motivation to develop home care skills, the first recall visit should be set at 1 to 2 months; alternatively, if good oral hygiene skill development and motivation are manifested, the first recall can be set at 2 to 3 months. If the patient has no areas of compromise, evidence of oral hygiene skill and motivation can be used to set the first recall interval. If the patient's efforts have been minimally successful, a first recall visit might be set at 2 to 3 months; with greater success the interval could be increased to 3 months or more.

B Further recall visits are easier to schedule in a behaviorally successful manner. At each recall visit, evaluate plaque control, gingival inflammation status, and pocket depths, and use this measure of the patient's "success" to determine the next recall interval. Patient behavior over the years is rarely consistent. Many factors in patient's lives influence their efforts at oral hygiene. Periods of stress or illness affect their ability to deal with plaque. If plaque control has been inadequate, shorten the recall interval. If much inflammation is present or pocket depths are increasing, shorten the intervals even more. If the patient's efforts do not improve, alternative approaches (even extraction of poor risk teeth that can endanger adjacent abutments) may be necessary. If efforts improve after several recall visits, an increase in the time between recalls is an appropriate reward. Maintain the current recall interval for a patient whose efforts are fair or adequate. Reward a patient whose efforts have given excellent results by increasing the time between recalls.

References

Chace R: The maintenance phase of periodontal therapy, *J Periodontol* 22:23, 1951.

Lindhe J: *Textbook of clinical periodontology*, ed 2, Copenhagen, 1989, Munksgaard, pp 615, 626.

Parr RW: *Periodontal maintenance therapy*, Berkeley, Calif, 1974, Praxis Publishing, p 1.

Ramfjord SP, Knowles JW, Nissle RR et al: Longitudinal study of periodontal therapy, *J Periodontol* 44:66, 1973.

Ramfjord SP, Morrison EC, Burgett FG et al: Oral hygiene and maintenance of periodontal support, *J Periodontol* 53:26, 1982.

Schluger S, Yuodelis R, Page RC, Johnson RH: *Periodontol diseases*, ed 2, Philadelphia, 1990, Lea & Febiger, p 732.

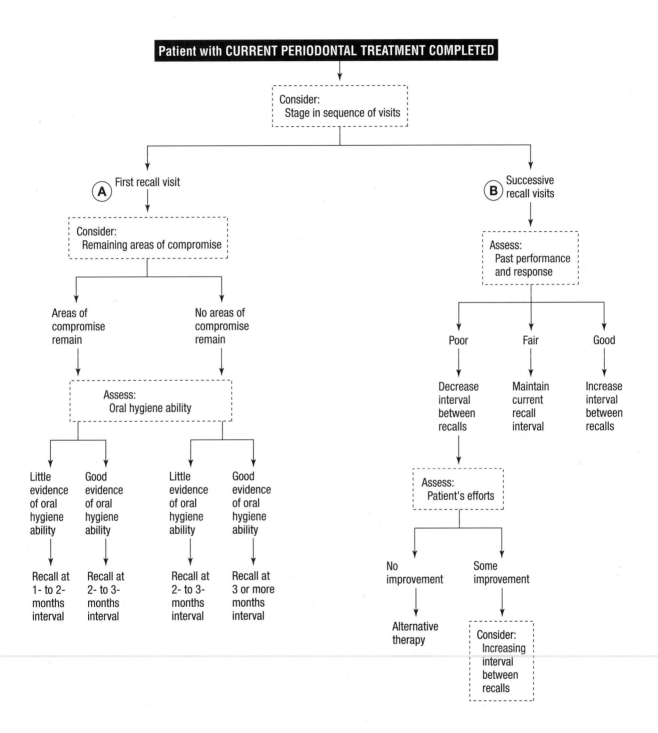

Patient with CURRENT PERIODONTAL TREATMENT COMPLETED

Consider:
Stage in sequence of visits

(A) First recall visit

Consider:
Remaining areas of compromise

Areas of compromise remain

No areas of compromise remain

Assess:
Oral hygiene ability

Little evidence of oral hygiene ability

Good evidence of oral hygiene ability

Little evidence of oral hygiene ability

Good evidence of oral hygiene ability

Recall at 1- to 2- months interval

Recall at 2- to 3- months interval

Recall at 2- to 3- months interval

Recall at 3 or more months interval

(B) Successive recall visits

Assess:
Past performance and response

Poor

Fair

Good

Decrease interval between recalls

Maintain current recall interval

Increase interval between recalls

Assess:
Patient's efforts

No improvement

Some improvement

Alternative therapy

Consider:
Increasing interval between recalls

48 Treatment Planning for the Patient with Human Immunodeficiency Virus

Gene A. Gowdey

The pharmaceutical industry has recently received Food and Drug Administration (FDA) approval to introduce a new class of drugs known as protease inhibitors. Whether or not these drugs can hold the human immunodeficiency virus (HIV) in check for long periods remains to be seen.

Advances have also been made in developing tests that measure the progression of disease, most notably, the blood test that determines the viral load. This blood assay provides a measure of the number of copies of HIV in circulating blood plasma, which may be a more accurate measure of disease activity than the CD4(+) T-lymphocyte count.

There are approximately 12 approved antiretrovirals to treat HIV infection. None of these drugs singly or in combination can cure or eliminate HIV infection. The virus rapidly develops resistance to most of the drugs that are currently available.

Recent epidemiologic data show overall reductions in the death rate of HIV-infected persons. Treatment planning objectives must be adapted to this changing state. Treatment plans should always lean toward a long-term dental management plan unless specific patient variables indicate the contrary.

A Before treatment planning, perform a thorough medical evaluation, and if necessary, obtain a physician consultation regarding specific issues of concern. Obtain additional patient information, as follows:
- History of HIV- or AIDS-related opportunistic conditions (Fig. 48-1, *A-F*)
- List of current medications and purpose of each
- Complete blood count with differential (blood laboratory report), including the following:
- CD4(+) T-lymphocytes (absolute number)
- Viral load
- Platelets

When in doubt about the long-term prognosis, consult with the patient's primary care physician.

Many times the dentist will have to coordinate medical management issues into the treatment plan. An example of this is thrombocytopenia, or a low platelet count, which is sometimes encountered with HIV patients. Primary care physicians may need to be called to assist with boosting counts (below 60,000 cells/cc) to adequate levels for dental therapy to proceed. Prednisone is often prescribed by primary care physicians to boost platelet counts, but sometimes a platelet infusion is necessary immediately preceding invasive procedures.

Another example of medical management needed in conjunction with dental therapy is the consideration of neutropenia (low neutrophil count) or granulocytopenia (low white blood cell count) during periods of chemotherapy (for malignancies). The dentist must consult with the medical oncologist to determine which times are safe for invasive procedures (usually between chemotherapy sessions or just before the next cycle).

B Make a judgment regarding the patients prognosis, as follows (Table 48-1):

1. Poor prognosis: terminally ill patients or deteriorating health with a short life expectancy
2. Moderate prognosis: patients having significant expressions of AIDS-related conditions but are currently stable
3. Good prognosis: patients with few complications of HIV who are relatively healthy

Individuals who have not responded well to the multiple drug therapies and who are having major opportunistic conditions may fall into the poor prognosis category. Provided that the blood laboratory values are within acceptable limits, no specific contraindications to dental therapy may exist. However, because a poor prognosis exists, most of the treatment planning should be palliative only. The patient should be offered diagnostic, preventive, restorative, and removable prosthetic services. Refrain from offering crown and bridge services or root canal work. The treatment plan should be centered around patient comfort and the control of dental infections.

In the moderate prognosis case, offer the full range of comprehensive dental services. Such patients may achieve good prognosis status in the future. The treatment planning decisions should be made with specific concern for individual circumstances. HIV disease or AIDS by itself should not be a reason to curtail treatment planning recommendations for persons with a moderate prognosis or better.

In the case of good prognosis offer the full complement of comprehensive dental services; the myth that because someone has HIV, he or she cannot safely undergo invasive dental therapy should be dispelled. HIV patients respond to dental therapy in a similar manner as any other non-HIV patient.

With the proper interventions of medical management, all HIV patients can be offered dental care in a safe and predictable manner.

References

Carpenter CC, Fischl MA, Hammer SM, Hirsch MS, Jacobsen DM, Katzenstein DA et al: Antiretroviral therapy for HIV infection in 1996: recommendations of an international panel. International AIDS Society—USA. *JAMA* 276:146, 1996.

Greenspan D, Greenspan JS: HIV-related oral disease, *Lancet* 348:729, 1996.

Pindborg JJ: Classification of oral lesions associated with HIV infection, *Oral Surg* 67:292, 1989.

Sande MA, Volberding PA, editors: *The medical management of AIDS*, Philadelphia, 1997, WB Saunders.

Silverman, Jr, S, Migliorati CA, Lozada-Nur F et al: Oral findings in people with or at high risk for AIDS: a study of 375 homosexual males, *J Am Dent Assoc* 112:187, 1986.

Volberding PA: HIV quantification: clinical applications, *Lancet* 347:71, 1996.

Weinert M, Grimes RM, Lynch DP: Oral manifestations of HIV infection, *Ann Intern Med* 125:485, 1996.

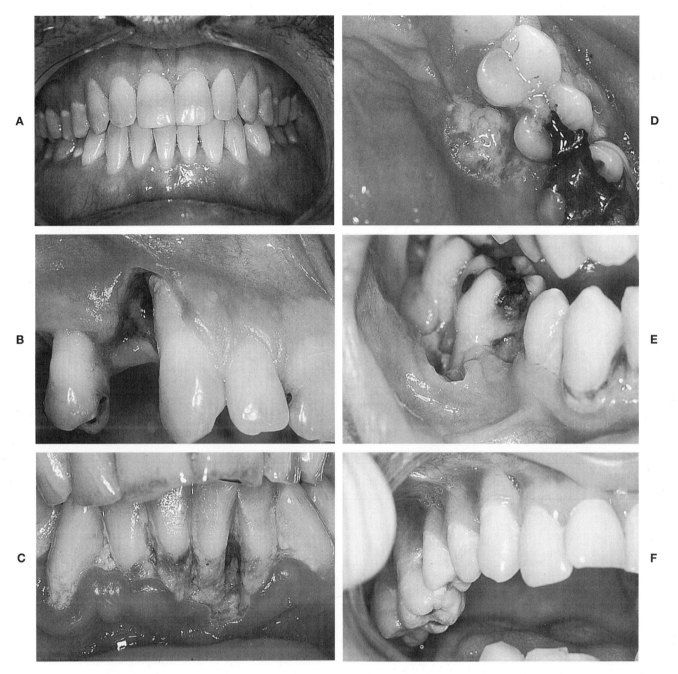

Fig. 48-1 **A,** Perfect health. **B,** HIV periodontitis. **C,** HIV periodontitis with gingival necrosis. **D,** Necrotizing stomatitis. **E,** HIV periodontitis with alveolar bone necrosis. **F,** Vanishing bone phenomenon (total alveolar process disintegration within 8 months). Note the extreme variance from perfect health to advanced debilitation. (Courtesy Dr. Gene A. Gowdey, San Francisco.)

TABLE **48-1**   **Determination of Level of Prognosis**

	CD4(+) T-Cells	Opportunistic Conditions	Response to Drugs	Viral Load
Poor prognosis for 5-year survival	0-100	Currently experiencing AIDS-defining deteriorating opportunistic conditions	Poor response to combination antiretroviral	(High) 30,000 or greater
Moderate prognosis for 5-year survival	100-200	History of AIDS-defining opportunistic conditions; currently not experiencing deteriorating opportunistic conditions	Moderate response to combination antiretroviral	(Medium) 5,000-30,000
Good prognosis for 5-year survival	200 or greater	History of minor opportunistic conditions; no AIDS defining conditions	Responding favorably to combination antiretroviral	(Low) 5,000 or less

PART TWO

Endodontics

Alan H. Gluskin, Editor

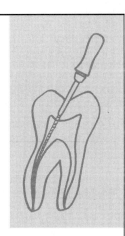

49 Sequence of Treatment for the Asymptomatic Patient

Alan H. Gluskin

The asymptomatic patient who requires comprehensive dental care to restore oral health may require endodontic procedures in the course of treatment.

Endodontic therapy is indicated for three main reasons: (1) the asymptomatic tooth has a failing or inadequate root canal filling, (2) testing or radiographs may disclose an asymptomatic or mildly symptomatic tooth with pulpal or periapical pathology, (3) endodontics in conjunction with periodontal or restorative procedures may be required on teeth to restore and rehabilitate oral function.

A Proper timing of comprehensive patient care is critical for proper treatment planning. A priority in comprehensive care is a thorough medical history and evaluation. A patient's physical condition and medications can influence endodontic treatment and the ability to heal. As a consequence, a medical history is imperative before any treatment (emergency or otherwise) is initiated.

Comprehensive care is the expected standard of care for the patient of record. The scope of care includes evaluation of the medical and dental history as described and a thorough head and neck examination, including soft and hard oral structures.

B Diagnostic aids (e.g., radiographs, pulp tests, periodontal probing, fiberoptics, percussion and palpation, and additional clinical and laboratory tests) should enable the dentist to diagnose the patient's hard and soft tissue oral problems and develop a problem list. Prioritizing a problem list for the specific task of determining the sequence of treatment is a fundamental principle in comprehensive care. The problem list should also have an underlying organizational efficiency so that more than one procedure in a quadrant can be attempted if this is acceptable to both the dentist and patient.

C In finalizing the treatment plan the dentist should determine a specific treatment needed for each tooth and the surrounding area. It must also be decided what specialty services might be required. Surgical procedures, such as extractions and ridge alterations, have first priority. Then any mobile and weakened teeth can be splinted before periodontal or endodontic therapy.

Usually, periodontal therapy such as scaling, root planing, and surgery precedes final endodontic procedures; however, performing endodontics before specific procedures, such as a proposed hemisection or root amputation, offers a much more reliable prognosis. With endodontics completed, the variables in surgical procedures are much more controllable. This is always true for periapical surgery.

Finally, restorative and prosthetic procedures can be initiated when the patient is free from active pathology in the teeth and supporting structures. A short time may be required before final restoration to clinically and radiographically evaluate periodontal and endodontic healing.

The patient must be maintained in a healthy state and monitored with follow-up care at regular intervals, including oral prophylaxis, radiographic recall, and clinical evaluation to monitor continuing health.

In summary, endodontic therapy is an integral part of comprehensive patient care. It must be done early, before restorative work, to evaluate healing and the prognosis of each tooth. It should be integrated in the treatment plan with periodontal therapy because one condition can affect the prognosis of the other.

References

Cohen S, Burns R: *Pathways of the pulp,* ed 7, St Louis, 1997, Mosby, p 60.

Walton RE, Torabinejad M: *Principles and practice of endodontics,* ed 2, Philadelphia, 1997, WB Saunders, p 52.

Weine RS: *Endodontic therapy,* ed 5, St Louis, 1995, Mosby, p 28.

Patient with a COMPLEX DENTAL PROBLEM who is ASYMPTOMATIC

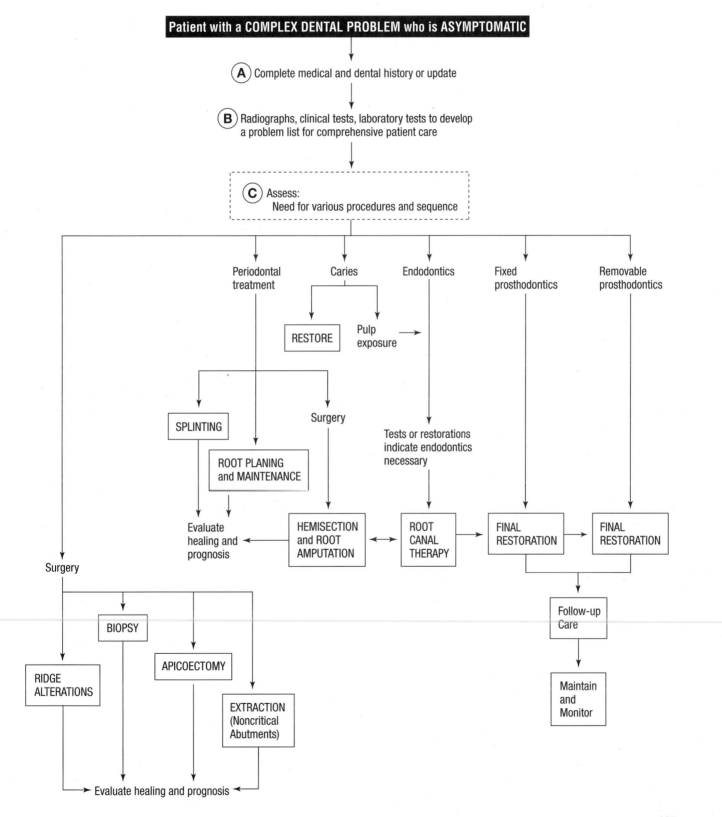

(A) Complete medical and dental history or update

(B) Radiographs, clinical tests, laboratory tests to develop a problem list for comprehensive patient care

(C) Assess:
   Need for various procedures and sequence

Periodontal treatment — Caries — Endodontics — Fixed prosthodontics — Removable prosthodontics

RESTORE — Pulp exposure

SPLINTING

ROOT PLANING and MAINTENANCE

Surgery

Tests or restorations indicate endodontics necessary

Evaluate healing and prognosis ← HEMISECTION and ROOT AMPUTATION ↔ ROOT CANAL THERAPY → FINAL RESTORATION — FINAL RESTORATION

Surgery

BIOPSY

RIDGE ALTERATIONS

APICOECTOMY

EXTRACTION (Noncritical Abutments)

Follow-up Care

Maintain and Monitor

Evaluate healing and prognosis

50 Sequence of Treatment for the Patient in Pain

Alan H. Gluskin

For many patients new to a dental practice or for patients seeking treatment after many years of neglecting their dental care, the overriding reason for a visit to the dentist is often oral pain or toothache.

Whether the etiology of a patient's pain is periodontal, endodontic, or of another origin, the acute emergency treatment is the first therapy the patient receives from the dentist. The treatment plan for comprehensive dental care usually follows.

A In making a diagnosis of tooth pain the dentist evaluates the patient's history, reviewing both the medical and dental records. The medical record should suggest any predisposing factors that might contribute to nonodontogenic pain in the head and neck area. Sinus disease, vascular pain syndrome such as migraine, circulatory insufficiencies, trigeminal neuralgia, psychogenic pain, myofascial pain dysfunction, or temporomandibular joint dysfunction all cause radiating pain to the jaws and teeth. In making a differential diagnosis of toothache the practitioner must understand that nonodontogenic etiologies may coexist with confirmed endodontic and periodontal pathology. This probability must be considered along with any possible odontogenic cause of pain in the patient.

B In developing a strategy for restoring the patient to optimal oral health, the practitioner must first deal with the patient's acute circumstances and emergency therapy. This may include oral surgery for the extraction of unrestorable or nonsalvageable teeth and initiation of endodontics for acute pulpal and periapical inflammation.

C For deep lesions, which may compromise pulp vitality, caries control should be a priority equal to an emergency if early on it is felt that the tooth can contribute to the overall treatment goals.

D If pulps are exposed or degenerating, then pulpotomy or pulpectomy techniques should be used with intermediate restorative materials to bridge the time gap between these procedures and the definitive therapy of endodontics. Unexposed caries control of vital teeth requires pulpal sedation and intermediate restorative materials if the therapy is provided before the treatment plan is finalized.

E Subsequent to these acute circumstances, an evaluation must be made regarding the periodontal attachment and bony support of teeth. Because periodontal health is the key element in tooth retention and the overall prognosis for teeth, periodontal assessment should be of primary importance in the early stages of the treatment plan.

Once hopeless teeth are identified, those with a better prognosis can be evaluated for worth in the final treatment plan. On occasion, temporary splinting may be required to evaluate salvageability of some mobile teeth while periodontal procedures to manage soft tissue disease is initiated and evaluated. Most complex and varied treatment plans require periodontal therapy as an integral part of the treatment regimen.

Some time should pass after the emergency therapy is rendered, during which the patient is monitored for healing. Then the prognosis for individual abutments in the comprehensive treatment plan can be ascertained.

In summary, endodontic therapy is an integral part of comprehensive patient care. Emergency treatment is initiated early to eliminate acute pulpal and periapical symptoms. Once diagnosis and emergency therapy are accomplished, the teeth can be restored with intermediate materials to evaluate healing and develop a treatment plan for comprehensive patient care.

References

Cohen S, Burns R: *Pathways of the pulp,* ed 7, St Louis, 1997, Mosby, p 60.

Walton RE, Torabinejad M: *Principles and practice of endodontics,* ed 2, Philadelphia, 1997, WB Saunders, p 52.

Weine RS: *Endodontic therapy,* ed 5, St Louis, 1995, Mosby, p 28.

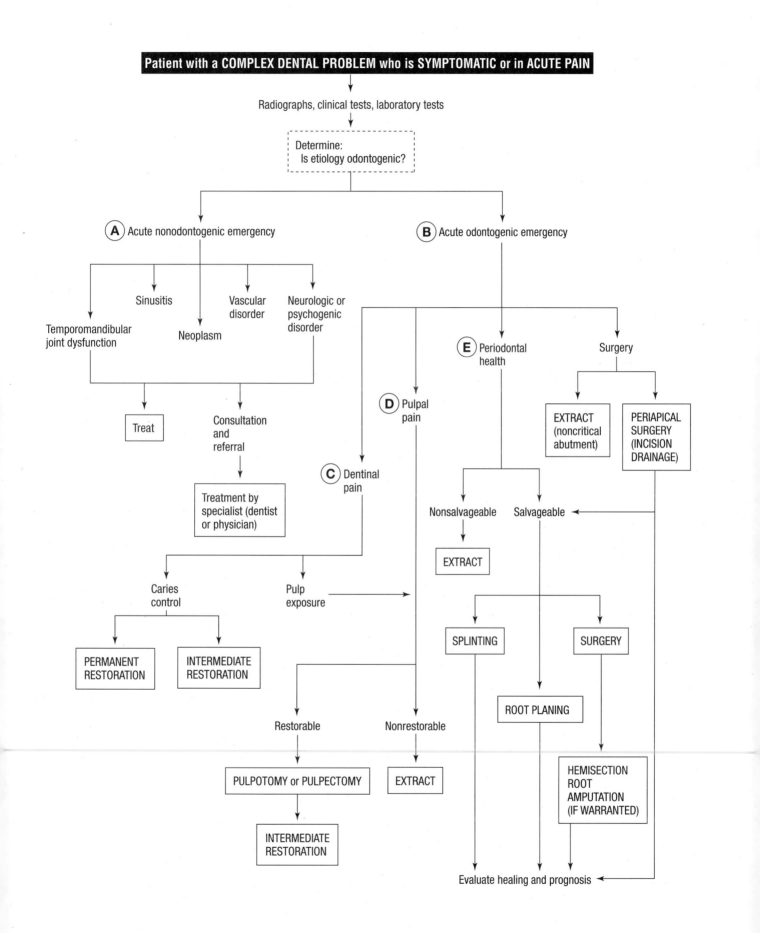

Patient with a COMPLEX DENTAL PROBLEM who is SYMPTOMATIC or in ACUTE PAIN

Radiographs, clinical tests, laboratory tests

Determine:
Is etiology odontogenic?

A Acute nonodontogenic emergency

B Acute odontogenic emergency

Sinusitis

Vascular disorder

Neurologic or psychogenic disorder

Temporomandibular joint dysfunction

Neoplasm

E Periodontal health

Surgery

Treat

Consultation and referral

D Pulpal pain

EXTRACT (noncritical abutment)

PERIAPICAL SURGERY (INCISION DRAINAGE)

Treatment by specialist (dentist or physician)

C Dentinal pain

Nonsalvageable

Salvageable

EXTRACT

Caries control

Pulp exposure

PERMANENT RESTORATION

INTERMEDIATE RESTORATION

SPLINTING

SURGERY

ROOT PLANING

Restorable

Nonrestorable

HEMISECTION ROOT AMPUTATION (IF WARRANTED)

PULPOTOMY or PULPECTOMY

EXTRACT

INTERMEDIATE RESTORATION

Evaluate healing and prognosis

51 Referral to an Endodontist

Alan H. Gluskin

The decision to refer a patient to an endodontist for therapy is made by the general dentist and is an integral part of the delivery of professional care. The thought process in making a referral should involve both technical and nontechnical considerations. Technical factors relate to the difficulty in accomplishing endodontic treatment relative to the biomechanical aspects of therapy. The dentist must consider his or her own level of training and experience, as well as his or her diagnostic judgment, before proceeding with any endodontic procedure. Nontechnical factors involve the patient's desires and include management difficulties and health complications that might impact therapy and postoperative repair and healing.

An underlying factor in all decision making is the principle of standard of care, defined as the care that a reasonably prudent practitioner would perform under the same or similar circumstances. When endodontic treatment is provided, all practitioners, whether they are general dentists or specialists, are judged by the same criteria and must render care to the same standards, namely that of the endodontist. Hence general dentists should select and treat only those cases for which they have the training and experience and should refer all others.

Once the clinician and patient determine that the problem tooth can be saved by endodontic therapy, the practitioner should consider a list of criteria in determining whether referral is indicated. The patient's best interest is always primary.

A wide range exists in the types of cases a dentist might refer. The potential for an adverse reaction or a procedural mishap in endodontics is high. Severe pain and prolonged suffering can quickly ruin a doctor-patient relationship, which may have taken years to develop.

A If the patient has a dental emergency, immediate attention is required. Such cases include toothache, pulpal exposures, swelling, and trauma. The dentist with a busy schedule may have little or no time to handle this scenario and maintain the standard of care; thus the patient should be referred.

B The patient has a complex case involving one or more of the following difficulties: a toothache for which the cause is difficult to determine; calcified canals or pulp chambers or complex root and canal morphology; teeth that have had prior procedural accidents, such as perforations or separated instruments; retreatment cases with silver cones or hard pastes; traumatized teeth with resorption or immature apices; critical abutments or teeth requiring access through crowns; and complex surgical cases. Dentists must decide if their experience and training are adequate to treat the problem. Referral of such cases allows the patient to benefit from the greater experience of the endodontist.

C Although there are almost no medical contraindications to endodontic therapy, medically compromised patients who have circulatory disease, bleeding disorders, pulmonary or liver disease, diabetes, adrenal insufficiency, pregnancy, allergies, or are receiving radiation or chemotherapy for an immunologic impairment (e.g., caused by HIV or cancer) can be treated quickly and efficiently by the endodontist, making interappointment complications less likely.

D In addition, a general dentist may wish to refer patients who exhibit management problems (e.g., those who are mentally compromised by phobias about dentistry or have true psychologic or mental disorders). Fearful patients can become impossible to calm or even anesthetize if they sense that the general dentist is unfamiliar or uncomfortable with an endodontic procedure. Sedation may be indicated in such a patient, with therapy rendered by a specialist. Many of these psychologic conditions can be overcome by the practitioner who shows a compassionate and caring manner and can develop the patient's trust. In this capacity a general dentist may have as much ability as the endodontist; however, to put the patient at ease and remove stress from the dentist, these patients should be referred to specialists to expedite treatment.

In summary, the prudent general dentist should attempt to select cases that will proceed smoothly and routinely and refer those who may present biomechanical or management difficulties.

The wisest time to make a referral of a potentially problematic case is before the case has been started. The dentist-patient relationship can be quite fragile and have litigious consequences if there is a perceived or real lack of diagnostic or clinical expertise on the part of the dentist. Patients have little to do with decision making in the referral process and must place a great deal of trust in the general dentist and the proposed specialist to provide the highest quality of treatment to correct their problems.

References

Cohen S, Burns R: *Pathways of the pulp*, ed 7, St Louis, 1997, Mosby, pp 21, 376.

Dietz, Sr, GC, Dietz, Jr, GC: The endodontist and the general dentist, *Dent Clin North Am*, 36:459, 1992.

Walton RE, Torabinejad M: *Principles and practice of endodontics*, ed 2, Philadelphia, 1997, WB Saunders, p 75.

Weine FS: *Endodontic therapy*, ed 5, St Louis, 1995, Mosby, p 203.

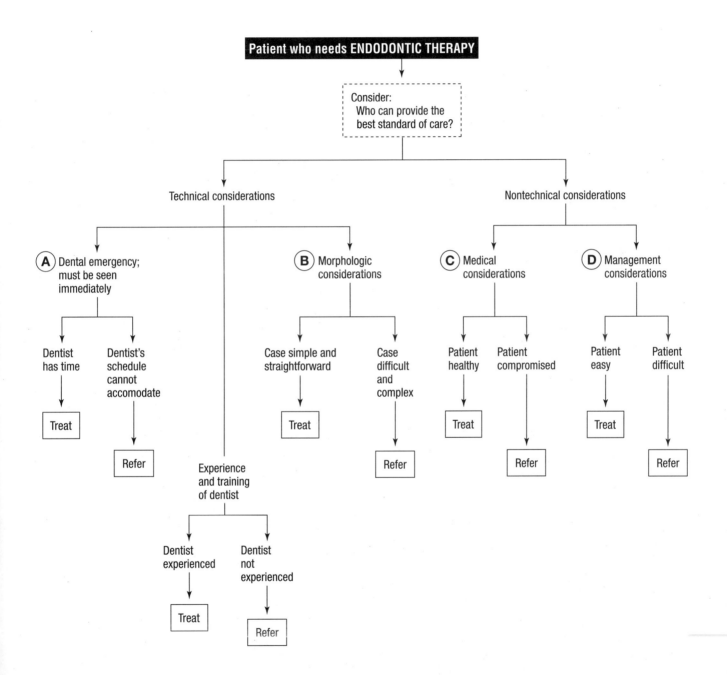

Patient who needs ENDODONTIC THERAPY

Consider:
Who can provide the
best standard of care?

Technical considerations

Nontechnical considerations

(A) Dental emergency;
must be seen
immediately

Dentist
has time

Treat

Dentist's
schedule
cannot
accomodate

Refer

Experience
and training
of dentist

Dentist
experienced

Treat

Dentist
not
experienced

Refer

(B) Morphologic
considerations

Case simple and
straightforward

Treat

Case
difficult
and
complex

Refer

(C) Medical
considerations

Patient
healthy

Treat

Patient
compromised

Refer

(D) Management
considerations

Patient
easy

Treat

Patient
difficult

Refer

52 Transdentinal Therapy Versus Conventional Endodontics

Alan H. Gluskin

A common occurrence in dental practice is the patient with nonurgent odontogenic pain. For the doctor to triage care, an understanding of the physiology of pulpal pain is paramount.

The sensibility of the dental pulp is controlled by myelinated A-delta and unmyelinated C afferent nerve fibers. While both sensory nerve fibers conduct pain signals to the brain, the differences between the two sensory fibers enable the patient to discriminate and characterize the quality, intensity, location, and duration of the pain response.

A The A-delta fibers course coronally through the pulp. These nerve endings branch onto and through the odontoblastic cell layer, into dentinal tubules, and contact odontoblastic processes, creating a pulpodentinal complex. Disturbances of the pulpodentinal complex in a vital tooth initially affect low threshold A-delta fibers by disruption of fluid or cellular processes in dentinal tubules. Dentinal pain or dentin sensitivity is provoked A-delta fiber pain and is immediately perceived as a quick, sharp momentary pain. The sensation dissipates quickly when the provoking stimulus is removed. The stimulus is most commonly cold liquids or biting against a dentinal fracture.

It is a common understanding that clinical symptoms correlate poorly with the health status of the pulp. However, symptoms of A-delta fiber pain (dentinal pain or sensitivity) warrant consideration of pulp preservation (transdentinal or sedative measures) as a primary treatment option because reasonable decisions regarding pulp vitality and repair can be made if degenerative changes are not exhibited clinically.

B C fibers are small, unmyelinated nerves that course centrally in the pulp. They are high threshold fibers and unlike A-delta fibers are not easily provoked. C fiber pain predominates with irreversible tissue injury. The pain is more diffuse and lingering and can escalate to an intensely prolonged episode or a spontaneous, constant, throbbing pain. Often the pain is referred to other teeth. C fiber pain is an ominous symptom that signifies that degenerative changes have occurred. In the absence of endodontic intervention the rapidly deteriorating condition will most likely progress to a periapical abscess.

C Pulpal pain symptoms are not mutually exclusive, and thus treatment recommendations for a vital tooth must carefully consider the clinical circumstances leading to a decision to attempt pulp preservation procedures or initiate endodontic therapy. Often symptoms are of both A-delta and C fiber origin. In the presence of irreversible inflammation the pulpal response is exaggerated and disproportionate to the stimulus. Exaggerated A-delta fiber pain may remain and be perceived as a dull, throbbing ache. This second pain overlay signifies the irreversible inflammatory involvement of deeper C fibers.

D The dentist attempting to identify treatment options must consider specific etiologic factors such as caries, fractures, periodontal disease, trauma, and a history of restorations. In addition to pain complaints, these etiologic factors will determine whether a decision to undertake pulp preservation procedures is reasonable.

E A number of pulpal insults can provoke a quick, sharp, momentary tooth pain. Dentinal hypersensitivity, recurrent caries, recession, or fractures can initiate A-delta fiber pain. Dentin therapy in the absence of degenerative symptoms is indicated. Chemical (desensitizing agents) or physical blockage of tubules (resins, varnishes, grafts) and conservative restorative techniques will all resolve A-delta fiber pain, which is reversible.

F An inescapable sequela of irreversible pulp inflammation is its eventual spread throughout the confines of the tooth and into the periapical tissues. Management of the degenerating pulp exhibiting the spontaneous, dull, throbbing ache of C fiber involvement necessitates initiating endodontic therapy and accomplishing thorough débridement of the pulpal tissues.

References

Brännström M: The hydrodynamic theory of dentinal pain: sensation in preparations, caries, and the dentinal crack syndrome, *J Endodon* 12:453, 1986.

Cohen S, Burns R: *Pathways of the pulp*, ed 7, St Louis, 1997, Mosby, p 20.

Kim S: Neurovascular interactions in the dental pulp in health and inflammation, *J Endod* 16:48, 1990.

Takahashi K: Changes in the pulp vasculature during inflammation, *J Endod* 16:92, 1990.

Trowbridge HO: Intradental sensory units: physiological and clinical aspects, *J Endod* 11:489, 1985.

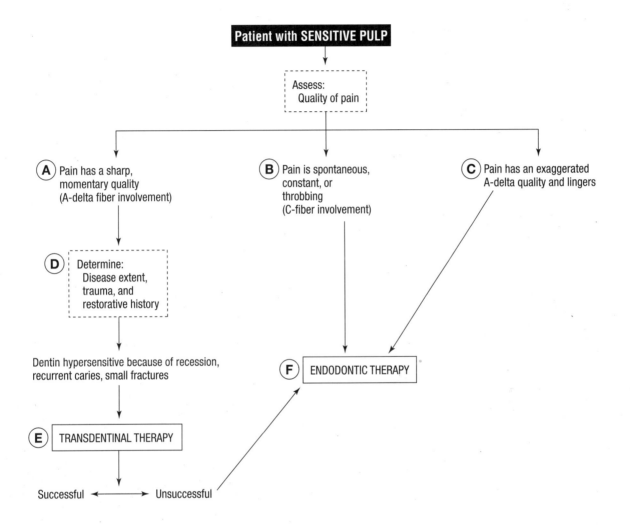

Patient with SENSITIVE PULP

Assess:
Quality of pain

A Pain has a sharp,
momentary quality
(A-delta fiber involvement)

B Pain is spontaneous,
constant, or
throbbing
(C-fiber involvement)

C Pain has an exaggerated
A-delta quality and lingers

D Determine:
Disease extent,
trauma, and
restorative history

Dentin hypersensitive because of recession,
recurrent caries, small fractures

E TRANSDENTINAL THERAPY

Successful ⟷ Unsuccessful

F ENDODONTIC THERAPY

53 Single Visit Versus Multiple Visit Endodontics

A. Scott Cohen

With proper case selection, most teeth can be treated endodontically in a single appointment. There are certain factors that the practitioner must consider before deciding how many appointments are necessary for completing root canal therapy.

A If the patient has an intraoral or extraoral swelling, the tooth should be temporized after cleansing and shaping the canals. Swellings often drain through the tooth and root canals should never be obturated in the presence of exudate.

B When a patient is experiencing acute pain from a necrotic tooth, the tooth should be temporized after cleansing and shaping. Such teeth are more prone to flare-ups, and it may be necessary to open the tooth for drainage should swelling develop subsequent to treatment.

C Certain teeth present challenges that require extra time to treat well. Most cases that involve retreatment are more complex because posts and other canal obstructions can be time consuming to remove. Calcified canals may be difficult to locate and enlarge. Anatomic root anomalies, such as dilacerations or severe root curvatures, usually require extra time for instrumentation. Any of these situations may require additional appointments to achieve ideal results.

One common cause of root canal failures is the inability to locate, clean, and obturate the fourth canal (second mesial-buccal) in maxillary molars. Approximately 75% of first molars and 50% of second molars contain four canals. Additional treatment time should be allocated for finding these canals. Two or more appointments may be appropriate for maxillary molars.

D Once a tooth is completely cleansed and shaped, the practitioner must decide if obturation is appropriate. All canals must be completely dry for ideal results. Blood or exudate will compromise the apical seal and can lead to failure. In such cases the tooth should be temporized and the patient scheduled for obturation several days later.

Filling a tooth in a single appointment is biologically superior to multiple appointments because there is no chance for resistant bacteria to regrow between treatment visits. In fact, obturation of root canals with gutta-percha is associated with fewer flare-ups and a decrease in postoperative pain.

Some patients may become tired or uncomfortable during an extended treatment visit. The clinician must not hurry to complete a case because it is at these times when mistakes are likely to happen. The practitioner must consider his or her case selection and clinical expertise when deciding if single-visit endodontics is best for the patient.

References

Cohen S, Burns R: *Pathways of the pulp*, ed 7, St Louis, 1997, Mosby, p 73.

Sundqvist G: Ecology of the root canal flora, *J Endodon* 18(9):427, 1992.

Torabinejad M, Kettering JD, McGraw JC, Cummings RR, Dwyer TG, Tobias TS: Factors associated with endodontic interappointment emergencies of teeth with necrotic pulps, *J Endodon* 14(5):261, 1988.

Torabinejad M, Dorn SO, Eleazer PD, Franson M, Jouhari B, Mullin RK, Soluti A: Effectiveness of various medications on postoperative pain following root canal obturation, *J Endodon* 20(9):427, 1994.

Walton R, Fouad A: Endodontic interappointment flare-ups: a prospective study of incidence and related factors, *J Endodon* 18(4):172, 1992.

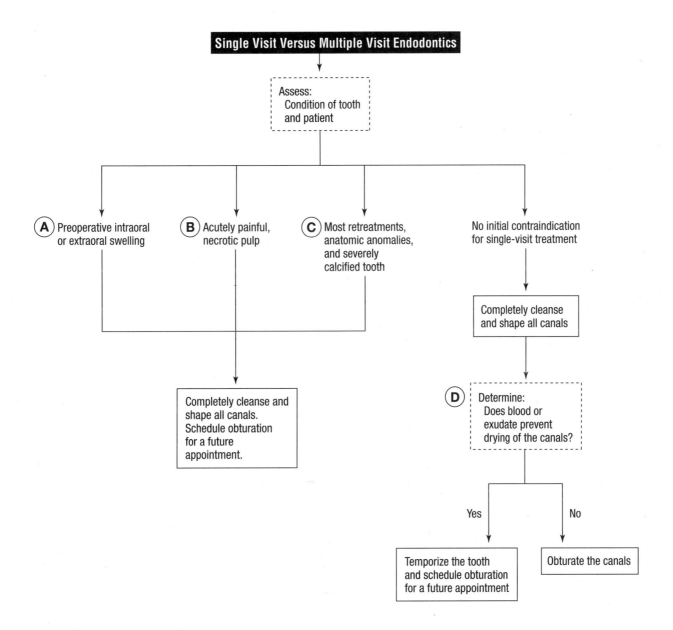

Single Visit Versus Multiple Visit Endodontics

Assess:
Condition of tooth
and patient

(A) Preoperative intraoral
or extraoral swelling

(B) Acutely painful,
necrotic pulp

(C) Most retreatments,
anatomic anomalies,
and severely
calcified tooth

No initial contraindication
for single-visit treatment

Completely cleanse and
shape all canals.
Schedule obturation
for a future
appointment.

Completely cleanse
and shape all canals

(D) Determine:
Does blood or
exudate prevent
drying of the canals?

Yes

No

Temporize the tooth
and schedule obturation
for a future appointment

Obturate the canals

54 Clinical and Radiographic Considerations before Planning Endodontics in Complex Cases

Hipolito Fabra-Campos, Jose Manuel Roig-Garcia

In deciding whether a tooth merits endodontic treatment as part of an overall treatment plan, the amount of existing tooth structure remaining, its restorability, the existence of fractures, and especially its periodontal status must be determined before proceeding.

A The initial step is radiographic and clinical evaluation of the amount of tooth structure available and the adequacy of the remaining portion to support a restoration that is part of the overall treatment plan. If the tooth is unrestorable (e.g., decay, tooth structure loss extends into a furcation, remaining root structure is insufficient to support crown), it should be extracted. If it is judged to be restorable, its endodontic status should be assessed.

B If the tooth is not endodontically involved, prosthetic preparation may necessitate pulpal exposure to meet demands for parallel abutment preparation or to reduce the crown height sufficiently to allow an adequate thickness of restorative material. If the pulp must be exposed to permit restoration of the tooth as an important part of the treatment plan, the possibility of performing root canal therapy should be assessed.

C Should the tooth appear to be fractured, the extent of the fracture(s) should be assessed. Fiberoptic and radiographic evaluation should be included in the decision regarding treatment options. A crack that is restricted to the crown should not influence the potential usefulness of the tooth. If the crack extends into the root and appears to involve only the coronal third, elimination of the coronal portion of the fracture may not endanger the continued usefulness of the tooth. Crown lengthening (see Chapter 11) or orthodontic extrusion (see Chapter 83) may permit its restoration. A more extensive fracture or a vertical fracture throughout the root would make the tooth unrestorable, and it should be extracted.

D The periodontal status of the tooth must be considered before proceeding with endodontic treatment. As attachment loss approaches 50%, the possibilities of successful periodontal treatment decline dramatically; however, the presence of periodontal lesions amenable to guided tissue regeneration (e.g., a deep three-walled osseous defect, a severe Class II furcation involvement, a deeper interdental crater) should not limit efforts to retain the tooth (see Chapters 27, 29, and 30). If the tooth is periodontally maintainable or can be made so, proceed with the indicated root canal therapy.

Should periodontal treatment result in a pulpal problem, which is a possible consequence of furcation surgery, proceed with endodontics, if feasible. With some molars, root amputation or hemisection and endodontic treatment permit retention of strategically important parts of molars (see Chapters 72 and 73).

E If all of the previous considerations indicate that the tooth will be useful when endodontically treated, the feasibility of root canal therapy should be considered next. Other factors such as the ability to access, internal and external resorption problems, and unsatisfactory earlier root canal therapy must be evaluated. When conventional endodontics cannot be used, root resection or apicoectomy may permit retention of the tooth (see Chapter 60). If these procedures cannot be performed or if they fail to be accomplished successfully, the tooth should be extracted.

References

Guilbert P, Rozanes SO, Tecuciano JF: Periodontal and prosthetic treatment of patients with advanced periodontal disease, *Dent Clin North Am* 32:331, 1988.

Kalwarf KL, Reinhardt RA: The furcation problem, *Dent Clin North Am* 32:243, 1988.

Lindhe J: *Textbook of clinical periodontology*, ed 2, Copenhagen, 1989, Munksgaard, p 569.

Nyman S, Lindhe J: A longitudinal study of combined periodontal and prosthetic treatment of patients with advanced periodontal disease, *J Periodontol* 50:163, 1975.

Trabert KC, Cooney JP: Endodontically treated teeth, *Dent Clin North Am* 28:923, 1984.

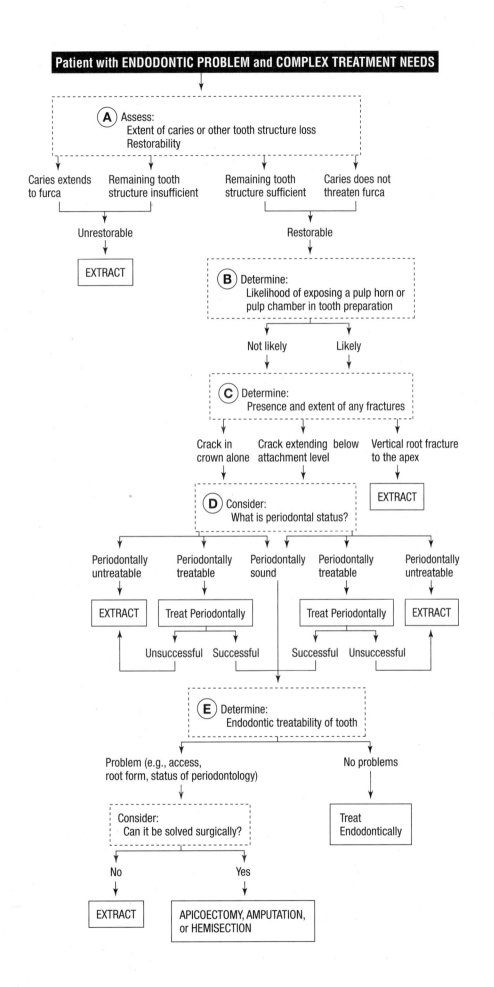

55 The Difficult Anesthesia Case

Alan H. Gluskin

Urgent care of an endodontic emergency often requires more than routine regional anesthesia of dental structures. Profound local anesthesia for these stressful interactions between doctor and patient is mandatory. Only with a complete lack of sensation can definitive treatment be rendered at a stress level that is acceptable. An anesthetic regimen that is specific for pulpal and periapical emergencies is required, and a strategy must be planned in advance to assure success.

Suppression of the pain signal is hampered by the numerous inflammatory pathways that are operating in the area. As inflammation increases and spreads, local tissue pH falls precipitously. The acidic environment prevents the anesthetic molecule from dissociating into ion form and migrating through the neural sheath. In addition, the inflamed nerve fibers are morphologically and biochemically altered throughout their length by neuropeptides and other neurochemicals. In a state of hyperalgesia, nerve block injections at sites associated with pain and swelling may be rendered less effective.

The clinician must gain an advantage by thoughtfully selecting alternate and supplemental sites for injecting anesthetic solution. Consideration must be given to the type and amount of anesthetic solution required for the conditions. There may be anatomic limitations such as dense bony plates, aberrant nerve distributions, or accessory innervations, especially in the mandible.

A The nerve block injection of a nerve trunk central to an area for a tooth is the standard intraoral approach for achieving initial regional anesthesia. A block injection anesthetizes a wider area while avoiding soft tissue areas involved in the inflammation and infection.

In difficult cases to block, depositing a greater volume of anesthetic in the region increases the likelihood of achieving pain control.

B The infraorbital nerve block (for anterior teeth) and the posterior superior alveolar (PSA) nerve block (for molars) are standard injections for the maxillary teeth. If swelling or gross infection is present, the anterior palatine canal injection (for anterior teeth), middle superior alveolar (MSA) nerve block (for mesiobuccal root of an infected maxillary first molar and premolars), and a maxillary nerve block through the greater palatine canal can be used to supplement the infraorbital nerve block in achieving greater anesthesia. In the absence of swelling and infection, local infiltration anesthesia can supplement the block injections to attain a satisfactory level of local anesthesia.

C Regional nerve blocks for the mandible include the inferior alveolar nerve block, Gow-Gates, Akinosi, and incisive blocks. However, the inferior alveolar nerve block is the most common, and it provides regional anesthesia to all the mandibular teeth. Profound anesthesia is often elusive with this injection and can be attributed to three basic errors.

First, an insufficient amount of anesthetic solution is deposited and cannot produce the effect required for the conditions. Second, the anesthetic is deposited distant from (i.e., too high, too low, too deep, too superficial) the mandibular foramen where the mandibular nerve bundle enters into the lower jaw. Third, supplemental adjunctive injections into the long buccal, mylohyoid, and mental nerve sites are given too soon. Intensive soft tissue anesthesia is produced and masks the sensations of a marginally effective nerve block. Pain is noticed as soon as treatment is attempted.

D Three supplemental injections are available to attain a reasonable depth of anesthesia when all other block techniques have been insufficient. Intraligamentary injections into the periodontal ligament space at the four interproximal line angles of the tooth can produce a short-lived anesthesia blocking cervical innervation to the teeth. This usually will permit the clinician to continue and to expose a pinpoint area of the pulp.

E When the pulp is exposed, an intrapulpal injection is immediately given with a short 30-gauge needle inserted tightly through the small opening. To be effective, the anesthetic solution must be forced into the pulp space with little or no back flow out of the tooth. The intrapulpal injection is extremely painful, if given ineffectively. Also, this injection must not be used in necrotic or infected teeth because toxic material may be forced into the periapical tissues.

F Anesthesia for the necrotic or infected canal or still painful vital tooth can be safely attained with an intraosseous injection under slow pressure into the adjacent interproximal crestal bone. The intraligamentary and intraosseous injections into the highly vascularized alveolar tissues and cancellous bone can produce an adverse cardiac response with solutions containing epinephrine. Care should be taken not to exceed recommended dosages.

References

Byers MR et al: Effects of injury and inflammation on pulpal and periapical nerves, *J Endodon* 16:78, 1990.

Childers M, Reader A, Nist R, Beck M, Meyers WJ: Anesthetic efficacy of the periodontal ligament injection after an inferior alveolar nerve block, *J Endodon* 22:317, 1996.

Cunningham CJ, Mullaney TP: Pain control in endodontics, *Dent Clin North Am* 36:393, 1992.

Dunbar D, Reader A, Nist R, Beck M, Meyers WJ: Anesthetic efficacy of the intraosseous injection after an inferior alveolar nerve block, *J Endodon* 22:481, 1996.

Wong MKS, Jacobsen PL: Reasons for local anesthesia failures, *J Am Dent Assoc* 123:69, 1992.

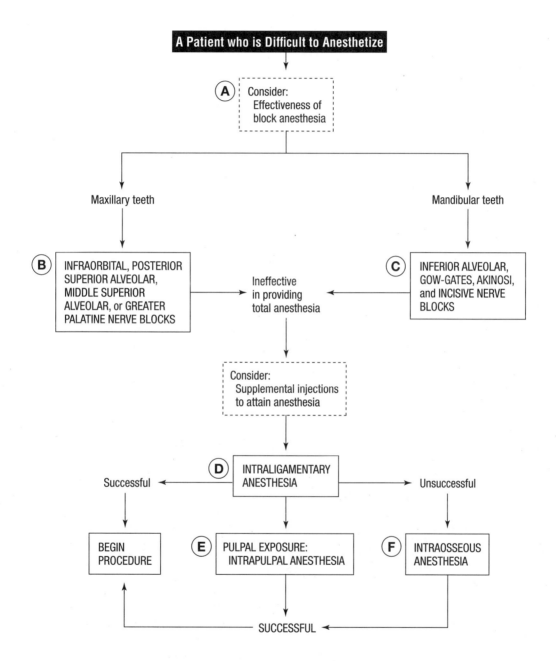

A Patient who is Difficult to Anesthetize

(A) Consider:
Effectiveness of
block anesthesia

Maxillary teeth

Mandibular teeth

(B) INFRAORBITAL, POSTERIOR
SUPERIOR ALVEOLAR,
MIDDLE SUPERIOR
ALVEOLAR, or GREATER
PALATINE NERVE BLOCKS

Ineffective
in providing
total anesthesia

(C) INFERIOR ALVEOLAR,
GOW-GATES, AKINOSI,
and INCISIVE NERVE
BLOCKS

Consider:
Supplemental injections
to attain anesthesia

(D) INTRALIGAMENTARY
ANESTHESIA

Successful

Unsuccessful

BEGIN
PROCEDURE

(E) PULPAL EXPOSURE:
INTRAPULPAL ANESTHESIA

(F) INTRAOSSEOUS
ANESTHESIA

SUCCESSFUL

56 Management of Endodontic Swellings: Local Versus Diffuse

A. Scott Cohen

Localized and diffuse endodontic swellings occur in predictable anatomic locations, according to the orientation of the root apex and the muscle attachments that surround the offending tooth.

A Determining the origin of a swelling is the most important step. A swelling may be an extension of pulpal disease or it may be of periodontal origin. It is also possible for a swelling to be nonodontogenic, unrelated to the tooth and attachment apparatus.

The basic method for diagnosing the source of the problem is to perform vitality testing on all teeth in question. A nonvital tooth is often the cause of intraoral and extraoral swellings.

After vitality testing, the periodontal attachment should be measured with a probe to check for any abnormalities. A periodontal abscess will generally manifest as a broad pocket, compared with endodontic abscesses that tend to form a narrow probing defect.

B Once it is established that a swelling is associated with a diseased pulp, the offending tooth should be accessed and a complete débridement of all canals performed. All canals must be cleansed and shaped because the swelling cannot resolve until all bacterial pathogens are removed from the root canal system. A method known as the *crown-down technique* is preferred because the coronal portion of the root canals are cleansed before apical instrumentation, which minimizes the amount of debris extrusion and reduces the occurrence of postoperative sequelae.

C Drainage frequently occurs through a tooth once it has been opened. Apical patency must be maintained during the cleansing and shaping process to ensure that drainage will continue. In most cases the drainage will stop after 20 minutes. Occasionally, drainage will continue to flow from a tooth for an extended period. During these rare occasions, the tooth should not be closed with a temporary filling material. Instead, a cotton ball should be placed in the pulp chamber, and the patient may then be dismissed. This will permit pus or exudate to escape from the tooth while preventing food impaction. The patient should be recalled the next day for irrigation, instrumentation, and closing of the tooth with a temporary filling such as Cavit or IRM. It is best to leave the tooth open for as short a time as possible because of contamination from the oral environment.

D Most teeth that are cleansed and shaped will not continue to drain for more than 20 minutes. The root canals of these teeth should be filled with a calcium hydroxide dressing followed by placement of a cotton ball in the pulp chamber and a temporary filling material, such as Cavit or IRM, to close the access. Calcium hydroxide preparations help dissolve and disinfect any remaining debris in the root canal system.

Calcium hydroxide also has therapeutic effects as a result of its ability to inactivate certain inflammatory mediators.

E Fluctuance, the sensation on palpation that there is fluid movement under the tissue, indicates that pus is present. Fluctuant swellings should be incised to allow pus to escape.

F Swellings that are localized but indurated do not need to be incised because no drainage will occur. These swellings will soon disappear once the root canal system of the offending tooth is cleansed and shaped.

G Diffuse swellings, also known as cellulitis, are the most serious because they have the greatest potential to spread to adjacent areas. Incising these swellings infrequently produces drainage. It is most important to completely cleanse and shape the root canal system of the offending tooth and to prescribe bactericidal antibiotics.

H One of the safest and most effective antibiotics to prescribe is penicillin (or amoxicillin). If the swelling to be treated is not responding well to penicillin, metronidazole can be prescribed concurrently on the same dosing schedule. For patients allergic to penicillin, clindamycin should be the next choice because it is bactericidal. Erythromycin is bacteriostatic and may prove less effective. Cephalosporins, such as Keflex, are not recommended because their spectrum is not as well suited for dental infections as penicillin or clindamycin.

I Patients should be treated for their pain and their infections. Nonsteroidal antiinflammatory drugs (NSAIDs) are excellent for mild to moderate pain. A maximum dose of 800 mg of ibuprofen can be prescribed every 6 hours. For severe pain, patients should take an additional 1000 mg of acetaminophen with a narcotic, such as two Tylenol 3 or two Vicodin, alternately with their NSAIDs. The patient should alternate these medications every 3 hours so that the dosing schedules remain unchanged.

References

American Association of Endodontists: *Management of acute pain*, Chicago, Spring/Summer 1995, Colleagues for Excellence, American Association of Endodontists.

Cohen S, Burns R: *Pathways of the pulp*, ed 7, St Louis, 1997, Mosby, p 35.

Harrington GW, Natkin E: Midtreatment flare-ups, *Dent Clin North Am* 36:409, 1992.

Laskin DM: Anatomic considerations in diagnosis and treatment of odontogenic infections, *J Am Dent Assoc* 69:38, 1964.

Safavi KE, Nichols FC: Alteration of biological properties of bacterial lipopolysaccharide by calcium hydroxide treatment, *J Endodon* 20:127, 1994.

Patient with ENDODONTIC SWELLINGS: LOCAL Versus DIFFUSE

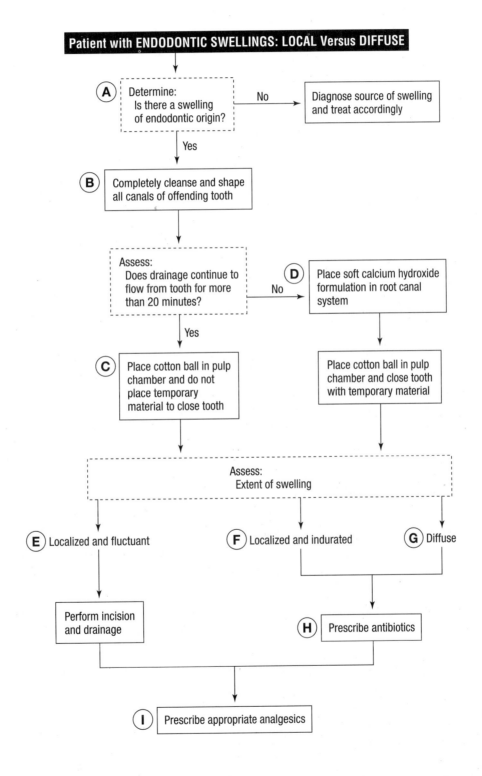

57 Management of Midtreatment Endodontic Flare-Ups

A. Scott Cohen

The American Association of Endodontists defines a flare-up as an acute exacerbation of periradicular pathosis after the initiation or continuation of root canal treatment. Flare-ups are stressful for the patient who is overcome by pain and for the dentist who must diagnose and treat the source of the problem.

A It is critical to properly diagnose the source of pain or swelling based on signs and symptoms. A tooth in midtreatment of root canal therapy is often the source of pain, but sometimes another tooth is simultaneously symptomatic. Similarly, a dentist may find that a particular tooth is involved even though the patient is convinced it is a different one because of the phenomenon of referred pain. For these reasons, the dentist needs to carefully assess which tooth is responsible.

B Thorough cleansing and shaping of all canals should ultimately eliminate all associated symptoms. A technique called the crown-down method of instrumentation allows for removal of all coronal debris before performing apical shaping. This results in less debris extrusion through the apex and fewer flare-ups in general.

C After thorough cleansing and shaping, nearly all teeth will show an absence of drainage after 20 minutes. At this time, the root canal system should be filled with a soft formulation of calcium hydroxide to disinfect and dissolve any remaining debris, as well as to reduce the inflammatory response.

D On the rare occasion when drainage persists after 20 minutes, a cotton ball may be placed in the pulp chamber with no temporary filling covering it. The patient should return the next day so that the root canal system can be irrigated, cleansed, and closed. It is best to leave the tooth open for as short a time as possible because of contamination from the oral environment.

E If the tooth has not yet been crowned then the occlusion should be reduced. If there is a coronal restoration then the dentist may decide to adjust the occlusion selectively on certain cusps.

F Soft tissue swellings associated with the tooth should be managed with incision and drainage procedures (see Chapter 56).

G Antibiotics are generally appropriate when there is a swelling. For pain without swelling, analgesics alone should make the patient comfortable. It is important for dentists to explain the likely duration and course of the acute episode so that the patient knows what to expect. It is the uninformed patient that will often call after hours because of questions and concerns.

For mild to moderate pain, nonsteroidal antiinflammatory drugs (NSAIDs) are usually sufficient. For severe pain, opioid analgesics may be taken alternately with NSAIDs, switching every 3 hours from one to the other. In this scenario, the opioid analgesic should be an acetaminophen product, such as Tylenol 3 or Vicodin, so that the patient does not exceed the daily NSAID dose.

References

Cohen S, Burns R: *Pathways of the pulp*, ed 7, St Louis, 1997, Mosby, p 35.

Goerig AC, Michelich RJ, Schulz HH: Instrumentation of root canals in molars using the step-down technique, *J Endodon* 8:550, 1982.

Harrington GW, Natkin E: Midtreatment flare-ups, *Dent Clin North Am* 36:409, 1992.

Torabinejad M, Cymerman JJ, Frankson M, Lemon RR, Maggio JD, Schilder H: Effectiveness of various medications on postoperative pain following complete instrumentation, *J Endodon* 20(7):345, 1994.

Torres JOC, Torabinejad M, Matiz RAR, Mantilla EG: Presence of secretory IgA in human periapical lesions, *J Endodon* 20:87, 1994.

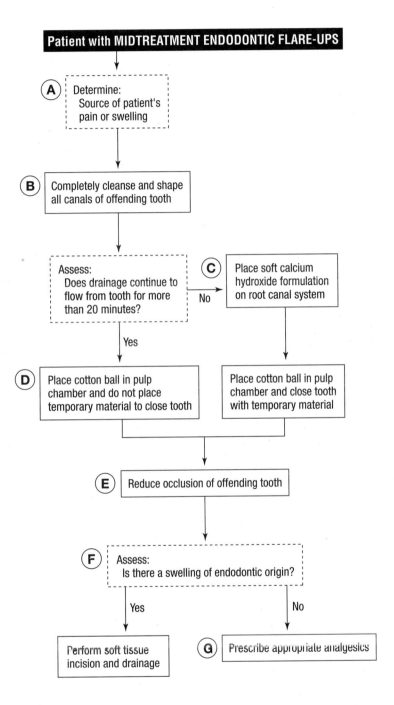

Patient with MIDTREATMENT ENDODONTIC FLARE-UPS

A Determine:
Source of patient's pain or swelling

B Completely cleanse and shape all canals of offending tooth

Assess:
Does drainage continue to flow from tooth for more than 20 minutes?

C Place soft calcium hydroxide formulation on root canal system

No

Yes

D Place cotton ball in pulp chamber and do not place temporary material to close tooth

Place cotton ball in pulp chamber and close tooth with temporary material

E Reduce occlusion of offending tooth

F Assess:
Is there a swelling of endodontic origin?

Yes

No

Perform soft tissue incision and drainage

G Prescribe appropriate analgesics

58 Surgery Versus Retreatment for Endodontic Failures

David C. Brown

A Endodontic failures associated with pathosis are occasionally symptomatic, which necessitates an additional treatment strategy. Several factors influence the decision in determining whether a case is a success or a failure. The criteria for determination of treatment failure include the following:
- Presence of pain or swelling
- Presence of a sinus tract
- Radiographic evidence of a nonhealing lesion of endodontic origin

B The selection of treatment for endodontic failures depends on the feasibility of establishing coronal access to the apical terminus of the root canal system. If the root canal system is properly cleaned, shaped, and obturated, the endodontic failure rate is extremely low and the need for surgical procedures is minimal. A first attempt should be made to retreat the root canal system. Of paramount importance is the requirement to three-dimensionally reclean, shape, and pack the entire root canal system in cases of failure. Surgery should be the choice only when these attempts have failed (Fig. 58-1). Once the practitioner is certain that no improvement in the result can be achieved by providing a nonsurgical treatment, only then should the surgical option be considered.

When the chances to negotiate the canal(s) are poor, surgery may be preferred over the option of retreatment. On occasions, disassembly of restorations such as well-fitting posts and cores and coronal restorations may endanger the integrity of the remaining tooth structure. Cost of restoration replacement may also be a consideration. Surgery is indicated if there is clinical evidence of canal blockages, ledges, apical perforations, fractured instruments that cannot be removed or bypassed, or calcifications that cannot be negotiated in retreatment.

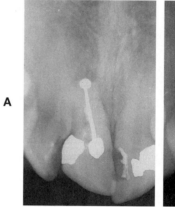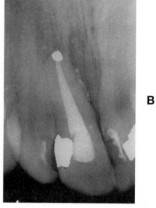

Fig. 58-1 **A,** Failure of surgical procedure after silver cone obturation. **B,** Successful conventional retreatment with gutta-percha shows importance of good three-dimensional obturation.

References

Arens DE, Adams WR, DeCastro RA: *Endodontic surgery*, Philadelphia, 1981, Harper and Row.

Carr GB, Bentkover SK: Surgical endodontics. In Cohen S, Burns R: *Pathways of the pulp*, ed 7, St Louis, 1997, Mosby.

Gutmann JL, Harrison JW: *Surgical endodontics*, Boston, 1991, Blackwell Science.

Patient who Requires a Decision of Surgery Versus Retreatment for an Endodontic Failure

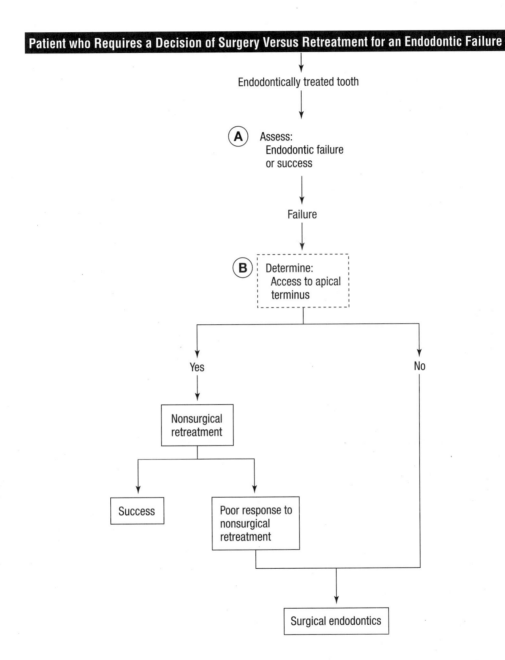

Endodontically treated tooth

A Assess:
Endodontic failure
or success

Failure

B Determine:
Access to apical
terminus

Yes

No

Nonsurgical
retreatment

Success

Poor response to
nonsurgical
retreatment

Surgical endodontics

59 Conventional Versus Surgical Endodontics for an Asymptomatic Tooth

Joseph H. Schulz

Whether pulpal pathosis is confined within the tooth structure or spreads into the periodontal tissue and alveolar bone, a tooth that is proven to be nonvital is a candidate for endodontic therapy. *Conventional endodontics* consists of thoroughly removing the pulp, shaping the root canal system, and sealing the débrided space to prevent toxic by-products of cellular degeneration from irritating the vital tissues of the alveolar housing. *Surgical endodontics* is an alternative to be used sparingly and only in those cases where conventional therapy cannot be done or has not been successful. Root-end resection and root-end filling are the basis of surgical endodontics. No existing seal is effective for a lifetime. Accessory canals can also enable products of pulpal degeneration to gain access to the alveolus. Conventional endodontics therefore has a greater chance of long-term success than does the surgical approach.

A Once the tooth has been diagnosed as nonvital, the patency of the canal from the pulp chamber to the apex must be assessed. If it is patent, conventional endodontics should be performed before restoration.

B If it is not patent to the apex because of calcifications, severe curvatures that cannot be negotiated, instrumentation accidents, obstructions, perforations, or apical root fractures, then surgical endodontics should be performed after débridement and the pulp space sealed as close to the apex as possible.

C If the tooth has been restored previously, determine whether the restoration can be removed without damaging the structural integrity of the root. If so, conventional endodontics should be used.

D If the existing restoration cannot be removed safely (e.g., postcrown), surgical endodontics is indicated.

E If an existing endodontic procedure is failing, retreatment should be considered. If there are no compromising factors (e.g., root fracture or perforation) and the canals appear accessible for instrumentation, conventional endodontics is the retreatment choice.

F If retreatment does not seem promising for improvement of the conventional results, surgical endodontics should be considered.

G If conventional retreatment or the surgical approach is failing, extraction must be considered.

References

Cohen S, Burns R: *Pathways of the pulp,* ed 7, St Louis, 1997, Mosby, p 608.

Guttman JL, Harrison JW: *Surgical endodontics,* Boston, 1991, Blackwell Science, p 3.

Seltzer S: *Endodontic retreatment. Endodontology: biologic considerations in endodontic procedures,* Philadelphia, 1988, Lea & Febiger, p 439.

Walton RE, Torabinejad M: *Principles and practice of endodontics,* ed 2, Philadelphia, 1997, WB Saunders, p 401.

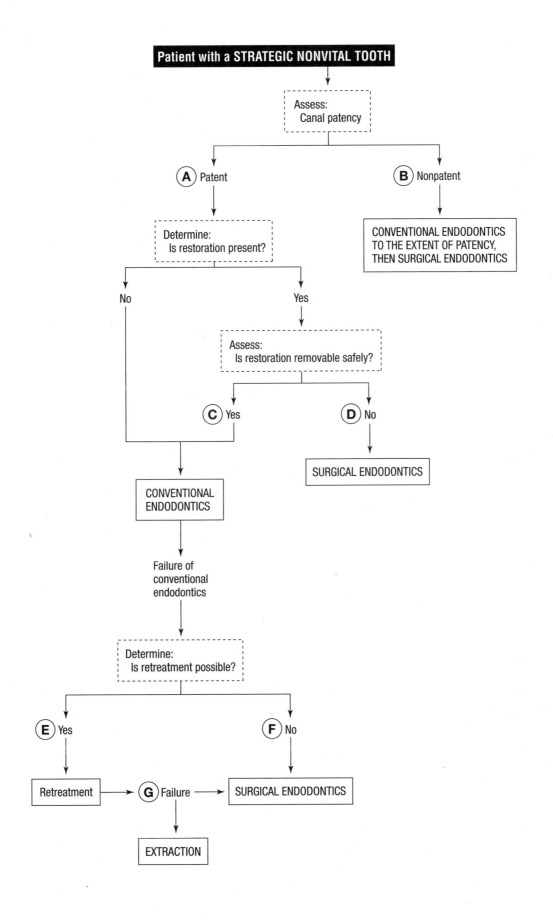

Patient with a **STRATEGIC NONVITAL TOOTH**

Assess:
Canal patency

A Patent   **B** Nonpatent

Determine:
Is restoration present?

CONVENTIONAL ENDODONTICS
TO THE EXTENT OF PATENCY,
THEN SURGICAL ENDODONTICS

No   Yes

Assess:
Is restoration removable safely?

C Yes   **D** No

SURGICAL ENDODONTICS

CONVENTIONAL
ENDODONTICS

Failure of
conventional
endodontics

Determine:
Is retreatment possible?

E Yes   **F** No

Retreatment → **G** Failure → SURGICAL ENDODONTICS

EXTRACTION

60 Root-End Resection and Root-End Filling: Apicoectomy and Retrograde Filling

Joseph H. Schulz

Whenever conventional endodontics is failing or is considered impossible, the use of surgical endodontics must be considered if retention of the tooth is critical. Necrotic pulp by-products are a site for bacterial growth and can cause inflammation in the alveolar housing when they escape from within the root. The failure of conventional therapy causes symptoms or pathoses to persist or develop over time.

Root-end resection (apicoectomy) is often used to remove the source of the inflammation (terminal branchings), to allow curettage of the diseased area, and to provide access to the site that must be sealed. If endodontic surgery compromises the crown-to-root ratio or is likely to result in a secondary endodontic-periodontal lesion, the prognosis may be adversely affected, and extraction may be the better choice.

To prevent future injury to the alveolar housing, a root-end (retrograde) filling seals the toxic by-products within the root. All accessible portals of exit should be sealed from the root canal system during surgical endodontic procedures.

A After the conventional endodontic approaches have been exhausted and there is persistence of periapical symptoms or the development of a lesion, surgical endodontics must be considered to retain a strategic tooth.

B If an existing periodontal condition has resulted in crestal bone loss, the dentist must evaluate whether sufficient bone would remain after surgical endodontics. An endodontic-periodontal lesion could dramatically worsen the prognosis.

C If surgical endodontics is required to seal a root surface near the gingival attachment, making the development of an unmanageable secondary endodontic-periodontal lesion likely, extraction should be considered.

D If the crown-to-root ratio would be compromised by surgical endodontics (e.g., to eliminate a severe curvature or to seal an apical perforation), the dentist might consider extraction.

E If the crown-to-root ratio is severely compromised by surgical endodontics and the tooth will be subjected to heavy occlusal forces, extraction should be considered.

F A root-end filling is recommended following all root-end resection procedures. If this cannot be done and conventional endodontics is inadequate, extraction should be recommended.

References

Dykema RW et al: *Johnston's modern practice in fixed prosthodontics,* ed 4, Philadelphia, 1986, WB Saunders, p 1.

Gartner AH, Dorn SO: Advances in endodontic surgery, *Dent Clin North Am* 36(2):357, 1992.

Guttman JL, Harrison JW: *Surgical endodontics,* Boston, 1991, Blackwell Science, pp 203, 338.

Pitts DL, Natkin E: Diagnosis and treatment of vertical root fractures, *J Endodon* 9(8):338, 1983.

Rapp EI et al: An analysis of success and failure in apicoectomies, *J Endodon* 17(10):508, 1991.

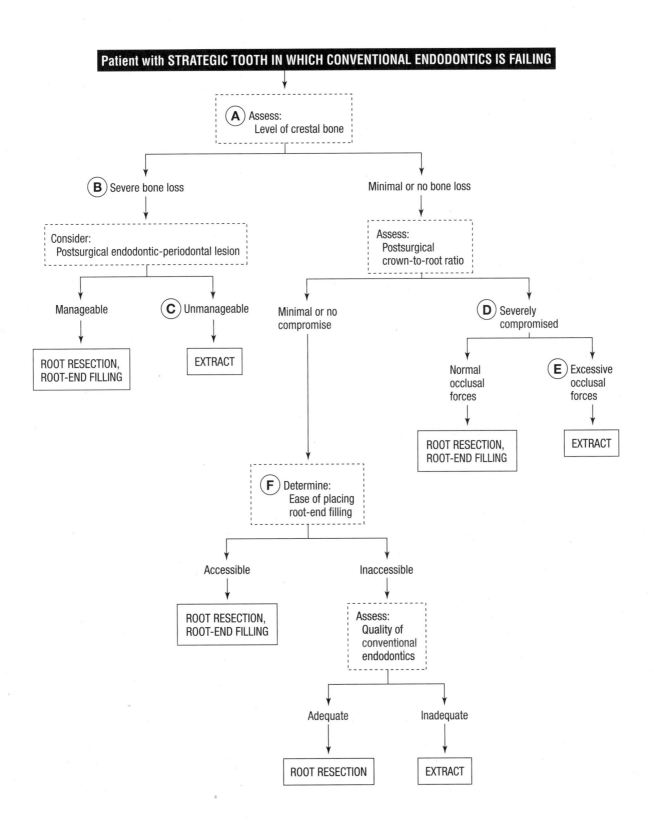

Patient with STRATEGIC TOOTH IN WHICH CONVENTIONAL ENDODONTICS IS FAILING

(A) Assess:
Level of crestal bone

(B) Severe bone loss

Minimal or no bone loss

Consider:
Postsurgical endodontic-periodontal lesion

Assess:
Postsurgical
crown-to-root ratio

Manageable

(C) Unmanageable

Minimal or no
compromise

(D) Severely
compromised

ROOT RESECTION,
ROOT-END FILLING

EXTRACT

Normal
occlusal
forces

(E) Excessive
occlusal
forces

ROOT RESECTION,
ROOT-END FILLING

EXTRACT

(F) Determine:
Ease of placing
root-end filling

Accessible

Inaccessible

ROOT RESECTION,
ROOT-END FILLING

Assess:
Quality of
conventional
endodontics

Adequate

Inadequate

ROOT RESECTION

EXTRACT

61 Coronal Mishaps on Endodontic Access: Recognition and Management

†William W.Y. Goon

Iatrogenic defects of the clinical crown can occur when attempting an endodontic access into the tooth. The failure to preplan the best approach to execute and the unwillingness to stop and reassess the alignment of the entry are common factors leading to damage to the crown. Also, full coronal coverage and calcific degenerative closure of the pulp space can handicap even the best attempts at direct access into the chamber of these teeth.

The procedural accident is preventable or can be minimized in the majority of cases. Preplanning is the key to avoiding this mishap. The tooth must be thoroughly assessed as to its general anatomy, cervical dimensions, arch, and occlusal alignments. The findings are supplemented with a radiographic assessment of the size, shape, and height of the pulp chamber within the crown. Mental imaging of the radiographic long axis of the submerged root against the clinical crown can give a better sense of root alignment for advantageous positioning of the operative bur.

Three supragingival defects are commonly produced by a misaligned bur. Although the prognosis for tooth retention is favorable, the severity of the defect requires careful consideration in the restoration of the crown.

A The crown that is gouged has been violated internally. If the root canal system can be located and treated, the crown should be restored with appropriate materials that can withstand the masticatory load for the tooth. An amalgam filling is less likely to flex and can allow the tooth to function without further impairment. The tooth should be monitored for stress fractures of the remaining tooth structure.

B The crown that is gouged extensively is mutilated internally. Treatment considerations involve the need for full coronal coverage and rehabilitation with a post once the endodontic procedure is completed. The tooth should be monitored for horizontal stress fracture of the crown and post.

C The crown that is perforated, regardless of size, should be temporarily patched to control salivary contamination of the root canal system. The extent of the internal defect (small gouges versus mutilation) governs how the crown is to be restored. The proximity of the defect to the interproximal soft tissue or the gingival sulcus may render the area inaccessible to effective oral hygiene and thus susceptible to caries. Before definitive restorative procedures, consideration of crowning lengthening procedures or orthodontic extrusion may facilitate the exposure of the defect for improved oral hygiene or enhance the longevity of the full coronal coverage (see Chapters 11 and 83).

References

Bakland LK: Endodontic mishaps: perforations, *Calif Dent Assoc J* 19(4):41, 1991.

Frank AL: Resorption, perforations, and fractures, *Dent Clin North Am* 18(2):465, 1974.

Torabinejad M: Endodontic mishaps: etiology, prevention, and management, *Alpha Omegan* 83:42, 1990.

†Deceased.

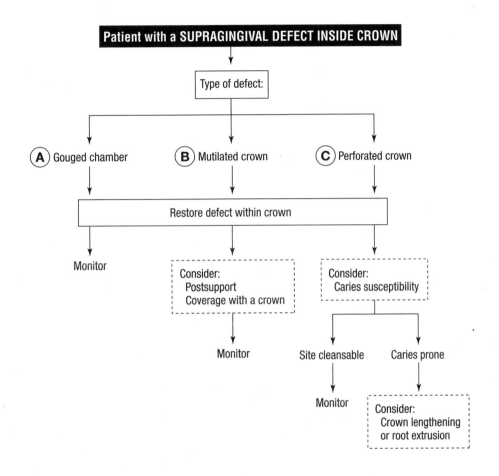

Patient with a SUPRAGINGIVAL DEFECT INSIDE CROWN

Type of defect:

A Gouged chamber **B** Mutilated crown **C** Perforated crown

Restore defect within crown

Monitor

Consider:
Postsupport
Coverage with a crown

Monitor

Consider:
Caries susceptibility

Site cleansable Caries prone

Monitor

Consider:
Crown lengthening
or root extrusion

62 Furcal Perforation Upon Endodontic Manipulation: Recognition, Management, and Prognosis for Tooth Retention

†William W.Y. Goon

A perforation into the furcation, also referred to as *cervical canal perforation*, is a significant injury to the periodontal apparatus. A misdirected bur, excessive or misguided postspace preparation, inappropriate widening of the canal orifice or flaring of the coronal canal space, and fruitless searches in a receded pulp chamber for heavily calcified root canal spaces are factors leading to perforations into the furcation. The size and location of the defect are unpredictable and vary according to the particular endodontic procedure attempted. Accessibility to and sealability of the defect can be troublesome. Inadequate management of the defect is an adverse event and is identified as the second greatest cause of endodontic failure.

A Upon detection, cursory triage must be initiated to evaluate the impact that the mishap may have on the original treatment plan and the strategic value of the tooth with and without corrective intervention. An extensive defect in a tooth with little strategic value should lead to consideration for extraction. Intact adjacent neighboring teeth should be used instead. A strategic tooth that is important to the overall success of the treatment plan must be evaluated for its long-term prognosis following corrective intervention and the successful completion of the intended endodontic treatment. The prognosis for tooth retention favors the multirooted tooth with a long root trunk. In the tooth with a short root trunk, root amputation or hemisection may be a more expeditious and predictable recourse.

B In considering corrective intervention, the configuration of the perforation determines the accessibility to and the ease and effectiveness of sealing the defect. A small defect or a narrow defect is more amenable to sealing by condensing Cavit, IRM, amalgam, or gutta-percha with sealer cement into the site. A large or broad defect exposes a wide surface wound with little or no retentive features. The placement of sealing materials over the defect must be balanced with sufficient condensing pressures to prevent gross extrusion of material into the furcation and to produce a tight seal of the defect.

C The tooth that is perforated should be immediately sealed up soon after discovery of the mishap. The objective is to prevent further irritation and deterioration of the exposed and still intact periodontal attachment tissues. Control hemorrhaging by lining the defect with calcium hydroxide, Cavit, tricalcium phosphate, or an absorbable collagen matrix as a necessary first step to regain direct visualization of the area to make a definitive assessment. The defect should be sealed with amalgam glass ionomer resin, Cavit, or gutta-percha and sealer at this time. Ultimately, an effective seal of the defect, rather than the material used, is decisive for a successful repair.

D The prognosis is favorable for the tooth with a newly discovered defect that is sealed immediately; however, early intervention may not preclude subsequent migration of gingival sulcular epithelium and periodontal pocket formation adjacent to the level of the sealed perforation within 24 months following corrective procedures. This complication is frequently associated with a short root trunk. Surgical curettage and perhaps retrograde sealing of the defect or root amputation are the remaining treatment options for salvaging the tooth.

E The prognosis is less favorable for the perforation that is discovered late and has significant breakdown of osseous supporting tissues. Although circumstances are less desirable, osseous breakdown does not necessarily preclude the salvageability of the tooth, especially one with a long root trunk. The defect should be sealed by filling the osseous cavity with tricalcium phosphate, an absorbable gelatin sponge, collagen, or hydroxyapatite to the level of the dental tissue to serve as a matrix for sealing. The tooth is closely monitored for osseous regeneration and reformation of the attachment apparatus. Gross extrusion of filling material into or nonresolution or further deterioration of the osseous tissues warrants consideration of the following treatment options: (1) osseous barrier induction with calcium hydroxide; (2) intentional replantation with direct sealing of the defect; (3) surgical curettage, retrograde seal, and perhaps a hydroxyapatite graft into the osseous defect; (4) root amputation; and (5) tooth extraction.

References

Bakland LK: Endodontic mishaps: perforations, *Calif Dent Assoc J* 19(4):41, 1991.

Balla R, LoMonaco CJ, Skribner J, Lin LM: Histologic study of furcation perforations treated with tricalcium phosphate, hydroxylapatite, amalgam, and life, *J Endodon* 17(5):234, 1991.

Benenati FW, Roane JB, Biggs JT, Simon JH: Recall evaluation of iatrogenic root perforations repaired with amalgam and gutta-percha, *J Endodon* 12(4):161, 1986.

Harbert H: Generic tricalcium phosphate plugs: an adjunct in endodontics, *J Endodon* 17(3):131, 1991.

Ibarrola JL, Bjorenson JE, Austin BP, Gerstein H: Osseous reactions to three hemostatic agents, *J Endodon* 11(2):75, 1985.

Roane JB, Benenati FW: Successful management of a perforated molar using amalgam and hydroxylapatite, *J Endodon* 13(8):400, 1987.

†Deceased.

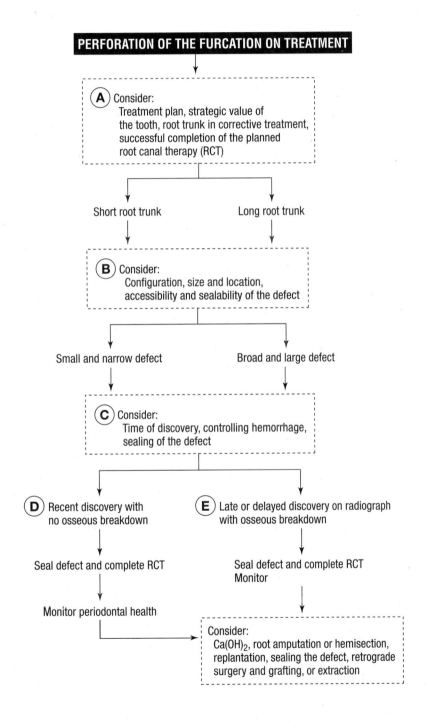

PERFORATION OF THE FURCATION ON TREATMENT

A Consider:
Treatment plan, strategic value of the tooth, root trunk in corrective treatment, successful completion of the planned root canal therapy (RCT)

Short root trunk

Long root trunk

B Consider:
Configuration, size and location, accessibility and sealability of the defect

Small and narrow defect

Broad and large defect

C Consider:
Time of discovery, controlling hemorrhage, sealing of the defect

D Recent discovery with no osseous breakdown

E Late or delayed discovery on radiograph with osseous breakdown

Seal defect and complete RCT

Seal defect and complete RCT
Monitor

Monitor periodontal health

Consider:
Ca(OH)$_2$, root amputation or hemisection, replantation, sealing the defect, retrograde surgery and grafting, or extraction

63 Managing the Perforated Root on Single-Rooted Teeth

An iatrogenic perforation of the single-rooted tooth can occur at any level of the root during endodontic and operative manipulations into or within the root canal space. Unexpected hemorrhaging and pain are the pathognomonic signs and symptoms heralding a perforation in the previously dry root canal of an asymptomatic tooth. The discussion that follows assumes that (1) completion of the planned endodontics is not problematic and (2) the periodontal supporting tissues are in optimum health.

A Perforations of the root are generally categorized according to the level of the root that is involved. Access preparation into the tooth and canal-widening procedures can result in perforations at the coronal level. Postspace preparation and conceptual deficiencies in managing the curved canal can lead to perforations at midroot level. The unskilled use of endodontic instruments can result in perforation of the apical foramen, or, laterally, through the side at the apex of the root.

B The coronal perforation can be identified through direct visualization into the tooth or confirmed by a misaligned endodontic instrument seen on the radiograph. The coronal defect is labeled as either at the supracrestal, crestal, or subcrestal bone level. Orthograde accessibility to the defect is usually not problematic; however, the sealing of the defect can be difficult. Periodontal complications are inevitably seen with an ineffective seal of the defect or with gross extrusion of sealing materials into the periodontal supporting tissues.

C An orthograde repair of the defect should be attempted for an area that is above or below the crestal bone level. With a large defect the root canal space is first blocked with a solid object such as a silver cone to ensure patency; this is followed by the circumferential insertion of repair materials such as amalgam glass ionomer resin, Cavit, IRM, or condensation of gutta-percha with sealer cement. Esthetic considerations and the need to surgically remove any extruded material determine the appropriate material to use.

D Surgical crown lengthening can expeditiously expose the defect for external sealing or inclusion under full coronal crown coverage. A solid object blocking the root canal space can serve as a matrix against which the reparative materials can be condensed and ensures reaccess into the root canal space. The procedure is indicated primarily for defects directly involving the crestal bone. Without crown lengthening, osseous breakdown often results from the irritating effects of the sealing materials and proximity of the defect to sulcular epithelium.

Although crown lengthening is a definitive treatment for the involved root, coronal coverage on a narrower root trunk may result in a marginally esthetic or disproportionately longer clinical crown. Also, the loss of osseous tissue support can adversely affect the periodontal health of the adjacent teeth. Consideration of these outcomes is necessary before a procedure is selected. However, for the perforated abutment tooth under a bridge the only acceptable treatment option is to surgically expose and seal the defect, leaving a residual periodontal pocket upon healing. The prognosis for tooth retention is favorable.

E Root extrusion is an option for exposing a defect that is inaccessible to a predictable orthograde repair or where crown lengthening is likely to compromise the periodontal support of the adjacent healthy root (teeth). The outcome of root extrusion must be viewed from the perspective of the involved root. Although root extrusion conserves the crestal bone level and maintains the periodontal support of adjacent teeth, the involved root loses root length, and the result is a restoration with compromised esthetics because of a narrower root trunk. The prognosis for tooth retention is favorable.

F Midroot perforations typically occur during preparation of space for a post or intracanal widening procedures. Unexpected pain and hemorrhage and radiographic evidence of an overly wide post within a narrow root or a post that courses through the root eccentrically are pathognomonic of a perforation. Persistent postcementation sensitivity can also herald a perforation by the post that had exited through an invaginated area of the root. The defect is not readily apparent on the radiograph, which may demonstrate a properly aligned post.

G A perforation on a postspace preparation can be caused by overwidening of the canal space or the creation of an artificial channel that is skewed off the long axis of the root canal. In either event the defect is usually accessible for orthograde repair. A matrix constructed from calcium hydroxide, tricalcium phosphate, or an absorbable gelatin sponge (Gelfoam) or collagen may be required to control hemorrhage and provide a surface for condensation of amalgam resin or gutta-percha with sealer cement. A direct surgical repair may be used in labial-buccal perforations where the osseous matrix is too thin or is completely destroyed. The potential for vestibular soft tissue discoloration may warrant the sealing of the defect with a nonstaining material like Super EBA, IRM, or resin, especially in the anterior regions of the mouth. Treatment options for the postrestored perforated root is limited by the surgical approach and accessibility.

H Aggressive or uncontrolled endodontic preparation can result in a large perforation through the lateral aspect of the root. In the single-rooted tooth, a lateral perforation is identical to a "stripped perforation" seen in the multirooted tooth. Accessibility to the midroot level is difficult, and con-

†Deceased.

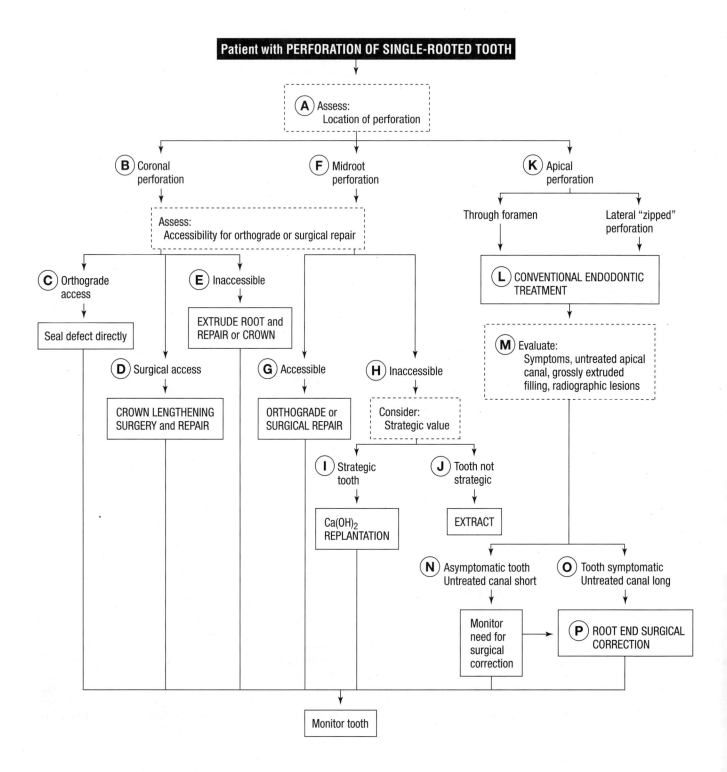

Patient with PERFORATION OF SINGLE-ROOTED TOOTH

A Assess: Location of perforation

B Coronal perforation

F Midroot perforation

K Apical perforation

Assess: Accessibility for orthograde or surgical repair

Through foramen

Lateral "zipped" perforation

C Orthograde access

E Inaccessible

L CONVENTIONAL ENDODONTIC TREATMENT

Seal defect directly

EXTRUDE ROOT and REPAIR or CROWN

M Evaluate: Symptoms, untreated apical canal, grossly extruded filling, radiographic lesions

D Surgical access

G Accessible

H Inaccessible

CROWN LENGTHENING SURGERY and REPAIR

ORTHOGRADE or SURGICAL REPAIR

Consider: Strategic value

I Strategic tooth

J Tooth not strategic

Ca(OH)$_2$ REPLANTATION

EXTRACT

N Asymptomatic tooth Untreated canal short

O Tooth symptomatic Untreated canal long

Monitor need for surgical correction

P ROOT END SURGICAL CORRECTION

Monitor tooth

trol of hemorrhaging can be problematic. The practical management of this mishap rests primarily on the strategic value of the tooth and whether the hemorrhaging can be controlled to permit the uncontaminated sealing of the entire root canal space.

I For the strategic tooth, treatment options may involve a prolonged and persistent attempt at using calcium hydroxide to control hemorrhaging or to induce the formation of an osseous barrier for condensation of sealing materials. Even with an osseous barrier the weakened condition of the root may predispose it to further treatment complications of root fracture on sealing procedures. Intentional replantation following the extraoral sealing of the defect may offer a more expeditious result but with attendant root complications of fracture or resorption. The prognosis for tooth retention is guarded.

J A tooth is deemed nonsalvageable if the defect is extensive, lacks a barrier matrix, cannot be adequately sealed by orthograde or surgical methods, has a weakened root, or cannot be managed without compromising the periodontal support around it and the adjacent teeth. The tooth should be extracted under these circumstances.

K An apical perforation sometimes is discovered on the radiograph(s) at the completion of root canal preparation. Perforation through the foramen is the most common mishap seen in the canal that is relatively straight. The perforation can also occur laterally alongside of the foramen. This mishap is called a *zipped perforation*, a transported foramen, or an apical tear or rip on the surface of the root. Both mishaps result from inexperience and inability to (1) maintain the working length between successive enlarging instruments and (2) control the penetration of each instrument within the confines of the canal terminus. Additionally, the frequency and severity of the zipped perforation are functions of the degree of root curvature and canal curvature. The defect, formed with overextended instruments, is seen in the curved canal as a result of (1) failure to properly bend and rebend the instruments throughout preparation, (2) forceful insertion of rigid instruments into an underprepared canal, and (3) deliberate rotation of fragile or weakened instruments within the canal space.

L Management of the apical perforation requires renegotiation of the canal, reestablishment of the correct length, and repair and sealing of the original canal space. For the curved canal that cannot be reentered, the instrument is withdrawn and preparation and sealing are confined to within the radiographic housing of the root. Extrusion of sealing material can be controlled by first constructing a barrier matrix by packing calcium hydroxide, tricalcium phosphate, or hydroxyapatite against the periapical tissues.

M The prognosis in apical perforations is adversely affected by (1) the inability to seal the defect and apex from leakage; (2) extrusion of sealing materials into the periapical tissues; and (3) in the curved root or canal, the length of the untreated original apical canal space.

N The tooth that remains asymptomatic and has no radiographic evidence of periapical breakdown should be monitored. This includes all teeth regardless of the result of the sealing procedure (filled adequately, overextended, or underextended).

O The tooth that is causing the patient severe discomfort or pain, is grossly overfilled, or radiographically demonstrates a periapical lesion should be considered for definitive surgical correction.

P The prognosis for tooth retention following surgical correction of the perforated apex is favorable. Postsurgical root-to-crown ratio should be 1:1 or greater. For a strategic tooth with poor periodontal osseous support, intentional replantation and extraoral sealing of the defect may conserve root length and salvage the tooth; however, postreplantation complications can result in a guarded to poor prognosis for the tooth.

References

Bakland LK: Endodontic mishaps: perforations, *Calif Dent Assoc J* 19:41, 1991.

Ingle JI, Abou-Rass M: Perforations and their management. In Ingle JI, Taintor JF, editors: *Endodontics,* ed 3, Philadelphia, 1985, Lea & Febiger, p 776.

Oswald RJ: Procedural accidents and their repair, *Dent Clin North Am* 23:593, 1979.

Torabinejad M: Endodontic mishaps: etiology, prevention, and management, *Alpha Omegan* 83.42, 1990.

Webber RT: Iatrogenic root perforations. In Gerstein H, editor: *Techniques in clinical endodontics,* Philadelphia, 1983, WB Saunders, p 185.

64 Pulpal Space Obliteration Following Trauma

Joseph H. Schulz

Dentin is produced by odontoblasts, derived from mesenchymal cells of the embryonic dental papilla. Odontoblasts form a lining of cells at the inner boundary of dentin and produce the hard dentin structure by secreting fibers and protein enzymes. This primary function diminishes when the tooth has reached its final development, approximately 1 to 4 years after erupting into the oral cavity. Any further addition of dentin (secondary dentin) results in a decreased pulp volume. This process may continue or eventually cease altogether. Pulpal cells, however, retain their dentin producing potential and may be provoked later into activity by injury and trauma.

A Continued deposition of dentin will occur in individuals throughout life, although imperceptibly slow. The result over decades can be a pulp space of greatly diminished volume. Such pulps may also appear histologically as "prematurely aged," characterized by a relative decrease in cellular content and an increase in collagen content. This effect will often be apparent in most teeth upon radiographic examination. In the absence of any signs and symptoms of pathosis, this should be considered a normal aging process. Pulpal assessment should reveal the teeth to be vital.

B Attrition, abrasion, and periodontal disease can cause pulpal cells to produce reparative dentin. If these are chronic irritations, the original odontoblastic cells respond to these inflammatory injuries by producing a form of dentin internally that resembles the original "tubular form" of dentin.

Moderate caries and restorative procedures may also result in the formation of reparative dentin. This dentin is the product of odontoblastlike replacement cells, and its structure may be quite amorphous, both in appearance and degree of mineralization. The pulp chamber will be decreased in size on the walls facing the injury. If no other signs or symptoms are reported, treatment is not indicated.

C More pronounced events such as deep caries, pulpal exposure, and fractures may cause inflammation leading to diffuse mineralization of the pulp beneath the injury and eventual necrosis. Such cases should be monitored and evaluated. Degenerative changes are an indication for immediate endodontic intervention.

D Mineralizations may also develop within the stroma of the pulp as discrete stones in the chamber or as diffuse islands in the canal(s). These are often associated with a nidus of injury or degeneration. Stones can be smooth or irregular, singular or multiple, and floating or attached to the dentin. If they are associated with symptoms of pulpitis, endodontic intervention is required.

E Traumatic injuries to anterior teeth can also lead to a pronounced mineralization of the entire pulp space. The crown may become noticeably darker with a yellow-brownish hue as the chamber closes or blood pigments are incorporated in the dentin. This mineralization is caused by cells from within the pulp as opposed to odontoblasts or their replacements. The pulp may eventually degenerate causing symptoms of pulpitis or evidence of periapical extension of disease. Some controversy exists whether to treat this condition of calcific metamorphosis prophylactically with endodontic therapy or wait until definite signs of necrosis are revealed. Research has shown that pulpal necrosis will occur after pulpal space obliteration in only 10% of traumatized teeth. Therefore endodontic intervention after evidence of pulpal calcific changes is not warranted in the absence of signs and symptoms of disease.

References

Jacobsen J, Kerekes K: Long term prognosis of traumatized permanent anterior teeth showing calcifying processes in the pulp cavity, *Scand J Dent Res* 85:588, 1977.

Seltzer S: *Endodontology*, ed 2, Philadelphia, 1988, Lea & Febiger, p 503.

Trowbridge HO, Kim S: Pulp development, structure and function. In Cohen S, Burns R, editors: *Pathways of the pulp*, ed 6, St Louis, 1994, Mosby.

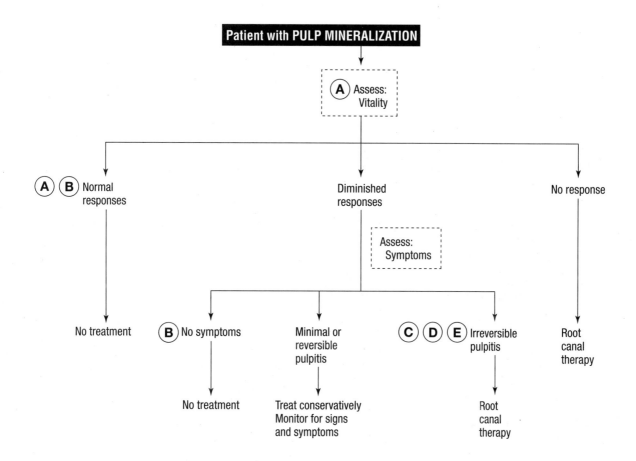

65 Management of Horizontal Root Fractures

Alan H. Gluskin

The primary goal in the practice of dentistry is preservation of the dental tissues. A serious challenge in achieving this goal is a traumatic injury to the teeth and supporting structures that causes a root to fracture in the alveolus. No two traumatic fractures are alike. Thus treatment planning requires a knowledge of the biologic principles of healing and an understanding of sequelae arising after traumatic injury.

Horizontal root fractures in the developed permanent dentition are reported to comprise just more than 5% of all traumatic injuries to teeth. Horizontal fracture after trauma is most likely in an adult where the root is solidly supported in bone and periodontal membrane. Avulsion or luxation is more probable in a younger patient with less attachment support. Horizontal root fractures occur most often in the maxillary central incisors, and while their incidence is not frequent, the treatment can be complex because of combined damage to pulp, dentin, cementum, bone, and periodontium.

A The clinical presentation of a horizontal root fracture may vary from a clinically normal presentation to an extruded or mobile crown depending upon the location of the fracture and the severity of the injury. An apical location usually results in little mobility. Coronal fractures exhibit significantly more movement. Clinical research has shown that if there is no communication or potential communication between the oral cavity and the fracture, the prognosis is not influenced by the location of the horizontal root fracture. Thus coronal, middle, and apical third fractures without oral contamination are treated in the same manner.

B The radiographic examination is important for identification and demonstration of the fracture. Radiographic identification is not always obvious immediately after the trauma. Root separation is seen when hemorrhage or proliferation of granulation tissue occurs between the segments. Multiple periapical radiographs are necessary to visualize coronal fractures. In addition, occlusal views aid in determination of apical fractures. Visualization of the root fracture will avoid a misdiagnosis.

Treatment at the time of injury depends on the following factors:
- Position of the tooth after it has been fractured
- Mobility of the coronal segment
- Status of the pulp
- Location of the fracture

C If the position of the tooth shows displacement or slight extension, it must be repositioned as soon as possible after the injury. This often involves pain management with local anesthetic to properly reduce the fracture and align the segments. The occlusion should be relieved, and stabilization is indicated when mobility is present. Splinting should be passively applied using an acid-etch technique for resin bonding. The fractured tooth and root should be stabilized for approximately 8 to 10 weeks.

D The mobility of the coronal segment is directly related to position of the fracture line. Repair across the fracture line is optimized by reduction and immobilization. On occasion, semipermanent splinting is indicated with more sturdy materials. Rigid orthodontic band splinting is contraindicated. Optimal oral hygiene care is essential. This is especially true in fractures close to the alveolar crest.

E Horizontally fractured teeth must be assessed for pulpal vitality in the same manner as any traumatically injured tooth. While the actual state of vitality cannot be obtained for many months, the patient's signs and symptoms are key indicators of pulp status. Pain, a sinus tract, or loss of attachment to the fracture line are all indicative of pulp necrosis. Mineralizations and obliteration of the pulp canal result in necrosis approximately 40% of the time. In a high percentage of instances of horizontal fracture, the apical segment remains vital. Thus treatment of the apical segment is rarely required, and endodontic therapy is confined to the coronal segment only.

F The position of the fracture line is an important consideration. Fractures in the apical one third of the root rarely require treatment or stabilization, and the doctor should watch and observe the clinical and radiographic outcomes.

Coronal fractures above the level of the alveolar bone require removal of the crown. Gingival recontouring or orthodontic extrusion should follow endodontic therapy. Restoration with a crown will protect the remaining tooth structure.

Middle third root fractures are the most problematic. Splinting is almost always mandatory. Fractures within 4 to 5 mm of the gingival crevice are at risk for apical migration of the sulcus and oral contamination or by unfavorable occlusal forces on the coronal segment.

If the coronal segment is lost, assuming the apical segment can be restored, the final restoration must consider periodontal cosmetics and an adequate crown-to-root ratio.

References

Andreasen FM: Pulpal healing after luxation injuries and root fracture in permanent dentition, *Endodon Dent Traum* 5:111, 1989.

Andreasen FM, Andreasen JO: Resorption and mineralization process following root fractures of permanent incisors, *Endodon Dent Traum* 4:202, 1988.

Andreasen FM, Andreasen JO, Bayer T: Prognosis of root-fractured permanent incisors: prediction of healing modalities, *Endodon Dent Traum* 5:11, 1989.

Andreasen JO: *Traumatic injuries of the teeth*, ed 2, Philadelphia, 1981, WB Saunders.

Hovland EJ: Horizontal root fractures—treatment and repair, *Dent Clin North Am* 36:509, 1992.

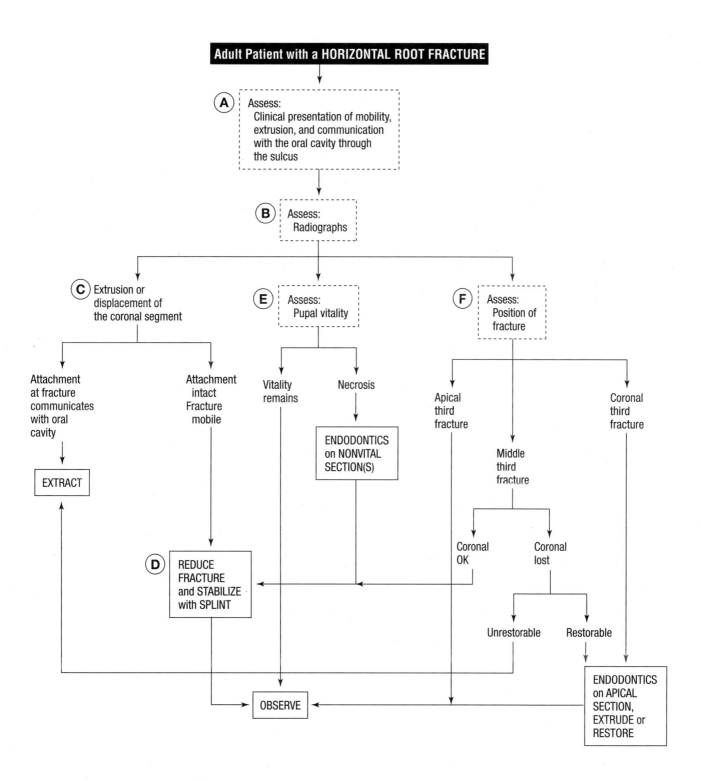

Adult Patient with a HORIZONTAL ROOT FRACTURE

A Assess:
Clinical presentation of mobility, extrusion, and communication with the oral cavity through the sulcus

B Assess:
Radiographs

C Extrusion or displacement of the coronal segment

Attachment at fracture communicates with oral cavity

EXTRACT

Attachment intact Fracture mobile

E Assess:
Pupal vitality

Vitality remains

Necrosis

ENDODONTICS on NONVITAL SECTION(S)

F Assess:
Position of fracture

Apical third fracture

Middle third fracture

Coronal third fracture

Coronal OK

Coronal lost

Unrestorable

Restorable

D REDUCE FRACTURE and STABILIZE with SPLINT

OBSERVE

ENDODONTICS on APICAL SECTION, EXTRUDE or RESTORE

66 Management of Dental Displacements

David C. Brown

A Displacement refers to an injury in which the tooth is moved from its position in the socket. The displacement may be lateral (buccal, lingual, mesial, distal), extrusive (out of socket), or intrusive (deeper into the bone).

Concussion is an injury to a tooth and its attachment apparatus without displacement from its position in the alveolus.

B Teeth should be repositioned as soon as possible following trauma that causes displacement. Teeth repositioned within 90 minutes from the time of injury exhibit less root resorption. Teeth that have been displaced long enough for the blood to be clotted around them should not be repositioned forcefully because of the possible initiation of root resorption. It is preferable to move the tooth orthodontically if repair has begun.

C Splinting should be nonrigid for 7 to 10 days. A flexible wire composite splint or a 20- to 30-pound monofilament nylon wire incorporated into bonded resin are advocated.

D Pulpal obliteration with mineralized tissue occurs approximately 20% of the time. It is a normal response to a moderate injury such as minimal displacement. Pulpal necrosis subsequent to pulpal obliteration occurs in approximately 10% of traumatized teeth. Therefore prophylactic pulp extirpation performed after evidence of pulpal mineralization is not justified.

E The pulp may not respond to vitality testing initially, but positive responses can return weeks or months later. Pulp tests for vitality should be repeated and compared with the initial appointment baseline at 1, 3, 6, and 12 months. If the pulp initially shows a vital response and subsequently responds nonvitally, this is a strong indicator of pulpal necrosis.

F Root resorption is usually seen after intrusive injuries. The next highest incidence follows extrusive injuries. Intrusions are also the injuries that have the highest incidence of pulpal necrosis. The presence of a necrotic pulp contributes to root resorption. Additionally an extended period of splinting is thought to contribute to root resorption.

G Pulpal necrosis occurs in 96% of intruded teeth. To prevent the onset of inflammatory resorption, the fully formed intruded tooth must have the pulp removed within 2 weeks of the time of injury. Subsequently calcium hydroxide therapy should be initiated soon after pulp removal. Any evidence of inflammatory root resorption would be justification for using calcium hydroxide therapy to assist in arresting the root resorption.

H The primary determining factor for endodontic treatment is the diagnosis of pulpal necrosis. This is based on previous sensitivity, marked discoloration, lack of pulpal responses to thermal and electric tests, and radiographic appearance. Traumatized teeth are unreliable in responding to pulp tests. A periapical radiolucency occurring without evidence of inflammatory resorption in a completely developed tooth would warrant endodontic treatment with gutta percha obturation. All intruded teeth and those showing root resorption should be therapeutically treated. Calcium hydroxide is used to fill the canal until the resorption has been arrested. The tooth can then be obturated with gutta-percha.

References

Andreasen JO: Luxation of permanent teeth due to trauma, a clinical and radiographic follow-up study of 184 injured teeth, *Scand J Dent Res* 78:273, 1970.

Andreasen JO: *Traumatic injuries of the teeth*, ed 2, Philadelphia, 1981, WB Saunders.

Andreasen JO, Andreasen FM: *Textbook and color atlas of traumatic injuries to the teeth*, Copenhagen, 1993, Munksgaard.

Oikarinen K, Gundlach FFH, Pfeifer G: Late complications of luxation injuries to teeth, *Endodon Dent Traumatol* 3:296, 1987.

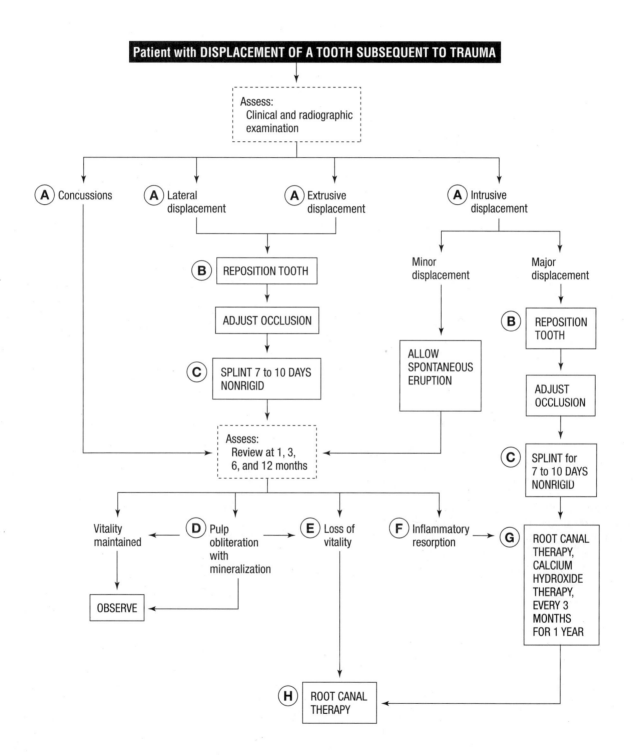

Patient with DISPLACEMENT OF A TOOTH SUBSEQUENT TO TRAUMA

Assess:
Clinical and radiographic examination

(A) Concussions

(A) Lateral displacement

(A) Extrusive displacement

(A) Intrusive displacement

(B) REPOSITION TOOTH

ADJUST OCCLUSION

(C) SPLINT 7 to 10 DAYS NONRIGID

Minor displacement

Major displacement

ALLOW SPONTANEOUS ERUPTION

(B) REPOSITION TOOTH

ADJUST OCCLUSION

Assess:
Review at 1, 3, 6, and 12 months

(C) SPLINT for 7 to 10 DAYS NONRIGID

Vitality maintained

(D) Pulp obliteration with mineralization

(E) Loss of vitality

(F) Inflammatory resorption

(G) ROOT CANAL THERAPY, CALCIUM HYDROXIDE THERAPY, EVERY 3 MONTHS FOR 1 YEAR

OBSERVE

(H) ROOT CANAL THERAPY

67 Management of Tooth Avulsion

David C. Brown

Complete avulsion occurs when a traumatic injury totally displaces a tooth from the socket. The emergency treatment for tooth avulsion is immediate replantation and splinting.

A Factors affecting the success of replantation are the following:
- *Extraoral time:* The shorter the extraoral time, the more certain is the prognosis of the replanted tooth. Extraoral time of less than 30 minutes gives a much-improved prognosis. If possible, the patient should be instructed to replace the tooth directly into the socket, or this can be done by a parent if the patient is a child. If the tooth is covered with debris, it can be flushed in milk or running cold tap water; it should not be scrubbed or chemically cleaned.
- *Storage media:* If the tooth cannot be immediately replanted, the storage media is critical. The tooth should be stored in a physiologic medium to prevent further injury to the periodontal ligament. The tooth should not be allowed to dry. Hank's balanced salt solution including a commercial "Save a Tooth" transport product is available, and this is an ideal storage medium. When immediate replantation cannot be achieved, and a more physiologic medium is not available, the tooth should be placed in the oral vestibule or under the tongue while the patient is transported to the dentist.

B The tooth should be replanted as soon as possible. The blood clot should be removed from the socket by gentle irrigation with Hank's solution. No attempt should be made to sterilize the tooth. The pulp should not be removed at this time. The socket should not be curetted.

C Splinting should be nonrigid for 7 to 10 days. Flexible wire composite splints or a 20- to 30-pound microfilament nylon wire in a bonded resin splint is advocated.

D The systemic administration of antibiotics at the time of and during the first week following replantation has been shown to prevent bacterial invasion of the necrotic pulp and subsequent inflammatory resorption. If the avulsed tooth or wound is contaminated with soil, the patient must receive a tetanus injection.

E If the tooth exhibits incomplete root formation, revascularization may occur following replantation.

F *All replanted teeth with complete root formation must be treated endodontically.* Endodontics should be instituted 10 to 14 days following replantation in an attempt to prevent the development of inflammatory root resorption. Nonsetting calcium hydroxide paste therapy to inhibit root resorption is currently the accepted therapeutic regimen.

G Calcium hydroxide is an absorbable material, and it is therefore necessary to reclean and repack the canal periodically, if there is a lengthy evaluation period.

References

Andreason JO: Effect of extra-alveolar period and storage media upon periodontal and pulpal healing after replantation of mature permanent incisors in monkeys, *Int J Oral Surg* 10:43, 1981.

Andreasen JO: *Traumatic injuries to teeth,* ed 2, Philadelphia, 1981, WB Saunders.

Camp JH: Diagnosis and management of sports-related injuries to the teeth, *Dent Clin North Am* 35:733, 1991.

Krasner P, Rankow HJ: New philosophy for the treatment of avulsed teeth, *Oral Surg* 79:616, 1995.

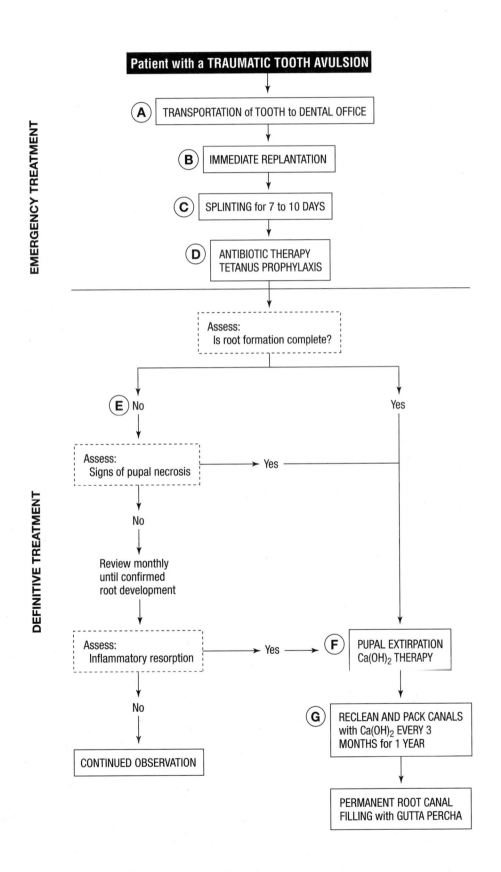

Patient with a TRAUMATIC TOOTH AVULSION

EMERGENCY TREATMENT

(A) TRANSPORTATION of TOOTH to DENTAL OFFICE

(B) IMMEDIATE REPLANTATION

(C) SPLINTING for 7 to 10 DAYS

(D) ANTIBIOTIC THERAPY TETANUS PROPHYLAXIS

DEFINITIVE TREATMENT

Assess: Is root formation complete?

(E) No

Yes

Assess: Signs of pupal necrosis → Yes

No

Review monthly until confirmed root development

Assess: Inflammatory resorption → Yes → (F) PUPAL EXTIRPATION Ca(OH)$_2$ THERAPY

No

CONTINUED OBSERVATION

(G) RECLEAN AND PACK CANALS with Ca(OH)$_2$ EVERY 3 MONTHS for 1 YEAR

PERMANENT ROOT CANAL FILLING with GUTTA PERCHA

68 Diagnostic and Treatment Considerations in the Management of Dental Resorption

Joseph H. Schulz

Resorption and deposition are the normal and dynamic responses of bone and cementum to forces bearing upon them throughout life. Resorption is a vital process. Whenever one of these counterbalancing forces goes awry, it may lead to extremely challenging situations.

Resorption proceeds after natural inhibitors, within the protein matrix in the cementum externally or the predentin internally, are lost. The cells and tissues causing the resorption originate from the pulp or the periodontal ligament. While minor surface repair and remodeling is normal, dentin once resorbed cannot be replaced. When it is resorbed grossly, the dentin is lost forever. Protecting and preserving tooth structure is imperative to the maintenance of healthy, functioning, natural dentition over a lifetime, and identification of pathologic resorption is key.

A Discovery of resorptive phenomena is usually made radiographically. If the resorption is external, occurring on the buccal or lingual surface, careful radiographic examination will reveal a "normal" pulp space running through the resorption, and an examination of horizontally varying views will divulge their three-dimensional positioning. Visual detection occurs when the granulation tissue becomes visible through the enamel. Symptoms usually occur late.

An initiating event or factor such as trauma, bacteria, pressure, chemicals, or necrotic debris is believed to be necessary to start the inflammatory events leading to resorption, and a driving force needs to be active to promote it. A seeming lack of causation is labeled idiosyncratic. Nonetheless, the end result is the same—loss of tooth or bone (Fig. 68-1).

Resorption of dentin and cementum has been described and named on the basis of several criteria: (1) the time of the effect (transient or progressive); (2) the location in the tooth where it is occurring (internal or external specifically cervical, lateral, or apical); (3) the nature of the action (invasive); and (4) the ultimate fate of the tissue (replacement or inflammatory).

B Transient surface resorption, if detectable, may warrant little more than recognition or comment. This may occur internally or externally involving just the cementum, the dentin or both. Histologically, repairs may appear as cementum, reparative dentin, or bone. No treatment is needed unless reactivation occurs.

C Progressive resorption is a profound attack on the dentin by forces continuing to drive the unbalanced process. The attacking front may be a surface phenomena or a burrowing effect dissolving the dentin. If the pulp tissue is normal and uninvolved in the process, then the proper avenue of treatment is to remove or reduce the driving force and repair the damage as required. The pulp may become involved during those efforts or subsequently, and hence root canal therapy may be necessary. Monitoring is advised not only for endodontic reasons but also to be vigilant against recurrence. It may be impossible to determine the driving force(s), to eliminate them or to repair the damage. Such cases present ethical dilemmas and commonly result in disappointment for the patient and the practitioner.

The categories of resorption are the following:

D *Internal resorption,* which may originate in a discrete locus or at multiple sites, is detectable on radiographs when small and visually later, as a pink spot, if occurring in the crown.

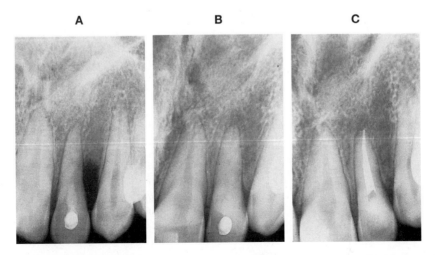

Fig. 68-1 **A,** The placement of calcium hydroxide 1 week after blunt trauma has devitalized the upper lateral incisor. After thorough cleaning and shaping, Ca(OH)$_2$ was placed to stimulate remineralization of the adjacent bone and to neutralize the acidic intracanal involvement. **B,** Remineralization of the alveolar matrix, 1 week later. **C,** Postobturation.

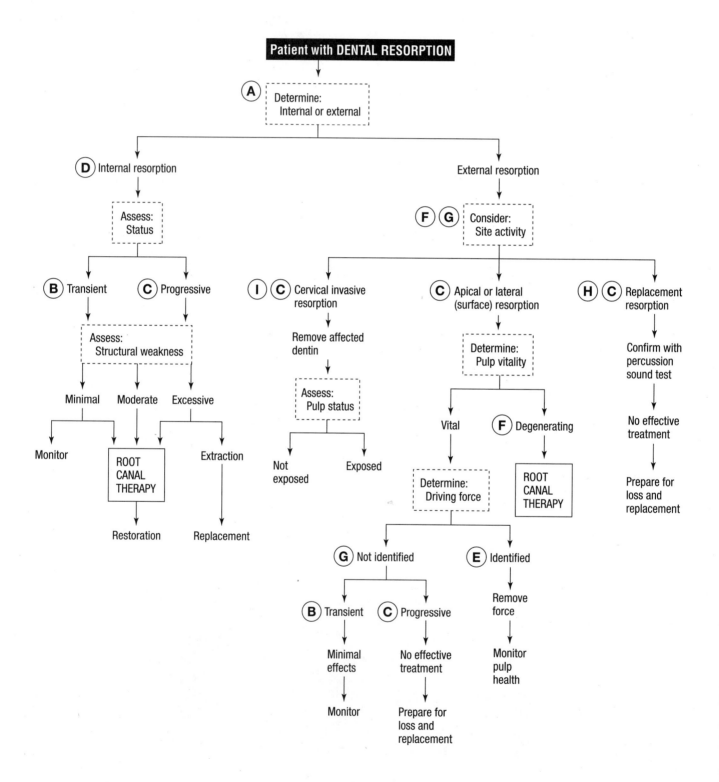

Patient with DENTAL RESORPTION

(A) Determine:
Internal or external

(D) Internal resorption

External resorption

Assess:
Status

(F)(G) Consider:
Site activity

(B) Transient

(C) Progressive

(I)(C) Cervical invasive
resorption

(C) Apical or lateral
(surface) resorption

(H)(C) Replacement
resorption

Assess:
Structural weakness

Remove affected
dentin

Determine:
Pulp vitality

Confirm with
percussion
sound test

Minimal   Moderate   Excessive

Assess:
Pulp status

Vital   (F) Degenerating

No effective
treatment

Monitor

ROOT
CANAL
THERAPY

Extraction

Not
exposed

Exposed

Determine:
Driving force

ROOT
CANAL
THERAPY

Prepare for
loss and
replacement

Restoration

Replacement

(G) Not identified

(E) Identified

(B) Transient   (C) Progressive

Remove
force

Minimal
effects

No effective
treatment

Monitor
pulp
health

Monitor

Prepare for
loss and
replacement

Symptoms occur late after the resorbing pulp tissue and the periodontal ligament or the external environment link. Discomfort may also originate from an adjacent area of inflamed pulp. Treatment is conventional root canal therapy, which has an anticipated high degree of success, if performed before the tooth is structurally weakened.

E *Apical resorption,* if caused by external pressure, may be arrestable by eliminating the source of that pressure (e.g., reduction of orthodontic forces or removal of an impinging tooth, tumor, cyst, or cancer). The pulp in such cases may be "normal," Endodontic therapy is indicated if the etiology is pulpal.

F *External resorption,* apical or lateral, resulting from noxious stimuli emanating from the degenerating or infected pulp may be terminated if root canal therapy is successful at eliminating the inflammatory pressure driving the process.

G *External resorption* caused by inflammatory pressure originating in the cementum or periodontal fibers is often associated with trauma to those elements. The pulp in such cases may be "normal" by all means of assessment currently available. Treatment such as root canal therapy alone or combined with calcium hydroxide therapy *may have some or no influence* on the course of the disease.

H *Replacement resorption* is rather unique in that the body substitutes another hard structure, bone, for the removed tooth substance. Theory suggests the triggering factor is necrosing periodontal fibers resulting from a traumatic episode. During the clearing and replacement of those fibers, the root and bone fuse (ankylose) and become one. Bone will eventually overcome the root structure entirely. Nothing can prevent it once initiated. The "replacement" does not restore the original shape or function of the root. Over time, the crown is supported directly by the alveolar bone and is eventually lost.

I *Cervical invasive resorption,* histologically, a burrowing effect, through a relatively small defect starts externally just apical to the gingival attachment. It invades the internal dentin, completely surrounding the pulp space, without directly communicating with the pulp. If detected early by radiographs and treated conservatively, by removal and repair, the practitioner may eliminate the problem without endodontic therapy.

Visual detection through the enamel (pink spot) and symptoms occurring late usually require conventional and surgical efforts. Cervical invasive resorption has been linked to chemical injury (heat activated internal bleaching), trauma, injury to the cementum apical to the attachment, and unknown causes. Continued monitoring is necessary because of possible recurrence or pulpal degeneration.

References

Andreason JO: *Traumatic injuries of the teeth,* ed 2, Philadelphia, 1981, WB Saunders.

Bakland L: Root resorption, *Dent Clin North Am* 36:2, 1992.

Tronstad L: Root resorption—etiology, terminology, and clinical manifestations, *Endodon Dent Traumatol* 4:241, 1988.

Trope M, Chivian N, Sigurdsson A: Traumatic injuries. In Cohen S, Burns R, editors: *Pathways of the Pulp,* ed 7, St Louis, 1997, Mosby.

69 Indications for the Treatment of a Vertically Cracked Tooth

Hipolito Fabra-Campos, Jose Manuel Roig-Garcia

A cracked tooth may have a longitudinal fracture at root level in an endodontically treated tooth. This fracture may extend from the root canal to the surrounding area, stretching along the length of the root either totally or partially. It may begin at the crown and continue along the length of the root toward the apex, or it may be localized along the root of the tooth with or without coronal effects.

Vertical root fractures can be caused by an excessive force produced within the root canal or in the pulp chamber as a result of root canal filling procedures, pin or post placement, seating of intracoronal restorations, or the reduction of the tooth's resistance following endodontic treatment.

A If the endodontically treated tooth is painful, the cause should be determined. The presence of a cracked tooth can be suspected if a separation of the root or fissure lines exists or if a clear lateral radiolucent image or areas of external resorption are observed on radiographs. Surgical inspection is necessary if this diagnosis is not certain.

B If there is no periodontal involvement and pain is present with or without an obvious periapical radiolucency, existing endodontics should be redone in case any contaminated pulp residue or unfilled canals are present. If the radiolucency is periapical, the fracture may be localized at the apex; thus periapical surgery with retrofilling is indicated.

C If there is periodontal involvement localized in a narrow infrabony pocket with limited depth in the surrounding area of the tooth, the prognosis is guarded because periodontal treatment is not a suitable solution for the lesion.

D If the fracture is localized in the coronal third of the root, the deepest area of the pocket is situated at the apical limit of the fracture. Eliminate the fractured fragment and surgically expose or orthodontically extrude the remaining portion. Crown lengthening may be used to expose the surrounding area of the root.

E If the fracture extends along the length of the root or the tooth has a fused root, it may be possible to preserve it by eliminating debris from the interior of the canal and then by filling with calcium hydroxide for a 9- to 12-month period. A full coverage temporary crown is indicated during this time. If after a few months the periodontal lesion disappears, the canal can be obturated with a fair prognosis. If time is not available, the tooth has no strategic value, or the periodontal damage does not resolve, extraction is indicated.

F If the affected tooth is multirooted and the crack only affects one root, the indicated treatment in the case of separated roots is hemisection or amputation of the affected root. If a molar has fused roots and strategic value, temporary refilling using calcium hydroxide can be attempted. If the lesion does not disappear, extraction is indicated. If the fracture is in one or both of the facial roots of an upper molar, amputation or hemisection with removal of both facial roots are guarded choices.

References

Ingle JI, Beveridge EF, editors: *Endodontics,* Philadelphia, 1976, Lea & Febiger, p 719.

Lin LM, Langeland K: Vertical root fracture, *J Endodon* 8:558, 1982.

Meister F, Lommel TJ, Gerstein H: Diagnosis and possible causes of vertical root fracture, *Oral Surg* 49:243, 1980.

Pitts DL, Natkin E: Diagnosis and treatment of vertical root fractures, *J Endodon* 9:338, 1983.

Polson AM: Periodontal destruction associated with vertical root fracture: report of four cases, *J Periodontol* 48:27, 1977.

Stewart GG: The detection and treatment of vertical root fractures, *J Endodon* 14:47, 1988.

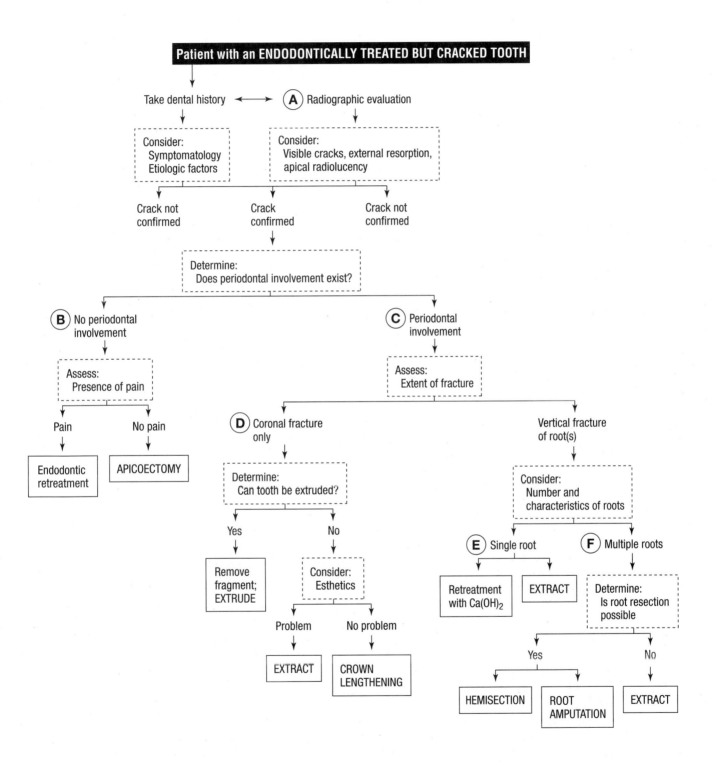

Patient with an ENDODONTICALLY TREATED BUT CRACKED TOOTH

Take dental history ⟷ (A) Radiographic evaluation

Consider:
Symptomatology
Etiologic factors

Consider:
Visible cracks, external resorption,
apical radiolucency

Crack not confirmed · Crack confirmed · Crack not confirmed

Determine:
Does periodontal involvement exist?

(B) No periodontal involvement

(C) Periodontal involvement

Assess:
Presence of pain

Assess:
Extent of fracture

Pain · No pain

Endodontic retreatment · APICOECTOMY

(D) Coronal fracture only

Vertical fracture of root(s)

Determine:
Can tooth be extruded?

Consider:
Number and characteristics of roots

Yes · No

Remove fragment; EXTRUDE

Consider:
Esthetics

(E) Single root

(F) Multiple roots

Retreatment with Ca(OH)₂ · EXTRACT

Determine:
Is root resection possible

Problem · No problem

EXTRACT · CROWN LENGTHENING

Yes · No

HEMISECTION · ROOT AMPUTATION · EXTRACT

70 Periodontal-Endodontic Ramifications of the Radicular Groove: Recognition, Diagnosis, and Practical Management

†William W.Y. Goon

Progressive localized periodontal disease inevitably develops alongside a radicular groove because of its intimate association with the periodontal sulcus. Maxillary incisors, in particular the lateral incisor, are predisposed to this developmental defect, which begins on or alongside of the cingulum and courses apically onto the root. A myriad of periodontal and endodontic manifestations, ranging from mild to severe, can arise as a result of this defect.

A A diagnosis of a radicular groove must begin with a thorough intraoral examination of the lingual aspects of all incisor crowns. The periodontal sulcus of incisors with a visually pronounced cingulum should be examined for the presence of localized periodontal disease and carefully probed in its entirety to help disclose any invagination on the tooth or root surface (Fig. 70-1).

B Radiographic discernment of parapulpal lines is diagnostic and should alert the astute clinician to search diligently for a grooved defect. The presence of a parapulpal line can easily be confused with an accessory root, an additional root canal, or a vertical root fracture yet often signifies a deeply invaginated defect (Fig. 70-2).

C A shallow groove and a short groove have the best long-term prognosis. Effective management consists of periodontal root planing, gingivectomy to the apical extent of the shallow groove, and plaque control.

D A moderately long groove or one that is invaginated are often associated with advanced periodontal disease. Periodontal manifestation is influenced by the defect's length and severity. Periodontal management may require a com-

bination of flap elevation, odontoplasty of the groove, filling or sealing the groove with restorative materials or sealants, osteoplasty, guided tissue regeneration, or repositioning the flap. Long-term plaque control is necessary in follow-up care. The success rate is enhanced when the groove is not excessively long and the pulp's vitality is not compromised by root alteration or filling procedures.

E An endodontic assessment of the vitality of the pulp is mandatory for any tooth with a deeply invaginated groove or one that radiographically demonstrates a parapulpal line. Some deeply invaginated grooves are defective, permitting direct bacterial entry into the root canal space. This can occur before or concomitantly with the insidious development of a localized periodontal pocket. Similarly, odontoplasty or groove-filling procedures can adversely affect the pulp's vitality, which must be continually monitored. The endodontic assessment of vitality can help to better sequence periodontal management by identifying and electively eliminating the endodontic factor before it becomes firmly established and a liability in the periodontal management.

F Some invaginated grooves are discovered late and have established endodontic-periodontal disease. Many of these

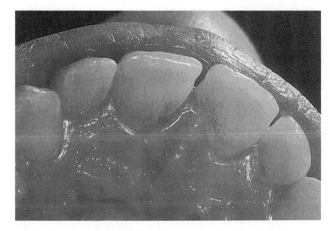

Fig. 70-1 Clinical presentation of the maxillary right central incisor with an invaginated defect that traverses from the cingulum of the crown and courses apically onto the root. The tooth is not fully erupted into the adult occlusion.

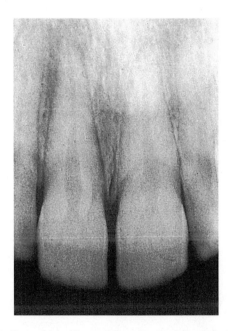

Fig. 70-2 Radiographic evidence of the radicular defect is demonstrated by a parapulpal line coursing mesioapically beyond the cervical level of the crown. Although the tooth is free from decay, the presence of the periapical lesion portrays the adverse endodontic-periodontal implications of the anatomic groove.

---

†Deceased.

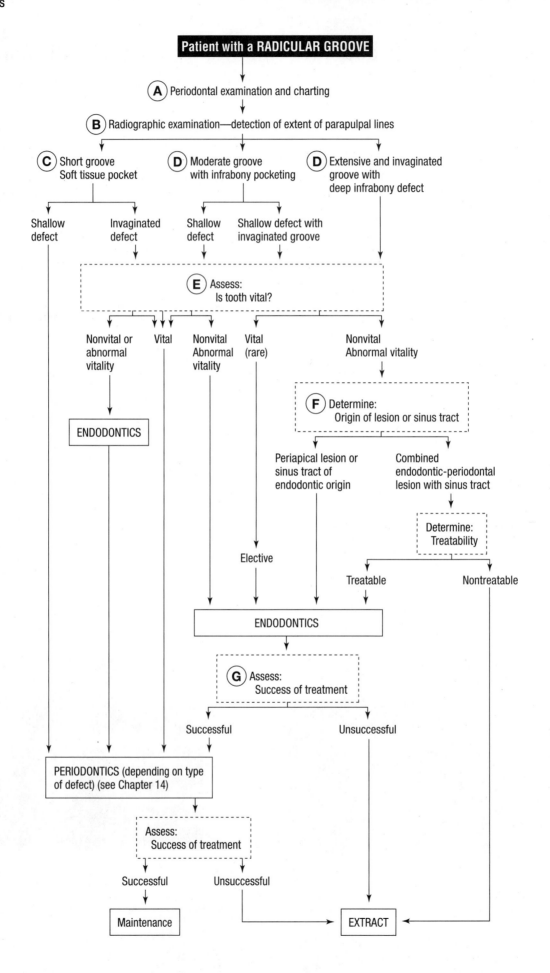

Patient with a RADICULAR GROOVE

(A) Periodontal examination and charting

(B) Radiographic examination—detection of extent of parapulpal lines

(C) Short groove
Soft tissue pocket

(D) Moderate groove
with infrabony pocketing

(D) Extensive and invaginated
groove with
deep infrabony defect

Shallow defect

Invaginated defect

Shallow defect

Shallow defect with invaginated groove

(E) Assess:
Is tooth vital?

Nonvital or abnormal vitality

Vital

Nonvital
Abnormal vitality

Vital
(rare)

Nonvital
Abnormal vitality

ENDODONTICS

(F) Determine:
Origin of lesion or sinus tract

Periapical lesion or sinus tract of endodontic origin

Combined endodontic-periodontal lesion with sinus tract

Determine:
Treatability

Elective

Treatable

Nontreatable

ENDODONTICS

(G) Assess:
Success of treatment

Successful

Unsuccessful

PERIODONTICS (depending on type of defect) (see Chapter 14)

Assess:
Success of treatment

Successful

Unsuccessful

Maintenance

EXTRACT

grooves involve most of the root's length. An infrabony pocket is associated with the defect, and a draining sinus tract of endodontic origin is not uncommon. The condition mimics genuine endodontic-periodontal disease, but, unless the radicular groove is detected and diagnosed, treatment will be ineffectual or compromised. Management of a groove with combined endodontic-periodontal disease is determined by the endodontic outcome. Without a favorable response to endodontic therapy, periodontal endeavors cannot be completely effective. A tooth with a radicular groove that is refractory to endodontic and periodontal treatment should be extracted.

G Occasionally, there is a need to assess a postendodontic failure and the nonresolution of an associated sinus tract and periapical lesion. It is common to find an incisor intact, except for the endodontic access preparation. A radicular groove may have been misdiagnosed as the underlying etiology. The ability to radiographically visualize a parapulpal line, however, is now seriously hampered by the overlapping root canal filling; therefore an intraoral inspection is mandatory. If a groove is detected, treatment should be terminated, and the patient should be advised of the poor prognosis for tooth retention.

References

Everett FG, Kramer GM: The distolingual groove in the maxillary lateral incisor; a periodontal hazard, *J Periodontol* 43:352, 1972.

Gao Z, Shir J, Wang Y, Gu F et al: Scanning electron microscopic investigation of maxillary lateral incisors with a radicular lingual groove, *Oral Surg* 68:462, 1989.

Goon WWY, Carpenter WM, Brace NM, Ahlfeld RJ: Complex facial radicular groove in a maxillary lateral incisor, *J Endodon* 17:244, 1991.

Lee KW, Lee EC, Poon KY: Palatogingival grooves in maxillary incisor: a possible predisposing factor to localized periodontal disease, *Br Dent J* 121:14, 1968.

Prichard JS: *A textbook of advanced periodontal therapy*, Philadelphia, 1965, WB Saunders, p 14.

Simon JHS, Glick DH, Frank AL: Predictable endodontic and periodontal failures as a result of radicular anomalies, *Oral Surg* 31:823, 1971.

71 Diagnosis and Treatment of Endodontic-Periodontic Lesions

David C. Brown

The diagnosis of an endodontic-periodontic lesion is directed toward determining whether the primary pathosis is of endodontic or periodontal origin. The primary etiology is the major determinant of treatment.

A *Primary endodontic lesion.* This is not a true periodontal lesion but exhibits a pseudo-pocket characterized by a sinus tract draining along the periodontal ligament into the sulcus. The defect usually involves only one aspect of the tooth, for example, in the furcation area. Pain is often not a feature, however, there may have been a history of pain in the past. *The pulp is necrotic.* Complete resolution is anticipated following endodontic treatment. These lesions do not require any periodontal treatment. Prognosis is good (Fig. 71-1).

B *Primary periodontal lesion.* Clinically there may be broad-based defects and bleeding on probing. Probing defects do not usually extend to the apexes of the involved teeth. Usually periodontal lesions are not isolated to a single tooth, although this can occur. There may be the presence of plaque and calculus and soft tissue inflammation associated with a purulent exudate. *The pulp is usually vital.* Treatment depends on the extent of the periodontal disease. The prognosis is totally dependent on the outcome of periodontal therapy and patient compliance with therapeutic recommendations. Root canal treatment is not indicated for resolution of such cases.

C *Endodontic-periodontic lesion (true combined lesion).* In cases where pulpal disease is long standing and periapical pathosis is chronic, plaque and calculus may develop in the defect. This results in periodontal pocket formation (i.e., primary endodontic lesion, with a secondary periodontal defect). In situations in which periodontal disease progresses sufficiently to expose the pulp to the oral environment via lateral canals, apical foramen, or dentinal tubules, pulpal inflammation and necrosis may occur (i.e., primary periodontic lesion with secondary endodontic involvement). This may follow periodontal treatment, after root planing has denuded the root of protective cementum. Teeth with combined endodontic-periodontic lesions have necrotic pulps, and periodontal examination reveals plaque, calculus, and a wide and conical periodontal pocket characteristic of chronic periodontitis. In the true combined endodontic-periodontic lesion, endodontic and periodontal treatment are required. After successful endodontic therapy, the prognosis is totally dependent on the periodontal outcome. In true combined lesions in which the primary etiology was periodontal in origin, the prognosis is guarded.

There are cases that do not fit a characteristic combined endodontic-periodontic lesion, or they do not respond as expected to treatment. Biopsy and histologic analysis are necessary for the differential diagnosis of a possible nonodontogenic origin.

References

Barkhordar RN, Stewart GG: The potential of periodontal pocket formation associated with untreated accessory root canals, *Oral Surg* 70:769, 1990.

Harrington GW: The perio-endo question: differential diagnosis, *Dent Clin North Am* Oct:673, 1979.

Seltzer S, Bender IB, Ziontz M. The interrelationship of pulp and periodontal disease, *Oral Surg* 16:1474, 1963.

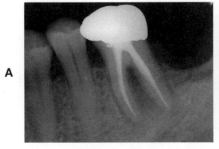 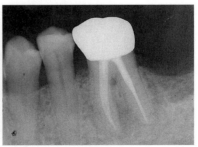

Fig. 71-1 **A,** Root canal therapy done on an endodontic-periodontic lesion diagnosed as having a necrotic pulp. **B,** The 1-year postoperative radiograph shows furcal and periapical healing demonstrating an endodontic etiology.

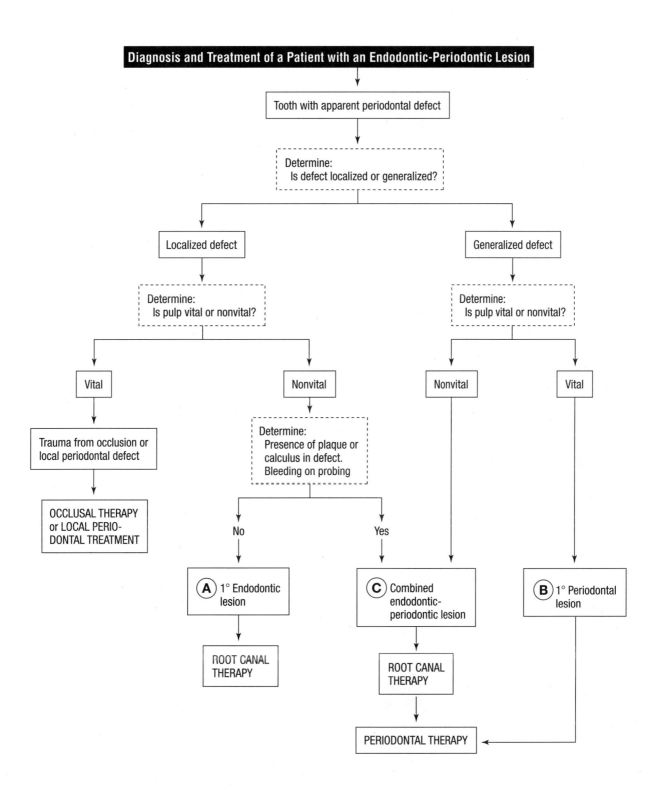

Diagnosis and Treatment of a Patient with an Endodontic-Periodontic Lesion

Tooth with apparent periodontal defect

Determine:
Is defect localized or generalized?

Localized defect

Generalized defect

Determine:
Is pulp vital or nonvital?

Determine:
Is pulp vital or nonvital?

Vital

Nonvital

Nonvital

Vital

Trauma from occlusion or local periodontal defect

Determine:
Presence of plaque or calculus in defect. Bleeding on probing

OCCLUSAL THERAPY or LOCAL PERIO-DONTAL TREATMENT

No

Yes

A 1° Endodontic lesion

C Combined endodontic-periodontic lesion

B 1° Periodontal lesion

ROOT CANAL THERAPY

ROOT CANAL THERAPY

PERIODONTAL THERAPY

72 Indications for Molar Tooth Radisection: Hemisection Versus Root Amputation

Jordi J. Cambra, Borja Zabelegui

Root radisection is a technique for maintaining a portion of a diseased or injured molar by removal of one or more of its roots. Radisection may be achieved by hemisection, in which the entire tooth is cut in half and one part is removed, or by root amputation, in which only one or two roots are amputated from the remainder of the tooth (Fig. 72-1). These surgical approaches may be useful in many situations. The indications for selecting hemisection or root amputation depend on the status of the individual molar and its relationship to other teeth. Guided tissue regeneration (GTR) may be a viable option instead of radisection (see Chapter 30).

A If a molar has fused roots, neither hemisection nor root amputation is possible. If a Class II furcation is present (see Chapter 26), GTR may be attempted. If a Class III furcation is present (see Chapter 25), extraction or maintenance with a hopeless prognosis should result.

B A maxillary molar with advanced involvement of a proximal furcation and separated roots where adjacent root proximity is a problem should be treated by root amputation to facilitate access for débridement by the dentist and the patient. Where root proximity is not a complicating factor, a Class II (definite) furcation involvement proximally could be treated by GTR or mucogingival-osseous surgery or maintained with frequent planing (see Chapter 10). The patient could enhance plaque control with an interproximal brush. The same is true when the facial furcation has a Class II involvement; however, if the furcations join one another (Class III), root amputation is indicated.

C A mandibular molar with advanced furcation involvement and separated roots that is an existing bridge abutment is a candidate for root amputation and retention of the existing bridge; a similarly involved mandibular molar that is not an existing bridge abutment is treated by hemisection and crowning. In either case if a Class II furcation is involved, GTR may be attempted. If a Class III furcation is present, hemisection or root amputation (if the tooth is part of an existing bridge) should be performed.

D If there is no endodontic involvement, periodontal considerations become of paramount importance. The roots to be amputated must be determined. If the root to be removed is clearly indicated, endodontics should be done before amputation; if there is a doubt, surgery and vital root amputation allow for clinical decisions to be made. If the molar is mandibular and is an abutment for an existing fixed bridge, root amputation may permit retention of that bridge. If it is not an existing abutment, hemisection and then crowning are indicated.

E When a necrotic pulp condition exists, endodontic treatment should be done before periodontal treatment. The differential diagnosis becomes difficult when the bone loss causing a deep pocket formation may be related to the failure of the root canal therapy as a result of technical errors (poor obturations). Perforations or vertical root fracture with no separation of fragments may cause bone loss defects that can mask primary periodontal conditions.

F If the molar being considered has a cracked or perforated root, part of it may be salvaged by radisection. If the tooth is asymptomatic, either maintenance with a guarded prognosis may be considered or a surgical approach could be used. If the tooth is symptomatic and not of strategic (long-term) value, it may be extracted; however, if the tooth has strategic value, it should be treated. If the tooth is mandibular and is an abutment for an existing bridge, root amputation should be considered if root canal therapy can be performed on the root to be retained. If it is not an abutment for an existing bridge, hemisection is a better option. If the molar is maxillary and a single facial root is cracked or perforated, root amputation is indicated if root canal therapy can be performed on remaining roots. If both facial roots are cracked or perforated, root amputation with removal of both facial roots is a guarded choice.

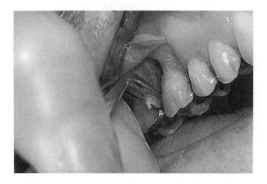

Fig. 72-1 The distal facial root of this first molar has been resected and is being withdrawn from the socket.

References

Basaraba N: Root amputation and tooth hemisection, *Dent Clin North Am* 13:121, 1969.

Grant DA, Stern IB, Listgarten MA: *Periodontics*, ed 6, St Louis, 1988, Mosby, p 935.

Hiatt WH, Owen CR: Periodontal pocket elimination by combined therapy, *Dent Clin North Am* 8:133, 1964.

Schluger S, Yuodelis RA, Page RC, Johnson RH: *Periodontal diseases,* ed 2, Philadelphia, 1990, Lea & Febiger, p 548.

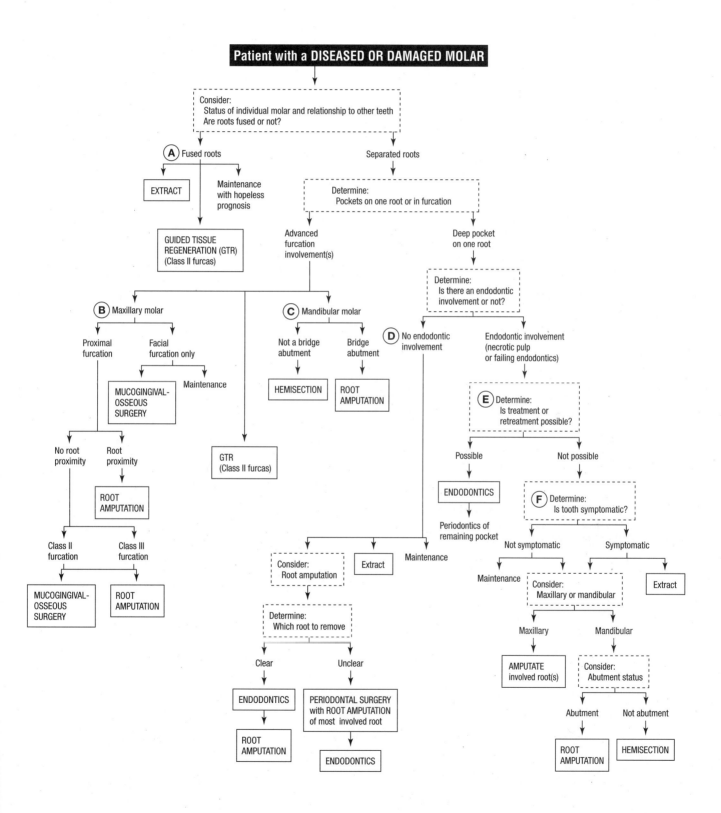

Patient with a DISEASED OR DAMAGED MOLAR

Consider:
Status of individual molar and relationship to other teeth
Are roots fused or not?

A Fused roots

Separated roots

EXTRACT

Maintenance with hopeless prognosis

Determine:
Pockets on one root or in furcation

GUIDED TISSUE REGENERATION (GTR) (Class II furcas)

Advanced furcation involvement(s)

Deep pocket on one root

Determine:
Is there an endodontic involvement or not?

B Maxillary molar

C Mandibular molar

D No endodontic involvement

Endodontic involvement (necrotic pulp or failing endodontics)

Proximal furcation

Facial furcation only

Not a bridge abutment

Bridge abutment

HEMISECTION

ROOT AMPUTATION

E Determine:
Is treatment or retreatment possible?

MUCOGINGIVAL-OSSEOUS SURGERY

Maintenance

No root proximity

Root proximity

Possible

Not possible

ROOT AMPUTATION

GTR (Class II furcas)

ENDODONTICS

F Determine:
Is tooth symptomatic?

Class II furcation

Class III furcation

Periodontics of remaining pocket

Not symptomatic

Symptomatic

MUCOGINGIVAL-OSSEOUS SURGERY

ROOT AMPUTATION

Consider:
Root amputation

Extract

Maintenance

Maintenance

Consider:
Maxillary or mandibular

Extract

Determine:
Which root to remove

Maxillary

Mandibular

Clear

Unclear

AMPUTATE involved root(s)

Consider:
Abutment status

ENDODONTICS

PERIODONTAL SURGERY with ROOT AMPUTATION of most involved root

Abutment

Not abutment

ROOT AMPUTATION

ENDODONTICS

ROOT AMPUTATION

HEMISECTION

73 Sequencing Endodontics and Root Radisection

Jordi J. Cambra, Borja Zabelegui

When a patient has a tooth requiring combined endodontic and periodontal treatment (root radisection), the sequencing of the treatment requires considerable thought. Whenever possible, endodontic treatment should be done before root radisection to avoid difficulty in obtaining adequate anesthesia for comfortable root canal therapy, which could complicate endodontics following vital root resection. Vital root resection rarely results in serious postoperative pain; however, as degeneration of the exposed pulp progresses, increasing acidity interferes with the efficacy of local anesthetic.

A In a nonvital tooth the problem may be only endodontic, even when probing suggests deep pockets are present; this is especially true if the problem is severe and acute. If this appears to be the case, endodontics should be done first because root radisection may not be needed if pockets resolve as a result of endodontic therapy.

B If root removal is needed, the first consideration is whether the roots to be resected are fused (Fig. 73-1). If so, the tooth must be extracted or maintained with a hopeless prognosis.

C If the roots to be amputated are not fused, the dentist must decide whether or not to perform root canal therapy. If an untreatable root would be retained, the tooth should be extracted or maintained with a hopeless prognosis if symptom-free.

D If endodontics can be done on all roots (or on all roots to be retained), determine which roots are to be resected. If doubt exists, periodontal surgery with vital resection of the root selected during surgery should be performed before endodontic treatment. If the roots to be amputated are clearly indicated, endodontic treatment should precede nonvital root radisection.

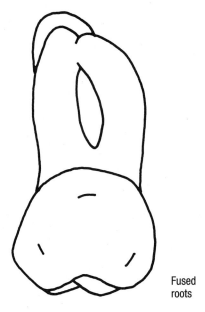

Fused roots

Fig. 73-1 Roots that are fused at their apices are not candidates for root amputation.

References

Basaraba N: Root amputation and tooth hemisection, *Dent Clin North Am* 13:121, 1969.

Grant DA, Stern IB, Listgarten MA: *Periodontics,* ed 6, St Louis, 1988, Mosby, p 916.

Hiatt WH, Amer CR: Periodontal pocket elimination by combined therapy, *Dent Clin North Am* 8:133, 1964.

Schluger S, Yuodelis RA, Page RC, Johnson RH: *Periodontal disease,* ed 2, Philadelphia, 1990, Lea & Febiger, p 549.

Simons HS, Glick DH, Frank AL: The relationship of endodontic-periodontic lesions, *J Periodontol* 43:202, 1972.

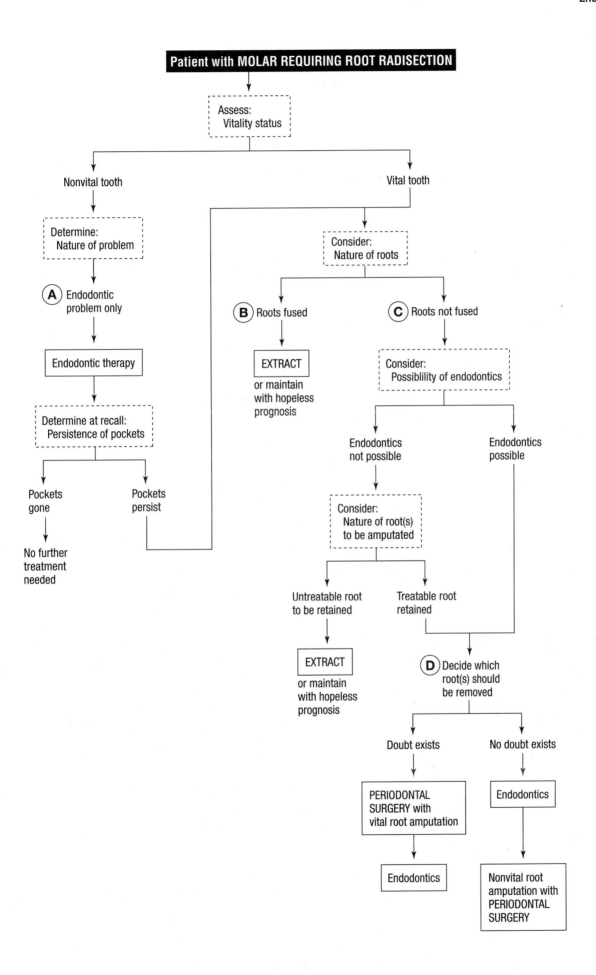

Patient with MOLAR REQUIRING ROOT RADISECTION

Assess:
Vitality status

Nonvital tooth

Vital tooth

Determine:
Nature of problem

Consider:
Nature of roots

(A) Endodontic
problem only

(B) Roots fused

(C) Roots not fused

Endodontic therapy

EXTRACT

or maintain
with hopeless
prognosis

Consider:
Possiblility of endodontics

Determine at recall:
Persistence of pockets

Endodontics
not possible

Endodontics
possible

Pockets
gone

Pockets
persist

Consider:
Nature of root(s)
to be amputated

No further
treatment
needed

Untreatable root
to be retained

Treatable root
retained

EXTRACT

or maintain
with hopeless
prognosis

(D) Decide which
root(s) should
be removed

Doubt exists

No doubt exists

PERIODONTAL
SURGERY with
vital root amputation

Endodontics

Endodontics

Nonvital root
amputation with
PERIODONTAL
SURGERY

74 Restorative Planning for Endodontically Treated Posterior Teeth

W. Paul Brown, Arun Nayyar

For restorative management of a tooth that has undergone root canal therapy, clinical reevaluation of remaining tooth structure is needed. Tooth strength is affected by the volume of intact tooth structure remaining after root canal treatment; thus it is imperative to minimize dentin removal. An endodontically treated tooth with a minimal access opening can be sealed with an amalgam or acid-etched composite resin. Most endodontically treated posterior teeth have lost one or both marginal ridges, and the access opening interrupts the integrity of the remaining dentin and enamel. Consequently, tooth strength, which had been provided by dentin and enamel, must be judiciously replaced. When a large volume of existing tooth structure has been lost, the restorative objective is to reinforce the remaining tooth structure to resist occlusal forces. This can be accomplished by a coronal radicular buildup, which provides needed retention and resistance form for the cast crown restoration.

A In deciding whether an endodontically involved posterior tooth can be saved, factors such as the extensiveness of caries, the nature and extent of cracks or fractures, the periodontal and combined periodontal-endodontic nature of the pathology, and the need for crown lengthening or for orthodontic forced eruption must be weighed. Before proceeding, decide whether the tooth can be restored once endodontics is done or redone.

B If the tooth can be treated endodontically and restoratively, a decision on the design of the restoration should be made. The amalgam dowel core buildup technique uses the pulp chamber for retention of the dowel and core segments. Most pulp chamber spaces are large enough to provide needed internal retention for the amalgam alloy.

Amalgam condensed against dentin has structural strength and margin-sealing ability and is one of the easiest materials to use, requiring no special setup. The less substantial the clinical crown, the greater the retention the alloy requires. This needed retention usually can be obtained by using the pulp chamber and, in those instances when the pulp chamber walls are minimal or missing, 2 to 4 mm of the diverging root canal space. A conservative approach to gain retention is critical. The removal of any healthy dentin greatly weakens the remaining structures and directly affects the life of the final restoration. Slow setting time for amalgam can be accelerated by increasing the trituration time (Fig. 74-1).

If an access opening is minimal, if endodontics are done through an existing crown, or if 20% or less of the clinical crown is missing, the amalgam dowel core can suffice as the final restoration.

C If 40% to 80% of the clinical crown is missing, a cast crown is needed after an amalgam core buildup.

D If 90% to 100% of the clinical crown is missing, a prefabricated or cast metal post can be used to provide better retention of the buildup material. The placement of a post does not significantly improve the strength of the amalgam buildup. Additional dentin must be removed from the canal walls to permit postinsertion, thus weakening the remaining tooth structure and increasing the likelihood of creating a crack or perforation. If crazing lines or near perforation indicate the need for better retention of the amalgam buildup, a resin liner may be used to increase the adhesion of alloy to dentin. The use of resin to bond amalgam to dentin also permits the size of the preparation to be minimized (which would further decrease the likelihood of fracture). A cast crown should be used to complete the restoration.

E If the tooth has been broken off at the gingival margin, a prefabricated cast dowel post may be used to serve as a scaffold and amalgam condensed around it. A cast gold post is indicated only if there is access difficulty. A cast crown is used to complete the restoration. Whenever a cast crown is used, its margins should reach 2 mm beyond the buildup material. Crown lengthening may be necessary to achieve this goal (see Chapter 11).

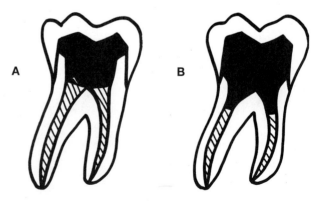

Fig. 74-1 **A,** A pulp chamber greater than 3 mm in depth or with significant undercuts has adequate retention for a buildup. **B,** When pulp chamber characteristics do not provide adequate retention, extending the buildup into the canals can provide retention.

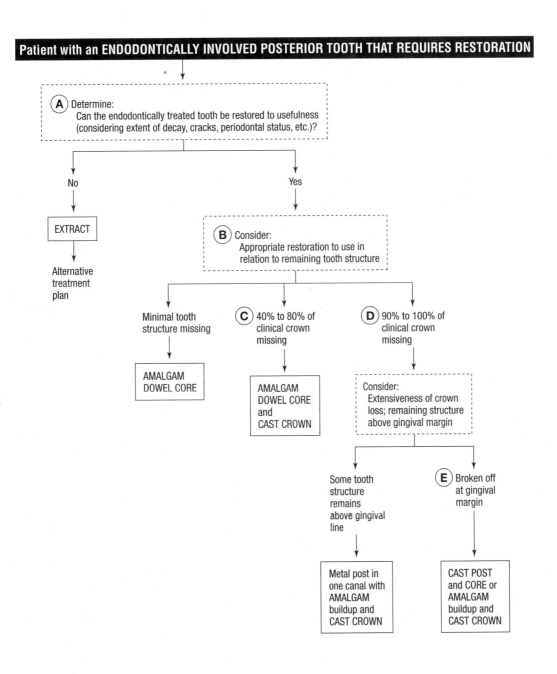

Patient with an ENDODONTICALLY INVOLVED POSTERIOR TOOTH THAT REQUIRES RESTORATION

A Determine:
Can the endodontically treated tooth be restored to usefulness (considering extent of decay, cracks, periodontal status, etc.)?

No → EXTRACT → Alternative treatment plan

Yes → **B** Consider:
Appropriate restoration to use in relation to remaining tooth structure

Minimal tooth structure missing → AMALGAM DOWEL CORE

C 40% to 80% of clinical crown missing → AMALGAM DOWEL CORE and CAST CROWN

D 90% to 100% of clinical crown missing → Consider:
Extensiveness of crown loss; remaining structure above gingival margin

Some tooth structure remains above gingival line → Metal post in one canal with AMALGAM buildup and CAST CROWN

E Broken off at gingival margin → CAST POST and CORE or AMALGAM buildup and CAST CROWN

References

Kanca J: The all-etch bonded technique/wet bonding, *Dent Today* 18:57, 1991.

Lacy AM, Staninec MA: The bonded amalgam restoration, *Quintessence Int* 20:521, 1989.

Nayyar A: Coronal-radicular restorations (technique and materials), *Clin Dent* 4:1, 1983.

Radke RA, Eissmann HF: Postendodontic restoration. In Cohen S, Burns RC, editors: *Pathways of the pulp,* ed 5, St Louis, 1991, Mosby, p 640.

Staninec M: Retention of amalgam restorations: undercuts versus bonding, *Quintessence Int* 20:347, 1989.

Staninec MA, Holt M: Bonding of amalgam to tooth structure: tensile adhesion and microleakage tests, *J Prosthet Dent* 59:397, 1988.

75 Structural Considerations in the Selection of a Dowel Design in Endodontically Treated Teeth

Alan H. Gluskin

Endodontically treated teeth are structurally compromised in a high percentage of cases that require restoration. It is important for the clinician to address structural considerations in determining which materials and techniques to use in restorative treatment.

Multiple factors must be considered in choosing a final restoration. Crucial considerations include the amount of remaining tooth structure, functional demands on the tooth, arch position and opposing occlusion, and length, width, and curvature of the root(s). It is a popular belief that endodontically treated teeth are more brittle from loss of moisture in dentin, yet research shows that moisture loss may only slightly affect the collagen of dentin and that an endodontically treated tooth's susceptibility to fracture is primarily caused by loss of tooth structure because of caries, previous restorations, fractures, or preparation of the root canal and access cavity. Therefore the strongest tooth is one that retains maximum structural integrity of dentin and enamel.

The primary purpose of a post or dowel is to support a core that can be used to retain the final restoration. Traditional post systems do not reinforce endodontically treated teeth and are not necessary when substantial tooth structure is present after teeth have been prepared.

Post systems belong in one of three main categories, each exhibiting different material or design characteristics. In the first system, the cast dowel closely reproduces the morphology of the root canal space. This is the morphologic dowel, and it requires the clinician to use a direct or indirect technique for its fabrication. A second system uses a preformed metallic dowel that corresponds to the instrumentation used in refining the dowel space. Once the dowel space is prepared, a matching dowel is selected and passively cemented. The third system incorporates the use of resin-bonding techniques and materials to adapt to the morphologically tapered, oval, or ribbon-shaped root and internally creates a resin reinforcement that can receive a metal or resin dowel, bondable reinforcement fabric, or bondable carbon fiber. Developmental invaginations, narrow mesial-distal width, and proximal concavities in the cervical and middle third of a high percentage of roots often influences the post system a clinician should choose. Restorative strategies must include considerations of structural loss in provision of any dowel post.

A The cast morphologic dowel restoration is recommended in teeth where conservation of dentin is important. The fracture potential of an endodontically treated tooth increases proportionately to the amount of dentin removed. In roots with narrow cross sections and ribbon-shaped or ovoid canals, the attempt to create a round diameter for a prefabricated post is contraindicated. The round preparation exposes the root to further structural loss and potential fracture, and hence morphologic dowels conserve structural integrity. Teeth that should be considered for the use of a morphologic dowel as evidenced by a narrow canal configuration include: mandibular incisors, maxillary and mandibular bicuspids, and the distal roots of lower molars.

B The standardized preformed dowel has a round cross section, and when designed with parallel walls, is considered to provide maximum retention. Additional variables that have been shown to increase retention include length (always retaining an effective apical seal), surface textures, and cementing materials. While conservation of dentin must be an overriding concern, roots with large cross sections and sufficient dentin are candidates for preformed dowel posts. These teeth include maxillary incisors, canines, and palatal roots of upper molars.

C The post systems that use dentin-bonded materials have the potential to bridge the gap between a morphologic dowel, which requires a laboratory fabrication and the preformed dowel systems. In oval or ribbon-shaped canal configurations, intraradicular resin bonding to dentin can eliminate the structural variable of root morphology and allow a bondable fabric or standard dowel to be resin cemented within all root configurations. Many of these systems are new, and hence long-term studies are lacking. However, dentin bonding is an accepted and practical procedure that, when incorporated with sound biologic reasoning for dowel placement, can provide both reinforcement and retention of the final restoration.

References

Gluskin AH, Radke RA, Frost SL, Watanabe LG: The mandibular incisor: rethinking guidelines for post and core design, *J Endodon* 21:33, 1995.

Kahn FH: Selecting a post system, *J Am Dent Assoc* 122:70, 1991.

Saupe WA, Gluskin AH, Radke, Jr, RA: A comparative study of fracture resistance between morphologic dowel and cores and a resin-reinforced dowel system in the intraradicular restoration of structurally compromised roots, *Quintessence Int* 27:483, 1996.

Shillingburg HT, Hobo S, Whitsett LD: *Fundamentals of fixed prosthodontics,* ed 2, Chicago, 1981, Quintessence Publishing, p 150.

Standlee JP, Caputo AA, Hanson EC: Retention of endodontic dowels: effects of cement, dowel length, diameter and design, *J Prosthet Dent* 39:400, 1978.

Tjan AHL, Whang SB: Resistance to root fracture of dowel channels with various thickness of buccal dentin walls, *J Prosthet Dent* 53:496, 1985.

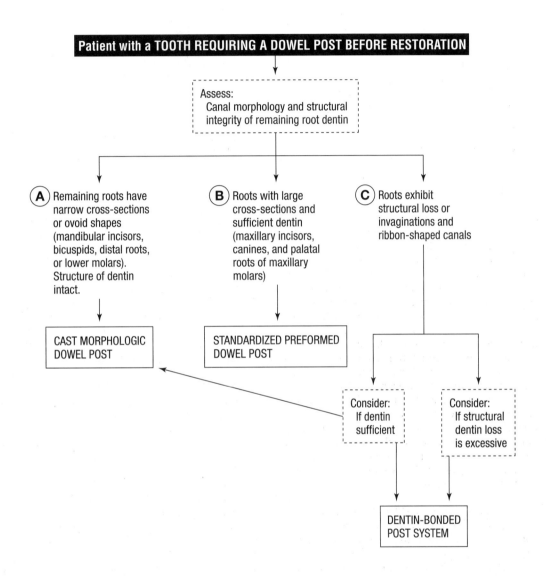

Patient with a TOOTH REQUIRING A DOWEL POST BEFORE RESTORATION

Assess:
Canal morphology and structural
integrity of remaining root dentin

A Remaining roots have
narrow cross-sections
or ovoid shapes
(mandibular incisors,
bicuspids, distal roots,
or lower molars).
Structure of dentin
intact.

B Roots with large
cross-sections and
sufficient dentin
(maxillary incisors,
canines, and palatal
roots of maxillary
molars)

C Roots exhibit
structural loss or
invaginations and
ribbon-shaped canals

CAST MORPHOLOGIC
DOWEL POST

STANDARDIZED PREFORMED
DOWEL POST

Consider:
If dentin
sufficient

Consider:
If structural
dentin loss
is excessive

DENTIN-BONDED
POST SYSTEM

76 Endodontic Considerations in Selecting Overdenture Abutments

†William W.Y. Goon

Adjunctive endodontic treatment may be required when the comprehensive treatment plan includes a tooth-supported complete denture. The primary beneficiary is the terminal dentition that is severely ravaged by tooth loss and advanced periodontal disease. Teeth in the terminal dentition can be salvaged by removal of the clinical crown, saving the residual root to serve as an abutment supporting the overdenture.

A Any tooth that is a potential overdenture abutment must undergo an endodontic assessment. The drastic reduction of the coronal tooth structure will unavoidably involve the root canal space.

An assessment of the patient is also required. The success of the overdenture favors the patient who is truly committed to restoring and maintaining optimum oral health. Patient compliance with the vigorous home care regimen is expected and must include strict oral hygiene of periodontal tissues and daily applications of topical fluoride on exposed natural tooth structure. Regular follow-up visits to review and revise the home maintenance measures and in-office application of silver nitrate in the patient with a high caries index are also necessary. Carelessness in assessing the patient can result in the oversight of a physical impairment, a systemic disease, or potential noncompliance in performing meticulous home care. Perhaps this is the reason for the present neglect and the consideration for denture.

Also, the dentist must assess his or her ability to render this type of service and the willingness to provide follow-up support and encouragement to the patient on home maintenance. The dentist who is unable to carry out this professional mandate should get additional training or refer the patient to a practitioner who is capable of overseeing the patient's health and welfare.

B The terminal status of teeth considered for overdenture abutments requires that the economic burden to the patient be kept to the absolute minimum. The ideal abutment is the single-rooted tooth whose root is structurally sound. The canine tooth is the ideal choice. Its "corner" location in the dental arch and the size and length of the root make it the most strategic tooth to retain. The premolar should be considered when the canine is not available. The incisors are a second choice.

Superseding the economic consideration are cases in which only a tooth-supported complete denture is the best option for rehabilitating the patient. Success of the overdenture may hinge on salvaging a less desirable tooth for abutment service, perhaps in the presence of a physical impairment or systemic disease. The overriding strategic value of having this abutment warrants a financial commitment to render a successful outcome. Less desirable abutments include the multirooted posterior tooth and a severely compromised root with poor bone support.

C Unfortunately, the patient requiring an overdenture seldom has ideal teeth readily available for abutment service. Often the vestiges of a neglected dentition are all that remain. To devise a functional treatment plan, priority in abutment selection is given first to the following:
1. A single-rooted tooth that can sustain the required coronal reduction without needing endodontic treatment. Roots with extensively receded or completely obliterated root canals are viable choices.
2. A single-rooted tooth that already has a successful endodontic filling is the next logical choice.
3. Finally, the single-rooted tooth that can be easily treated endodontically can be selected as an overdenture abutment.

D A single root of a periodontally compromised multirooted posterior tooth may be considered for abutment service following the same priority as for the single-rooted tooth. If indicated, root amputation of the least strategic root(s) can transform the salvaged root into an acceptable abutment. Consideration should be given to the posterior tooth with divergent roots that is amenable to root amputation. This abutment may require associated periodontal procedures to return the tissue to optimum health.

E The extreme case involves the heroic stabilization of a severely weakened root through an endodontic implant. The root so treated may require additional operative or periodontal procedures to retard the progression of periodontal and caries breakdown. An endodontic implant in roots with essentially a questionable prognosis involves the greatest monetary investment and risk of failure.

F The longevity of an overdenture abutment is significantly increased through a vigorous home care program. Recurrent decay and salivary percolation into the root canal space are the greatest liability to maintaining the integrity of the endodontic seal at the root end. The periodontium must be aggressively maintained in an optimum state of health with meticulous oral hygiene. The susceptibility of exposed root surface of the abutment to caries breakdown can be chemically controlled with daily applications of topical fluoride and fluoride oral rinses. Close supervision and reinforcement of home care techniques are parts of an ongoing process that is tailored specifically to each patient.

†Deceased.

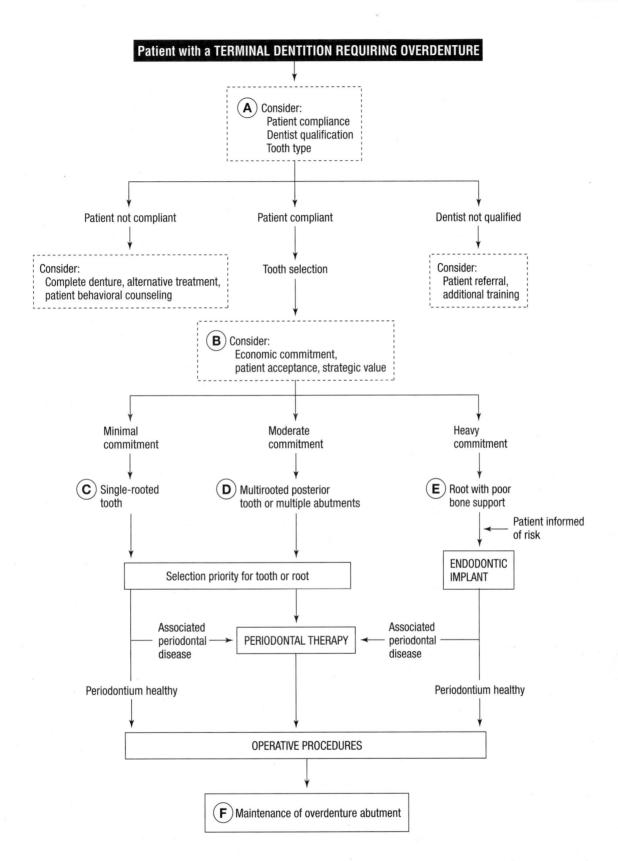

Patient with a TERMINAL DENTITION REQUIRING OVERDENTURE

(A) Consider:
  Patient compliance
  Dentist qualification
  Tooth type

Patient not compliant   Patient compliant   Dentist not qualified

Consider: Tooth selection   Consider:
Complete denture, alternative treatment,   Patient referral,
patient behavioral counseling   additional training

(B) Consider:
  Economic commitment,
  patient acceptance, strategic value

Minimal   Moderate   Heavy
commitment   commitment   commitment

(C) Single-rooted   (D) Multirooted posterior   (E) Root with poor
    tooth   tooth or multiple abutments   bone support

                                                   ← Patient informed
                                                     of risk

Selection priority for tooth or root   ENDODONTIC
                                                   IMPLANT

Associated   PERIODONTAL THERAPY ← Associated
periodontal   periodontal
disease   disease

Periodontium healthy   Periodontium healthy

OPERATIVE PROCEDURES

(F) Maintenance of overdenture abutment

References

DeFranco RL: Overdentures. In Winkler S, editor: *Essentials of complete denture prosthodontics*, Philadelphia, 1979, WB Saunders, p 581.

Grossman LI, Oliet S, Del Rio CE: *Endodontic practice*, ed 11, Philadelphia, 1988, Lea & Febiger, p 346.

Radke RA, Eissmann HF: Postendodontic restoration. In Cohen S, Burns RC, editors: *Pathways of the pulp*, ed 5, St Louis, 1991, Mosby.

Trabert KC, Cooney JP, Caputo AA et al: Preparations for overdentures. In Ingle JI, Taintor JF, editors: *Endodontics*, ed 3, Philadelphia, 1985, Lea & Febiger, p 847.

77 The Endodontically Adequate Abutment Tooth: A European View

Borja Zabelegui

When a patient has an endodontically involved tooth that is a strategic abutment in a complicated restorative case, the dentist must decide whether the tooth is endodontically treatable or not and whether the successfully treated tooth will be adequate for use in the planned restoration. The endodontic treatment may be surgical or nonsurgical.

A The involved tooth is first assessed radiographically and clinically. If root canal therapy can be completed successfully or the tooth can be retreated successfully, nonsurgical treatment is preferable (see Chapter 59). If root canal therapy has not or cannot be performed successfully, surgical endodontics (apicoectomy) may be used to resolve the problem (see Chapter 58).

B Next, the restorability of the tooth is assessed. If crown lengthening is needed to provide an adequate base for restoration, the dentist must decide whether the tooth can retain adequate support to function as an abutment. If so, proceed with endodontics and crown lengthening in sequence as appropriate (e.g., lengthening before endodontics so a rubber dam can be placed). If not, the tooth should be extracted.

C If apicoectomy is to be used, the remaining crown-root ratio must be adequate to function as an abutment. The crown-to-root ratio and the length of span must interrelate such that the abutment will not be traumatized in function.

If sufficient support would remain following apicoectomy or apicoectomy and crown lengthening, the appropriate sequencing of endodontics, crown lengthening, and apicoectomy can be developed. If both surgical procedures can be done at once, time and discomfort may be minimized. If the remaining tooth support following one or both of the surgical procedures is inadequate, an alternative restorative plan should be developed. The availability of additional abutments, so that double abutting can be used, would enhance the predictability of success as an abutment. If surgery or double abutments fail to provide adequate foundations, then the plan may evolve into extracting the tooth or incorporating the tooth in a way that it may still be useful (e.g., an overdenture abutment).

References

Hunter AJ, Feiglin B, Williams JF: Effects of post placement on endodontically treated teeth, *J Prosthet Dent* 62:166, 1989.

Lord JL, Teel S: The overdenture: patient selection, use of copings and follow-up evaluation, *J Prosthet Dent* 32:41, 1977.

Moffa JP, Rossano MR, Doyle MG: Pins—a comparison of their retentive properties, *J Am Dent Assoc* 78:529, 1969.

Radke RA, Eissmann HF: Postendodontic restoration. In Cohen S, Burns RC, editors: *Pathways of the pulp,* ed 5, St Louis, 1991, Mosby, p 640.

Ruddle CJ: Endodontic considerations for periodontal prostheses, *J Cal Dent Assoc* 41:17, 1989.

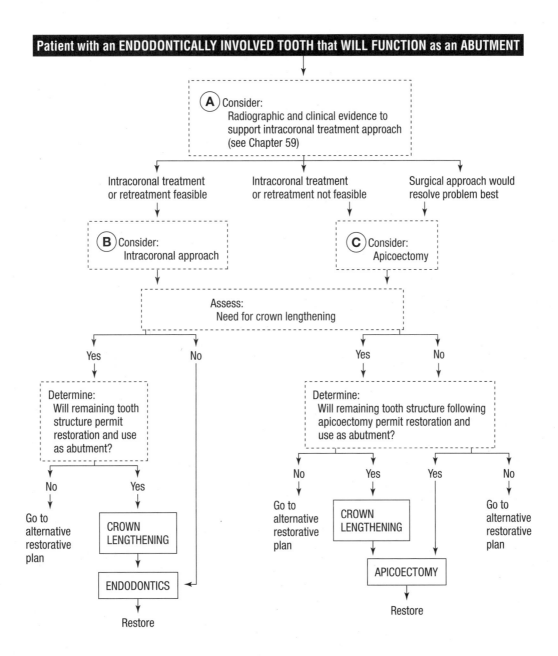

Patient with an ENDODONTICALLY INVOLVED TOOTH that WILL FUNCTION as an ABUTMENT

Ⓐ Consider:
Radiographic and clinical evidence to support intracoronal treatment approach (see Chapter 59)

Intracoronal treatment or retreatment feasible

Intracoronal treatment or retreatment not feasible

Surgical approach would resolve problem best

Ⓑ Consider:
Intracoronal approach

Ⓒ Consider:
Apicoectomy

Assess:
Need for crown lengthening

Yes   No

Yes   No

Determine:
Will remaining tooth structure permit restoration and use as abutment?

Determine:
Will remaining tooth structure following apicoectomy permit restoration and use as abutment?

No   Yes

No   Yes   Yes   No

Go to alternative restorative plan

CROWN LENGTHENING

Go to alternative restorative plan

CROWN LENGTHENING

Go to alternative restorative plan

ENDODONTICS

APICOECTOMY

Restore

Restore

PART THREE

Orthodontics

W. Eugene Roberts, Editor

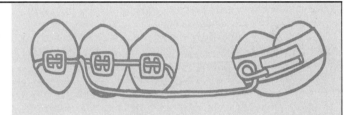

78 Assessment of Malocclusion

W. Eugene Roberts, Rafael Pasalodos Gibert, Maria Antonia Barcelo Puig

Esthetic and functional problems related to poor dental alignment are common concerns of prospective dental patients. All dentists should be aware of the expanding role of orthodontics in managing complex malocclusions. Depending on case selection, performing orthodontics in general practice can be a practice builder or a source of frustration. A sequence of critical questions is presented to help the practitioner decide which cases are in the scope of general practice and which should be referred to an orthodontist or multidisciplinary team.

Rigidly integrated dental implants have revolutionized the scope of orthodontic therapy for partially edentulous patients. Limited orthodontic therapy can help salvage malaligned abutments and stabilize periodontally compromised teeth, however, the patient can benefit only if the dentist has a thorough understanding of the importance of adjunctive orthodontic therapy in the cost-effective management of common malocclusions.

Diagnosis. Determine if the malocclusion is *dynamic* (e.g., growth, degeneration, active disease) or *static* (e.g., a relatively stable malocclusion in physiologic equilibrium).

A Dynamic problems are malocclusions superimposed on one or more physiologic variables: growing face, some forms of progressive systemic disease (e.g., arthritis, osteoporosis), and temporomandibular joint (TMJ) degeneration, all of which are common dynamic problems. Effective management of evolving or relatively unstable malocclusions usually requires the assistance of specifically trained specialists. Dynamic malocclusions have the potential to get much worse if inappropriately managed. Inadequate treatment of complex problems is frustrating for both the patient and doctor and may preclude more appropriate options.

B Static problems are relatively stable malocclusions (i.e., the occlusion responds to orthodontic treatment as a single variable)—usually dental alignment problems of varying complexity. Because orthodontic treatment of complex alignment problems can be technically demanding, careful assessment of the malocclusion is necessary. If the problems are outside or may be outside the range of expertise of the practitioner, the opinion of an orthodontist is indicated.

C The first anatomic consideration is the face. Compared with the facial midline, the frontal view should be symmetric. Average profile convexity for most ethnic groups is approximately 10° to 15° (i.e., the chin is posterior to a straight line tangent to the most prominent point on the forehead [glabella] and passing through the base of the nose [subnasale]). Convexity greater than 20° and less than 5° (especially concave profiles) is often associated with significant skeletal problems and should be analyzed cephalometrically.

D Lip evaluation is a critical functional consideration. The lips should be competent (touch or nearly touch in repose). Patients with incompetent lips, especially if associated with habitual mouth breathing, should be evaluated by a spe-

cialist. Lip protrusion for most European Caucasians is approximately 2- to 4-mm anterior to a line from subnasale to soft tissue pogonion (most prominent curvature of the chin). Other ethnic groups are usually more protrusive; lip protrusion itself is not a problem if the lips are competent.

E The centric relation to centric occlusion shift ($C_r \rightarrow Co$ shift) is measured in three directions: vertical, horizontal, and lateral deviation. Shifts of greater than 1 mm require referral.

F It is wise to correct Class I or III malocclusion as part of the treatment plan. However, asymptomatic patients with a buccal occlusion within 2 mm of Class I can often be maintained indefinitely. Class II problems greater than 3 mm usually require definitive orthodontic diagnosis and treatment.

G Habits in nongrowing adults are often difficult to correct and may be associated with skeletal malocclusions requiring surgical treatment.

H Crowding of less than or equal to 3 mm can usually be managed with interproximal stripping of enamel. It is important to monitor enamel thickness with radiographs and avoid greater than 0.25-mm stripping on any single tooth surface. Expansion of mandibular cuspids may require permanent retention.

I Overjets less than or equal to 3 mm usually can be maintained indefinitely if there is little or no $C_r \rightarrow Co$ shift; however, overbites that interfere with normal functional disclusion (usually >50% incisal overlap) should be corrected. Midline discrepancies of greater than 2 mm are often a manifestation of substantial occlusal asymmetry.

J Skeletal crossbites are manifested by an apical base discrepancy and may require surgical correction. Dental crossbites, not associated with a bone deficiency or excessive vertical dimension of occlusion, can often be corrected with cross elastics.

In summary, this chapter provides a step-wise procedure for determining the complexity of a malocclusion. Orthodontic considerations should be part of the differential diagnosis for all dental patients. The dashed lines (on the flow chart) track the types of problems that are most likely to be effectively managed in general practice. Problems beyond the expertise of the primary care practitioner should be referred to an orthodontist.

References

Proffit WR, Fields H, Ackerman JL, Sinclair PM, Thomas PM, Tulloch JFC: *Contemporary orthodontics,* St Louis, 1993, Mosby, p 1.

Roberts WE: Bone physiology, metabolism, and biomechanics in orthodontic practice. In Graber TM, Vanarsdall, Jr, RL, editors: *Orthodontics: current principles and techniques,* St Louis, 1994, Mosby, p 193.

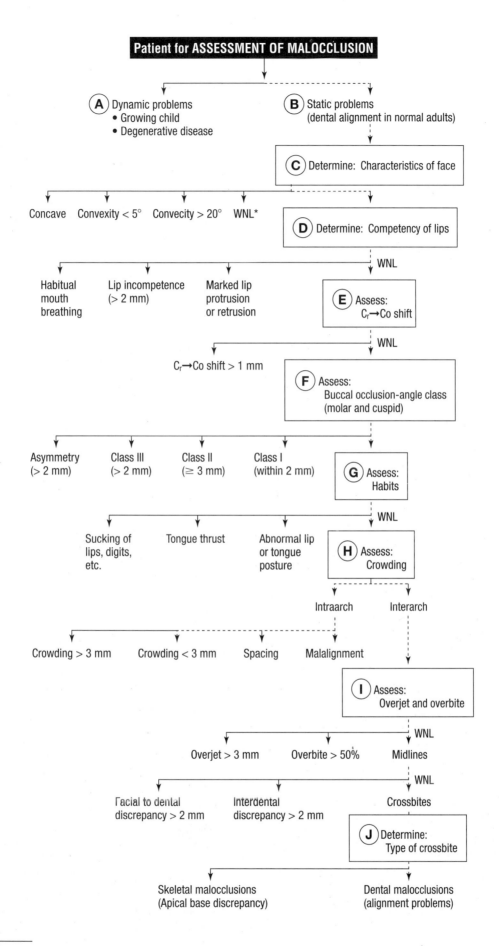

*WNL, within normal limits. Dashed lines indicate treatment may be within scope of general practice.

171

79   Molar Uprighting and Creating Space

†Gordon R. Arbuckle

The tooth that is most often lost as a result of caries or periodontal disease is the permanent first molar. Unless this condition is managed in a timely fashion, tipping, drifting, and rotation of the adjacent teeth will occur. Mesial tipping is usually the focus of attention, but correction of lingual inclination is of equal importance. Preprosthetic molar alignment is commonly indicated and can often be achieved with fixed orthodontic appliances. Careful periodontal and prosthodontic evaluation is essential before undertaking this orthodontic procedure. Orthodontic therapy in the presence of active periodontal disease can lead to rapid and irreversible deterioration of the periodontium. With careful diagnosis and treatment planning, this adjunctive procedure can significantly improve the final prosthetic restoration and create a periodontally manageable restored dentition.

A   Gingiva around tipped molars may appear pink, firm, and generally healthy; however, it may be fibrotic from repeated episodes of gingivitis. Inflammation may be present in the depths of the periodontal crevices. Therefore probing of the gingival pockets is an essential part of the pretreatment evaluation. Orthodontic uprighting would be ill advised in the presence of active periodontal disease. Bleeding on probing is one of the most reliable indicators of inflammation. If no bleeding occurs and the pocket depths are within acceptable limits, inflammatory disease is absent or minimal. In the presence of bleeding, a comprehensive periodontal evaluation is needed.

B   Periodontitis is characterized clinically by a loss of attachment (LOA). If the probing depth is 0 to 3 mm with no LOA and no bleeding noted on gentle probing, the gingiva may be assumed to be healthy and orthodontic treatment can be initiated. Pockets greater than 3 mm indicate the need for periodontal evaluation before and at regular intervals during orthodontic treatment. The periodontal treatment of choice for a prospective molar uprighting procedure is to maintain the area by nonsurgical means. If indicated, surgical procedures and more aggressive care should be accomplished 4 to 6 months before appliance placement.

C   The assessment of adequate attached gingiva varies considerably from tooth to tooth and even from surface to surface on the same tooth. It is a matter of clinical judgment as to the likelihood of a tooth remaining stable and healthy during an orthodontic procedure such as uprighting. It is suggested that areas with less than 2 mm of keratinized gingiva be considered as a potential problem because the resulting attached gingiva will probably be only 1 mm when the crevice depth is subtracted. Teeth having less than 1 mm of attached gingiva are potential candidates for grafting. These pretreatment decisions require full consideration of the potential additional insults that the ortho-dontic appliance, lack of accessibility for hygiene, and eruption of the tooth may cause.

D   The prognosis for orthodontically uprighting a molar with furcation involvement is guarded. In general, furcations are considered likely areas for recurrence of active bone loss from periodontitis. It is unwise to upright a molar and place a prosthesis in an area where the periodontium cannot be maintained. If an incipient furcation involvement is suspected, the patient should be referred for proper diagnosis, classification, and treatment. Furcation care is complex and requires regular periodontal maintenance during the orthodontic procedure.

E   If an edentulous space opposes the molar(s) to be uprighted, serious thought must be given as to the justification for an uprighting procedure. It is possible that either mesial or distal movement of the uprighted molar(s) may establish an opposing occlusion. Restoration of opposing edentulous areas requires a complete prosthetic evaluation and treatment plan.

F   If uprighting moves the tooth out of occlusion, a mesial-distal adjustment may be necessary to maintain contact with the opposing dentition. Such adjustments may be easily accomplished but often dictate the need for a more comprehensive course of orthodontic treatment.

G   Numerous techniques for molar uprighting or space closure have been presented in the literature. A typical segmental uprighting appliance is shown in Fig. 79-1.

The primary mechanical consideration is that control of the vertical extrusion of an uprighted tooth requires significant anchorage requirements, and therefore bonding or banding of additional teeth is obviously necessary. Use of cross-arch stabilization via a lingual or transpalatal arch is often needed.

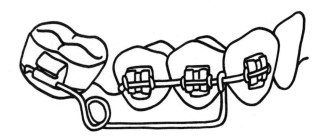

Fig. 79-1 Typical segmental uprighting appliance.

†Deceased.

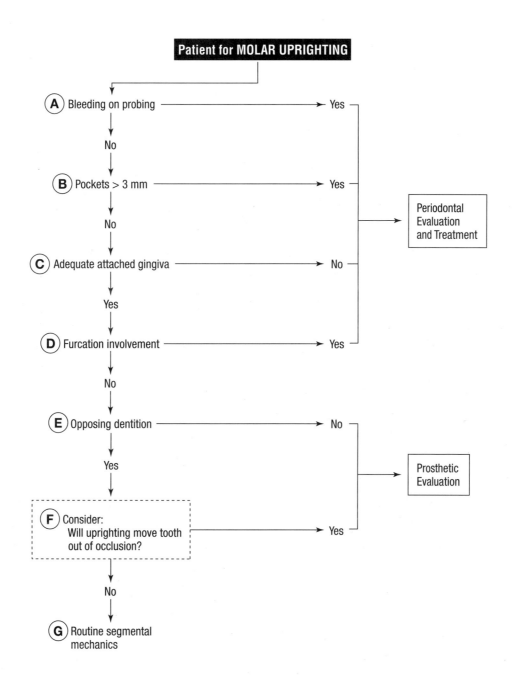

Patient for MOLAR UPRIGHTING

A Bleeding on probing ──────► Yes

No

B Pockets > 3 mm ──────► Yes

No

C Adequate attached gingiva ──────► No

Yes

D Furcation involvement ──────► Yes

No

E Opposing dentition ──────► No

Yes

F Consider:
Will uprighting move tooth
out of occlusion? ──────► Yes

No

G Routine segmental
mechanics

Periodontal
Evaluation
and Treatment

Prosthetic
Evaluation

References

Hall WB: *Decision making in periodontology,* Philadelphia, 1988, Mosby.
Moyers RE: *Handbook of orthodontics,* ed 4, Chicago, 1988, Mosby.
Proffit WR: *Contemporary orthodontics,* ed 2, St Louis, 1993, Mosby, p 558.

Roberts WE, Marshall KJ, Mozsary PG: Rigid endosseous implant utilized as anchorage to protract molars and close an atrophic extraction site, *Angle Orthod* 60:135, 1990.

80 Nonrestorable Space in the Maxilla

David B. Clark

Occasionally, patients have nonrestorable space in the maxillary arch. Generally, this space is insufficient for the placement of a pontic and yet too large to allow space closure through modest overcontouring of proximal contacts. Space problems develop as a result of early tooth loss, congenitally missing teeth, and tooth size anomalies. The permanent first molar is frequently lost to caries or periodontal disease. This often results in considerable mesial drift of the second and third molars while the premolars drift distally. Anteriorly, incisors are frequently lost as a result of trauma. Maxillary lateral incisors are among the teeth most often diminished in size, "peg shaped," or congenitally missing. Unmanaged space frequently leads to undesirable tipping, rotating, and drifting of teeth.

A The first consideration in management of maxillary anterior space is whether adequate overjet exists to allow for complete space closure. Inadequate overjet necessitates management of the space rather than space closure. A diagnostic setup should be used to determine the most ideal occlusion.

B Midline deviations are an important consideration. Once the best occlusion is determined, the specific tooth movements dictate if space should be opened for a pontic or equalized on the mesial and distal surfaces of one or several teeth. Several small interproximal spaces are often easier to restore than a large asymmetric one.

C Midline deviations and posterior dental symmetry should be considered conjointly when adequate overjet exists for space closure. Unilateral space closure may result in a midline deviation. A diagnostic setup is indicated to assess the optimum occlusion. Midline deviations toward the space usually worsen with space closure. A midline deviation away from the space may improve with space closure. In all cases a change in posterior symmetry involves consideration of interarch occlusal relationships.

D The first decision for management of posterior space involves posterior crown tipping. Uprighting molars facilitates oral hygiene, reduces mesial pseudopockets, and allows advantageous remodeling of the alveolar process. A diagnostic setup helps differentiate treatment options: (1) establishing a space the width of the missing tooth, (2) opening space less than the width of the missing tooth, (3) completing the space closure, or (4) equalizing the space mesially and distally for proximal restoration.

E Crossbites or rotations complicate treatment and may be difficult to retain. Comprehensive treatment is required to correct *skeletal crossbites*. Dental crossbites may be corrected orthodontically. Crossbite and rotation correction is often indicated for preprosthetic alignments.

F If the space is 1 mm or less and cannot be closed, equalizing space on the mesial and distal surfaces for restoration of proximal contacts should be considered. This option may also be viable for spaces greater than 1 mm if indicated by the diagnostic setup.

G Treatment options include: (1) space closure and retention, (2) reopening of the space for restoration with a fixed or removable partial denture, or (3) equalizing the space on the mesial and distal surfaces and restoring the proximal contacts. In most cases treatment is best performed with fixed appliances. Space closure is usually the most challenging technically and may involve comprehensive treatment. Conversely, opening space can often be accomplished with limited appliances. Alveolar ridge atrophy is unfavorable for space closure.

References

Moyers RE: *Handbook of orthodontics,* ed 4, Chicago, 1988, Mosby, pp 74, 233.
Proffit WR: *Contemporary orthodontics,* ed 2, St Louis, 1993, Mosby, pp 219, 553.

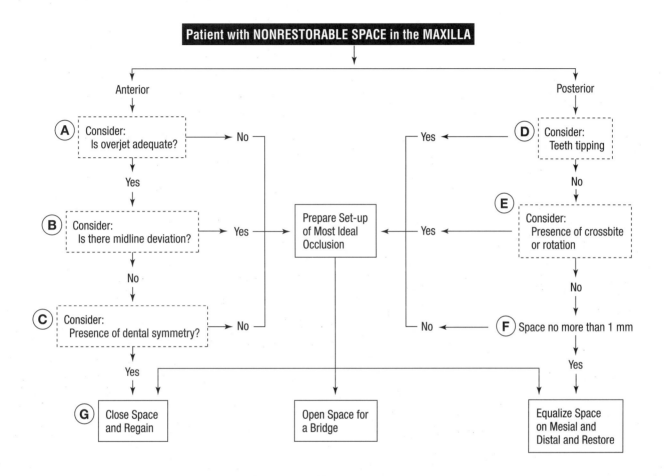

Patient with NONRESTORABLE SPACE in the MAXILLA

Anterior

Posterior

A · Consider: Is overjet adequate? → No

Yes

D · Consider: Teeth tipping → Yes

No

B · Consider: Is there midline deviation? → Yes

No

Prepare Set-up of Most Ideal Occlusion ← Yes

E · Consider: Presence of crossbite or rotation → Yes

No

C · Consider: Presence of dental symmetry? → No

Yes

F · Space no more than 1 mm → No

Yes

G · Close Space and Regain

Open Space for a Bridge

Equalize Space on Mesial and Distal and Restore

81 Edentulous Spaces in the Mandibular Posterior Segments

W. Eugene Roberts

Because of the decline in the incidence of caries and periodontal disease, the number of partially edentulous, but otherwise dentally healthy, adults is rapidly increasing. The most common missing teeth in the mandibular (Md) arch are first and second molars, respectively. Many patients delay definitive treatment, so adjacent teeth drift into a substantially compromised occlusion. Optimal restoration of esthetics and function is complicated by the following: (1) tipping of abutments into the extraction site, (2) extrusion of maxillary (Mx) molars into potential pontic space, (3) occlusal overload of the residual dentition, and (4) long-term hygiene problems. Preprosthetic alignment of abutments and occlusal antagonists is usually necessary. With a relatively modest extension of the treatment plan, orthodontic space closure is often a viable option.

Many patients with posterior missing teeth are adolescents or young adults. Based on average life expectancy, the functional service requirement for a restoration of occlusion is more than 50 years. Because of mechanical problems, secondary caries, and periodontal compromises, a routine "bridge" or more properly a fixed partial denture (FPD) often fails within 10 years in the mechanically challenging Md posterior segments. Replacing a FPD is usually a difficult and expensive problem because of deterioration of abutments and their periodontal support. If residual molars are present in the affected quadrant, orthodontics is a highly cost-effective option, compared with a series of increasingly compromised prostheses.

Treatment options for management of a Md first molar extraction site include: (1) three-unit FPD, (2) implant-supported single tooth replacement, and (3) orthodontic space closure. A removable partial denture (RPD) for restoration of a Md first molar extraction site is rarely indicated. Opposing an intact Mx arch, orthodontic space closure is a viable option if the third molar is present in the affected quadrant. However, space closure may still be the treatment of choice if there is only one opposing Mx molar. Because of heavy loading and hygiene problems during a lifetime, the orthodontic solution is functionally superior to prosthetics. No prosthesis can match well-aligned, healthy, natural teeth in optimal occlusion. Closing an 8- to 10-mm permanent molar extraction site usually requires approximately 24 months. This is not a disadvantage if preprosthetic orthodontics is necessary anyway; however, space closure should be initiated early in treatment to avoid extending the overall treatment time. After the implant is placed, an optimally positioned cuspid or premolar anterior to the extraction site is stabilized with an anchorage wire extending from the retromolar implant. Segmental uprighting and space closure is initiated as the first step in orthodontic treatment. A significant advantage for orthodontic space closure is that it is more likely to be a permanent solution to the problem.

A Adequacy of the dentition distal to the first or second molar extraction site is the initial consideration. Assuming the Mx first and second molars are present and in Class I occlusion, an adequate third molar on the affected side is necessary for an optimal orthodontic result.

B The key diagnostic questions are the following:
1. Is the third molar present?
2. If so, is it accessible for orthodontics?
3. If not, is it salvageable by uncovering, uprighting, or repositioning?

In the absence of an adequate third molar for exercising the orthodontic option, implant-supported or conventional prosthodontics to restore the missing molar is indicated. If only one Mx molar is present, and it is in or can be moved to the first molar position, a single molar terminal occlusion may be indicated.

C Adequate anchorage for conventional orthodontic space closure is the next consideration. Because molar spaces are usually greater than or equal to 10 mm, it is rarely possible to close the space without producing a skewing of the arch, deviation of the midline, and asymmetric occlusion. In the exceptional circumstance that adequate anchorage is available for an acceptable result (e.g., Class III cuspid, crowded Md incisors, anterior crossbite, favorable midline deviation), conventional orthodontics is indicated. In the absence of adequate anchorage, an orthodontically dedicated implant is a viable option.

D An adequate site for placing the implant outside the arch is the next consideration. The implant is usually placed in the retromolar fossa approximately 5 mm distal to the third molar; however, it is possible to use the medial aspect of the external oblique ridge or the ascending ramus as alternate sites. The retromolar site is preferred because complete space closure is precluded by placing the implant in the extraction site. The retromolar implant mechanism is also effective for aligning mesially tipped Md molars to serve as FPD abutments (Fig. 81-1).

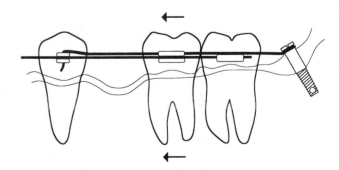

Fig. 81-1 Sagittal view of implant anchored orthodontic mechanism to achieve mesial space closure of second and third molars into a first molar extraction site. (From Roberts WE, Garetto LP, Katona TR: Principles of orthodontic biomechanics: metabolic and mechanical control mechanisms. In Carlson DS, Goldstein SA, editors: *Bone biodynamics in orthodontic and orthopedic treatment,* Ann Arbor, 1992, Center for Human Growth and Development.)

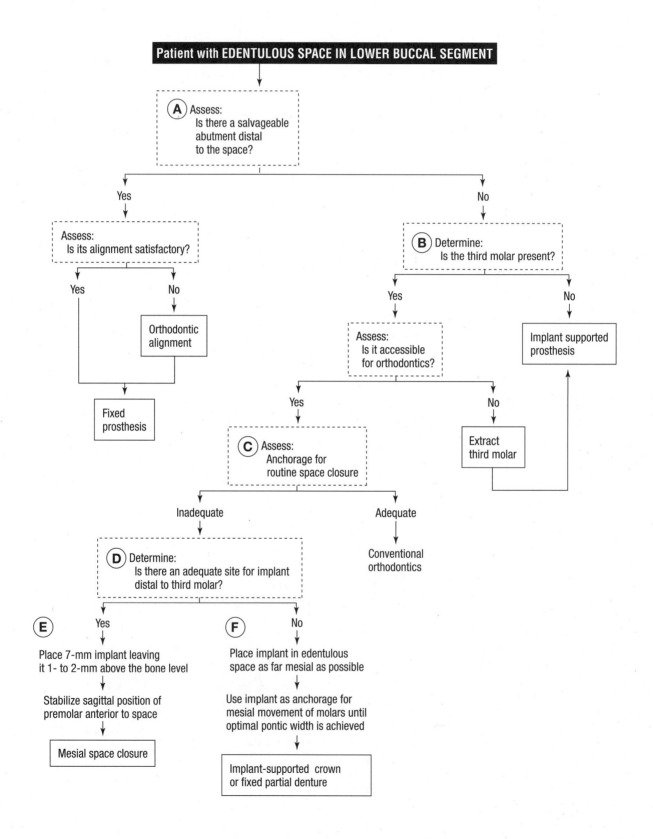

Patient with EDENTULOUS SPACE IN LOWER BUCCAL SEGMENT

A Assess:
Is there a salvageable abutment distal to the space?

Yes

Assess:
Is its alignment satisfactory?

Yes No

Orthodontic alignment

Fixed prosthesis

No

B Determine:
Is the third molar present?

Yes

Assess:
Is it accessible for orthodontics?

Yes

C Assess:
Anchorage for routine space closure

Inadequate

D Determine:
Is there an adequate site for implant distal to third molar?

E Yes

Place 7-mm implant leaving it 1- to 2-mm above the bone level

Stabilize sagittal position of premolar anterior to space

Mesial space closure

F No

Place implant in edentulous space as far mesial as possible

Use implant as anchorage for mesial movement of molars until optimal pontic width is achieved

Implant-supported crown or fixed partial denture

Adequate

Conventional orthodontics

No

Extract third molar

No

Implant supported prosthesis

E A 7.00 × 3.75 mm titanium implant (e.g., Nobel Biocare) is adequate for orthodontic anchorage. The implant should have a flat top for attachment of the anchorage wire with a cover screw. A longer implant is unnecessary and may impinge on the inferior alveolar nerve. The site is prepared with a 3.15-mm twist drill, and the implant is inserted as a self-tapping fixture. The implant is screwed into the site until the cervical flange contacts the periosteal surface. Thread engagement of the 2- to 3-mm thick cortical bone is the objective; countersinking of the implant in thin cortical bone may lead to instability. Because the indirect anchorage mechanism on a submerged implant delivers a relatively light load to the abutment, a healing phase before initiating orthodontic treatment is unnecessary. If the retromolar implant is in occlusion, a routine healing sequence of 4 months is needed before placing a prosthesis. At the initial surgery, the titanium alloy anchorage wire is attached directly to the endosseous base with a standard cover screw. An anchorage wire, extending from the abutment, is used to stabilize the sagittal position of the premolar anterior relative to the edentulous space (Fig. 81-2). Translation mechanics across the edentulous space results in unidirectional space closure (i.e., molars moving mesially to eliminate the space). Detailed discussions of the mechanics and physiologic rationale are in the literature.

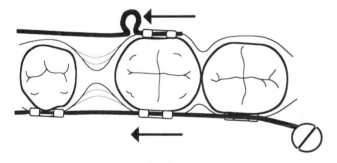

Fig. 81-2 Occlusal view of the implant anchored orthodontic mechanism shown in Fig. 81-1 demonstrates shielding of the periosteal surface to achieve space closure of an atrophic ridge. (From Roberts WE, Garetto LP, Katona TR: Principles of orthodontic biomechanics: metabolic and mechanical control mechanisms. In Carlson DS, Goldstein SA, editors: *Bone biodynamics in orthodontic and orthopedic treatment,* Ann Arbor, 1992, Center for Human Growth and Development.)

F In the event complete space closure is undesirable, orthodontic alignment of the distal abutment with or without some space closure may be indicated to decrease the mechanical demands on the subsequent FPD. To exercise this option, place the implant in the edentulous space as far mesially as possible. After a 4-month healing interval, the transmucosal abutment and a temporary, single tooth replacement prosthesis are placed. The implant-supported prosthesis is then used as anchorage for mesial movement of the molars. Once an optimal pontic width with acceptable opposing occlusion is achieved, there are two options for restoring the residual space: (1) place a single tooth implant-supported prosthesis or (2) remove the implant, cover the site with soft tissue, and restore with a conventional FPD. For the long-term, a relatively short-span FPD may be superior to an implant-supported prosthesis. Heavy occlusal loading during a lifetime may contribute to fatigue failure of the implant, prosthetic components, or supporting bone.

In summary, rigid (osseointegrated) bone fixtures offer a broad range of orthodontic possibilities for enhancing the long-term dental health of partially edentulous patients. Missing Md first molars are the most common application of implant anchorage to close space, but similar methods can be applied for other missing teeth in both arches. The most ideal use of an implant may be as an orthodontic anchorage to reposition the residual teeth for optimal esthetics and function.

References

Cronin RJ, Cagna DR: An update on fixed prosthodontics, *J Am Dent Assoc* 128:425, 1997.

Roberts WE: Bone physiology, metabolism, and biomechanics in orthodontic practice. In Graber TM, Vanarsdall, Jr, RL, editors: *Orthodontics: current principles and techniques,* ed 2, St Louis, 1994, Mosby, p 193.

Roberts WE: Adjunctive orthodontic therapy in adults over 50 years of age, *J Indiana Dent Assoc* 33, 1997.

Roberts WE, Nelson CL, Goodacre CJ: Rigid implant anchorage to close a mandibular first molar extraction site, *J Clin Orthod* 28:693, 1994.

Roberts WE, Arbuckle GR, Analoui M: Rate of mesial translation of mandibular molars utilizing implant-anchored mechanics, *Angle Orthod* 66:331, 1996.

82 Flared Maxillary Incisors

James J. Baldwin, †Gordon R. Arbuckle, William F. Hohlt

The esthetic problem of flared or spaced maxillary (Mx) incisors is a common concern of both adults and adolescents. Successful orthodontic correction of dentofacial form and function requires careful attention to the periodontium and perioral musculature. Both are important considerations in determining the etiology of the condition and its potential for correction. The position of the dentition is dictated by the biomechanic environment: occlusion, posture of the perioral musculature, swallowing patterns, and persistent habits. An abnormal biomechanic equilibrium, associated with a progressive loss of periodontal support, may result in pathologic drifting and migration of teeth. The practitioner must carefully evaluate the entire health picture of the patient in establishing an appropriate diagnosis. Treatment planning is directed at eliminating the etiology of the problem. The therapeutic goal is to establish a new, relatively stable incisor position that is consistent with the esthetic and functional desires of the patient. Maintenance of the desired result may require both orthodontics and behavior modification to establish a more ideal soft tissue equilibrium.

A   A comprehensive assessment of the patient's periodontal status is the initial consideration. From a routine orthodontic perspective, bleeding on probing is a reliable indicator of gingival inflammation that requires periodontal evaluation and treatment. Pocket depths in excess of 3 mm should be assessed before tooth movement. Modest recession (<2 mm) does not contraindicate orthodontics, but greater recession in the presence of minimal attached gingiva requires careful evaluation. Areas with less than 2 mm of keratinized gingiva are considered a potential problem and should be managed before orthodontic therapy is initiated. A tooth with less than 1 mm of attached gingiva is considered a candidate for grafting. Radiographic evidence of significant alveolar bone defects requires a complete periodontal evaluation before tooth movement. Once the inflammatory disease process is controlled, periodontally compromised teeth can be moved orthodontically. However, control of extrusion usually requires relatively light forces delivered with fixed appliances. Improving alignment and occlusion of periodontally compromised teeth can substantially benefit oral health.

B   Elimination of pernicious habits is essential to long-term success. Improper lip or tongue posture, thumbsucking, and pencil or pen biting are the most common disorders; however, many persistent postural problems (while sleeping or awake) can adversely affect the position of the teeth. A careful differential diagnosis is needed to establish the probable etiology so that specific orthodontic and behavior modification therapy can be designed. For example, flared Mx incisors with an anterior open bite may be secondary to interincisal tongue posture. An effective series of postural modification exercises begins with instructing the patient to find the anterior palatal rugae with the tip of the tongue and then swallowing while the tongue maintains contact with the rugae. The second exercise is to place a small piece of

candy or a mint on the dorsum of the tongue, instruct the patient to press the mint against the roof of the mouth, and then swallow with the tongue elevated as the mint dissolves. The third exercise is for the patient to use a hand mirror to demonstrate the normal tongue posture learned from the first two exercises. Tongue posture should be constantly monitored by the patient, who must understand that the success of the treatment depends on establishing and maintaining a normal soft tissue environment. Finally, *instruct the patient that the tongue is never postured between the teeth*. Although this latter command would appear to be all that is necessary, behavior modification is more effective as a series of finite steps with limited objectives.

C   Mandibular (Md) lip biting and posturing of the lip between the Mx and Md incisors ("lip trap") are common pernicious habits associated with incisal flaring. Reversal of these muscular imbalances is achieved by initiating lip posture exercises to position the Md lip anterior to the incisal edges of the Mx incisors. Lip posture training should be pursued progressively as the flared incisors are retracted orthodontically. Md lip posture on the labial surface of the Mx incisors creates a soft tissue equilibrium that aids in the correction of the problem and helps insure long-term stability of the result.

D   Increased overjet may be related to a discrepancy in tooth size between the Mx and Md incisors in an otherwise Class I occlusion. An anatomic tendency for overjet predisposes the patient to a lip-tongue seal during swallowing that is often associated with an interincisal posture of the Md lip. Reliable correction of this form of "flared incisors" necessitates both correction of the lip habit and reduction of the residual overjet. The latter requires intermaxillary treatment such as: (1) interproximal reduction (enamel stripping) of the Mx incisors or (2) creation of interproximal spaces between the Md incisors. Restorative resin can be used to close the interproximal spaces and achieve the desired tooth size. In a similar fashion, malformed teeth such as pegged or missing lateral incisors require a treatment plan that leaves adequate space for esthetic restorations or replacements. To properly assess such problems, a Bolton tooth size analysis is indicated followed by an orthodontic wax setup to evaluate therapeutic alternatives. A prosthetic evaluation is indicated when contemplating prostheses, esthetic bonding, or anterior laminates.

E   Flaring of the Mx incisors is often associated with occlusal compensations such as extrusion of Mx or Md incisors. Posterior tipping with a removable appliance is rarely a viable option because a lack of vertical control results in extruded incisors and excessive overbite. Fixed appliances are more effective because the vertical position and axial inclination of the incisors can be controlled as they are retracted. However, it is important to secure adequate anchorage, which usually requires a full fixed appliance from first molar to first molar.

---

†Deceased.

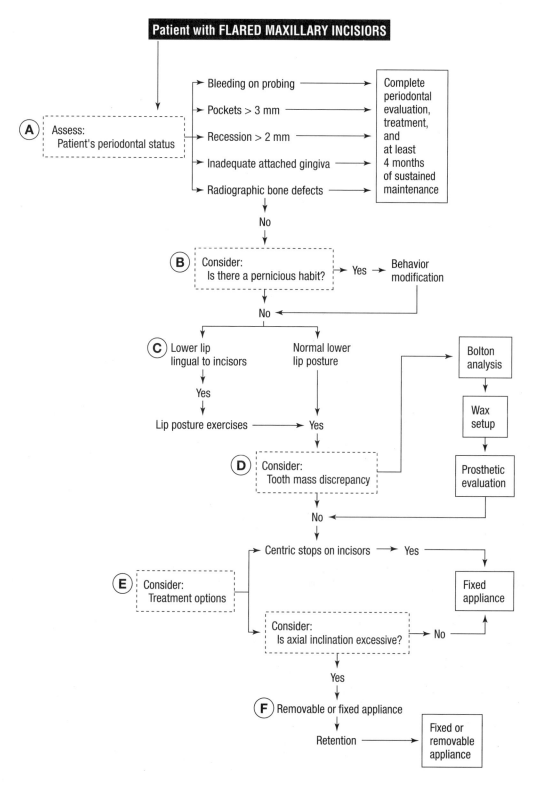

Patient with FLARED MAXILLARY INCISORS

F The stability of completed treatment depends on the accuracy of the diagnosis and the success in eliminating the specific etiology. Unresolved pernicious habits or tooth size discrepancies favor a return to the original malocclusion. With ideal alignment of the incisors and appropriate muscular equilibrium, the usual period of removable retention is approximately 6 months full time and nights only indefinitely. A permanent, fixed lingual retainer may be required to maintain the closure of diastemas.

References

Bolton WA: The clinical application of a tooth-size analysis, *Am J Orthod* 48:504, 1962.

Proffit WR: *Contemporary orthodontics,* ed 2, St Louis, 1993, Mosby, p 576.

Roberts WE: Bone physiology, metabolism and biomechanics in orthodontic practice. In Graber TM, Vanarsdall, Jr, RL, editors: *Orthodontics: current principles and techniques,* ed 2, St Louis, 1994, Mosby, p 193.

Vanarsdall, Jr, RL: Periodontal/orthodontic interrelationships. In Graber TM, Vanarsdall, Jr, RL, editors: *Orthodontics: current principles and techniques,* ed 2, St Louis, 1994, Mosby, p 712.

83 Orthodontic Crown Lengthening of a Fractured Tooth

William F. Hohlt

Trauma frequently fractures a natural tooth so that the remaining root surface is partially or completely below the crest of alveolar bone. Restorations requiring subcrestal finishing lines have been accomplished by using invasive flap procedures with subsequent removal of crestal alveolar bone below the intended finishing line. An alternative (usually more esthetic) approach is to orthodontically extrude the tooth to the point where the finish line is exposed. Extending crown preparations on extruded teeth helps prevent retentive failure and allows redevelopment of the 2-mm biologic width of attached gingiva. Restorative materials that impinge on the biologic width induce inflammation and periodontal pocket formation.

How far to extrude a tooth relates to its final use. For single crown restorations without a post and core, the projected crown length should not exceed the root length in bone. If a post and core restoration is planned, the projected crown length should equal the post length inserted into the tooth root. Ideal crown-to-root ratios are 1:1.5 or more, but as little as 1:1 is acceptable. When healthy teeth are extruded, the entire alveolar process follows in the direction of eruption. Light eruptive forces promote formation of crestal bone while strong eruptive forces cause supracrestal fiber tearing, and little or no bone is formed.

A In the absence of a subgingival fracture line or other defect that is likely to create a biologic width problem, the tooth should be restored without orthodontic extrusion. If any portion of the fractured root is within 2 mm of the alveolar bone crest, a partial periodontic crown lengthening procedure can be performed if there is adequate attached gingiva and the area is not esthetically sensitive. For oblique fractures with a fracture line that is at or below the alveolar crest, the best alternative is orthodontic extrusion.

B In cases where the tooth needing extrusion has had previous endodontic treatment, a small fabricated eyelet can be inserted in the prepared pulp canal and cemented in place with Durelon (ESPE, D-8301). The eyelet is constructed from 0.020-inch stainless steel wire in such a way as to have a corkscrew appearance. Alternatively, small cross members welded onto the axial wire also provide resistance from dislodgment. In cases where there is neither enamel to bond an appliance or no pulp canal for insertion of an eyelet, an attachment can be improvised using a custom-pinched band or temporary casting.

C Anchorage is defined as resistance to unwanted tooth movement. In general, extrusive movement occurs more quickly than intrusive movement; nevertheless, sound anchorage requirements must be observed to eliminate undesirable side effects. For extrusion of a single tooth, use adjacent anchorage units with two to three times the reactive root surface area. For example, two premolars and a canine are usually suitable anchorage to extrude a first molar. A central incisor is easily extruded using the adjacent central and both lateral incisors as anchorage units. A single osseointegrated implant is adequate anchorage for virtually any type of orthodontic tooth movement.

D Methods for extruding a fractured tooth may be simple, such as tying elastic thread between a tooth root and an anchor unit (wire bonded between adjacent teeth), or they may involve more sophisticated force systems. The method currently described requires little reactivation. It takes advantage of the torsion and bending properties of stainless steel wires to extrude teeth. The anchorage units are splinted together with a stiff rectangular wire, 0.018 × 0.025 inch (0.018-inch bracket slot), while the 0.014-inch erupting wire is tied in "piggyback" fashion to the heavier stabilizing segment. Fig. 83-1 demonstrates a spring designed to extrude a central incisor; note the 0.014-inch segment doubles back incisal to the bracket wings on teeth #7 and 10 to resist rotation. Fig. 83-2 demonstrates a common approach to premolar root extrusion where a rectangular loop configuration provides the eruptive force. The anchorage units are splinted together with a heavy rectangular arch wire. The active arch wire is attached to an auxiliary

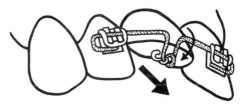

Fig. 83-1 Mechanics to extrude an incisor along its long axis.

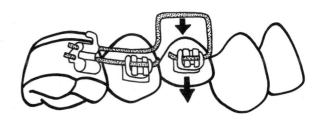

Fig. 83-2 Premolar extrusion to achieve a 1:1 crown-to-root ratio.

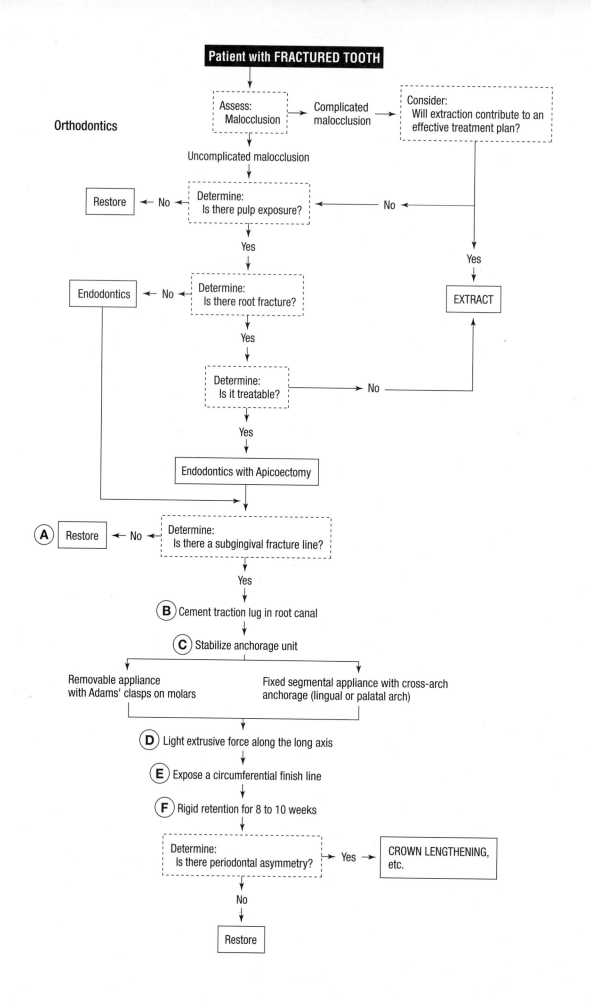

bracket tube on the first molar. Fig. 83-3 demonstrates extrusion of tooth #31 using teeth #30, 29, and 28 as anchorage units. A 0.014-inch round, stainless steel wire segment is fabricated so that the terminal segment of wire engages the bracket of tooth #28 by doubling back superior to the bracket wing. This doubled-back wire prevents the segment from rolling as the wire's other end is twisted and tied to the attachment of tooth #31. As the energy in the spring wire dissipates, the reactive end extrudes the molar root for the first 3 to 4 mm of the arc. It is wise to limit the activation of the wire to no more than 4 mm in case the patient fails to return for the scheduled adjustment 3 to 4 weeks later. Greater activation could result in excessive extrusion and buccal tipping.

E A selective supracrestal fiberotomy can be used to prevent crestal bone development in areas where the root should be extruded relative to the periodontium. If a tooth is fractured at the level of crestal bone, a supracrestal fiberotomy is advised to forcibly erupt the fractured root without stimulating crestal bone formation. If there is an oblique root fracture where part of the root is below the level of the crestal bone, a partial supracrestal fiberotomy should be performed on the root area that has normal attachment. Once

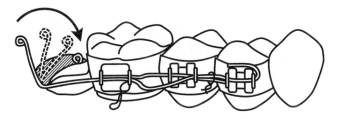

Fig. 83-3 Demonstration of how tooth extrudes for first 3° to 4° of arc. Note how erupting wire wraps back around occlusal of bracket wing on first premolar, providing resistance to torsion.

the oblique fractured root surface has erupted to the desired level of crestal bone, a weekly series of 360° fiberotomies can be performed. In cases involving oblique fractures, it is often necessary to equilibrate the erupting fragment if occlusal trauma is noted with the opposing arch. By severing the supracrestal fibers, the tooth root will quickly (in 3 to 4 weeks) extrude from the bone. When supracrestal fiberotomies are performed, archwire segments should be activated to ideal projected needs rather than be overactivated. Following a fiberotomy there is little resistance to tooth movement, and the tooth can be pulled out of its periodontal support.

F Once the tooth has been extruded satisfactorily, a brief stabilization period is needed. Activation should be discontinued and the tooth held in its new position for approximately 8 to 10 weeks. Stabilization can be achieved using either a passive wire or the deactivated extrusion spring. Initially, it is wise to place a temporary prosthesis because the extruded tooth may intrude somewhat. Once mobility returns to normal and the position of the tooth remains stable for an additional 8 to 10 weeks without retention, final restoration is indicated.

References

Dykema RW: *Johnson's modern practice in fixed prosthodontics,* ed 4, Philadelphia, 1986, WB Saunders, p 10.

Parma-Benfenati S, Fugazzoatto PA, Ruben MP: The effect of restorative margins on the postsurgical development and nature of the periodontium, Part 1, *Int J Periodont Restor Dent* 5(6):31, 1985.

Pontoriero R, Celenza F, Ricci G et al: Rapid extrusion with fiber resection: a combined orthodontic periodontic treatment modality, *Int J Periodont Restor Dent* 7(5):31, 1987.

Proffit WR: *Contemporary orthodontics,* ed 2, St Louis, 1993, Mosby, p 260.

Simons JHS, Kelly WH, Gordon DG et al: Extrusion of endodontically treated teeth, *J Am Dent Assoc* 97:17, 1978.

84 Orthodontics and Periodontal Needs

Timothy F. Geraci

The goal of orthodontic tooth movement in an adult is to improve both the periodontal and restorative environments. The adult orthodontic candidate who has preexisting periodontal involvement requires a dentist with critical diagnostic skills, rigid periodontal therapeutic skills, and a knowledge of the biomechanic movement of teeth. An adult has a static orthodontic environment; the growth period has been completed. Biomechanic intervention can either improve or worsen the periodontal status.

A When the oral hygiene level is not acceptable, the patient should not undergo orthodontic therapy. The inflammatory lesion must be controlled during orthodontic movement; otherwise, the case could be compromised or teeth lost as a result of the orthodontics. Thorough root planing and root débridement are basic preorthodontic requirements if pathology is present. Surgical intervention may be required to ensure clean roots or reduction of nonmaintainable pocket depth. A periodontal abscess during the active orthodontic phase can be disastrous.

B Interceptive mucogingival surgery should be performed in areas with potential problems. A compromised solution may result if the problem is not addressed until it is acute. Because of the position of the teeth in the alveolar housing, there may be a partial absence of bone over the facial or lingual root surface and a connective tissue attachment only. Failure to recognize this problem before treatment begins could result in severe root exposure during treatment or a tooth that is in a proper position but cannot be restored owing to lack of supporting bone.

C The patient's root form and length are important with respect to orthodontic suitability. Poor root form and length are unfavorable for orthodontic therapy.

D Teeth with preexisting furcation involvements of Class II or more are poor candidates for orthodontic movement. The chances of an abscess or increased bone loss are too great. The involved tooth may be endodontically treated and the root or roots removed if the tooth is critical to the case. A tooth with Class I furcation involvement requires the highest priority during orthodontic therapy, and it must be monitored and débrided constantly.

E Patients with preexisting crepitus, muscle tenderness, excessive occlusal wear, restricted mandibular opening, mandibular deviation on opening and closing, or subluxation of the mandible are not good candidates for orthodontic tooth movement. Their conditions may not improve with orthodontic treatment and, in fact, may worsen. Their dental findings should be documented before beginning tooth movement.

F If anterior teeth that have drifted labially and are going to be retracted to a functional position, sufficient overjet and overbite are required. Occlusal adjustment may be needed to place the mandible in a stable, retruded position. If a suitable overjet-overbite and stable occlusal position cannot be achieved, orthodontic movement is unfavorable. A diagnostic occlusal splint is indicated to determine if these objectives can be achieved.

G Before initiation of minor tooth movement procedures, the patient must be informed of the need to retain teeth in their new position via splinting or fixed bridgework and of the cost involved in restoring the case. If a tipped tooth is being placed in an upright position for fixed bridgework, occlusal reduction is required during treatment to gain space in an occlusal-apical direction for the tooth to move. Because of the "increase" in clinical crown during the uprighting and the reduction of the occlusal height to gain space, followed by crown preparation, a posterior tooth that has been uprighted may require an endodontic procedure (Figs. 84-1 and 84-2).

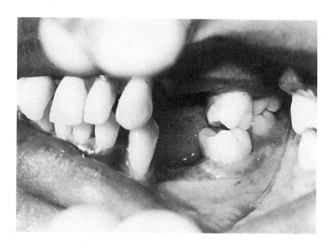

Fig. 84-1 Preoperative view of a tilted molar with a mesial osseous defect before uprighting.

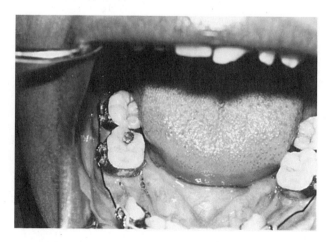

Fig. 84-2 The same teeth with the orthodontic appliance in place to bring the tilted teeth upright.

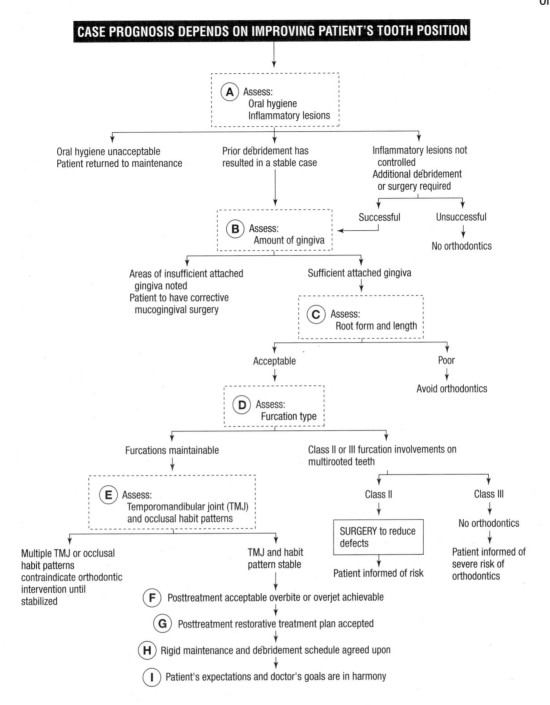

CASE PROGNOSIS DEPENDS ON IMPROVING PATIENT'S TOOTH POSITION

(A) Assess:
Oral hygiene
Inflammatory lesions

Oral hygiene unacceptable
Patient returned to maintenance

Prior débridement has
resulted in a stable case

Inflammatory lesions not
controlled
Additional débridement
or surgery required

Successful   Unsuccessful

No orthodontics

(B) Assess:
Amount of gingiva

Areas of insufficient attached
gingiva noted
Patient to have corrective
mucogingival surgery

Sufficient attached gingiva

(C) Assess:
Root form and length

Acceptable   Poor

Avoid orthodontics

(D) Assess:
Furcation type

Furcations maintainable

Class II or III furcation involvements on
multirooted teeth

Class II   Class III

SURGERY to reduce
defects

No orthodontics

Patient informed of risk

Patient informed of
severe risk of
orthodontics

(E) Assess:
Temporomandibular joint (TMJ)
and occlusal habit patterns

Multiple TMJ or occlusal
habit patterns
contraindicate orthodontic
intervention until
stabilized

TMJ and habit
pattern stable

(F) Posttreatment acceptable overbite or overjet achievable

(G) Posttreatment restorative treatment plan accepted

(H) Rigid maintenance and débridement schedule agreed upon

(I) Patient's expectations and doctor's goals are in harmony

H Because orthodontic tooth movement involves a breakdown of bone where pressure is applied and deposition of bone in areas of application of tension, the osseous topography of an area changes as a result of tooth movement. Infrabony defects can be reduced by deposition of bone on the tension side of the root and positioning of the root into an infrabony defect on the pressure side of the root. During the active phase of movement the roots should be débrided and the soft tissue lining the pockets curettaged every 2 weeks. As stated earlier, the inflammatory lesion must be controlled during the active phase. Constant débridement of an area increases the chances for reducing an infrabony defect and for successful resolution of a case. Patients with more severe infrabony lesions should be placed on a strict 3-month periodontal maintenance program during their orthodontic therapy.

I Finally, the patient should understand the objectives of minor tooth movement. The expectations of the patient and the goal of the doctor cannot be in conflict, and the dental objectives should be noted and discussed before treatment is initiated.

References

Lindhe J: *Clinical periodontology,* ed 2, Copenhagen, 1989, Munksgaard, p 564.

Sadowsky C, BeCole E: Long-term effects of orthodontic treatment on periodontal health, *Am J Orthod* 80:156, 1981.

Zachrisson B, Alnaes L: Periodontal conditions in orthodontically treated and untreated individuals, Part I, *Angle Orthod* 43:401, 1973.

Zachrisson B, Alnaes L: Periodontal conditions in orthodontically treated and untreated individuals, Part II, *Angle Orthod* 44:43, 1974.

85 Pure Mucogingival Concerns of Patients Scheduled for Orthodontics: A European View

Giovan Paolo Pini-Prato, Carlo Clauser, Giliana Zuccati

A Proper plaque control is crucial during orthodontic treatment. Orthodontic appliances are a factor in plaque retention; therefore the patient is required to use a more traumatic method of toothbrushing. Traumatic toothbrushing and plaque accumulation are etiologic factors for recession. Plaque removal may be impaired by anatomic (mucogingival) conditions. Pulling frena and shallow vestibules that affect toothbrushing should be corrected before orthodontic treatment.

B Deep intraosseus impacted teeth (usually upper canines) can be orthodontically guided to erupt in the center of the alveolar crest (where adequate keratinized tissue is physiologically available), thereby preventing mucogingival problems. A full-thickness flap must be raised to bind an attaching device to the tooth to achieve this goal. The flap is finally repositioned into its place and the traction chain remains submucosal. In the case of a persistent deciduous canine, its empty socket can be used as a path for the traction chain *(tunnel traction)* (Fig. 85-1).

C Teeth that erupt buccally entrap and destroy the gingiva between the erupting cusp and deciduous tooth (Fig. 85-2). It can be saved and used as donor material to create a satisfactory width of gingiva for the permanent tooth.

D The donor site for interceptive surgery is the area between the erupting cusp and deciduous tooth. The recipient site is the area immediately apical to the erupting cusp. A flap with two horizontal gingival pedicles is indicated if the tip of a cusp is erupting at the level of the mucogingival junction (MGJ) (see Fig. 85-2). An apically positioned flap with vertical releasing incisions or a free graft of the entrapped gingiva is indicated if the cusp is erupting apical to the MGJ.

E An appreciable amount of gingiva is needed to withstand effective toothbrushing and prevent recession in young orthodontic patients. The risk of recession is greater if the gingiva is thin and narrow and the tooth has to be moved buccally. In case of actual recession, reconstructive surgery is indicated (Fig. 85-3).

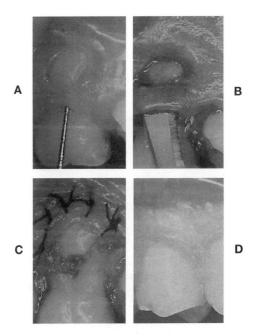

Fig. 85-2 **A,** A maxillary right premolar is erupting buccally. The buccal gingiva remains entrapped between the erupting cusp and the deciduous tooth. **B,** The entrapped gingiva is dissected and displaced apically (bipedicle flap). **C,** Sutures. **D,** Healing after 2 years.

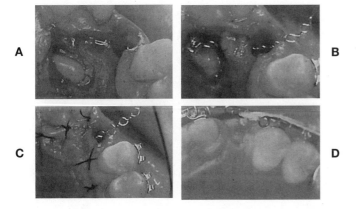

Fig. 85-1 **A,** A full-thickness palatal flap has been raised to expose the cusp of an impacted maxillary left canine. **B,** Submucosal traction. A hand-made chain is fixed to the cusp of the canine and passed through the empty socket of the deciduous canine. **C,** The flap is sutured. **D,** The permanent impacted canine is erupting at the center of the alveolar ridge. (Courtesy Dr. A. Crescini.)

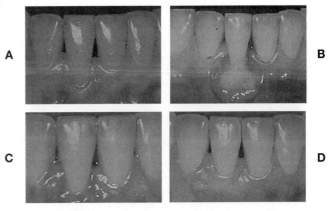

Fig. 85-3 A recession on a mandibular central incisor is treated by free gingival graft before orthodontic treatment.

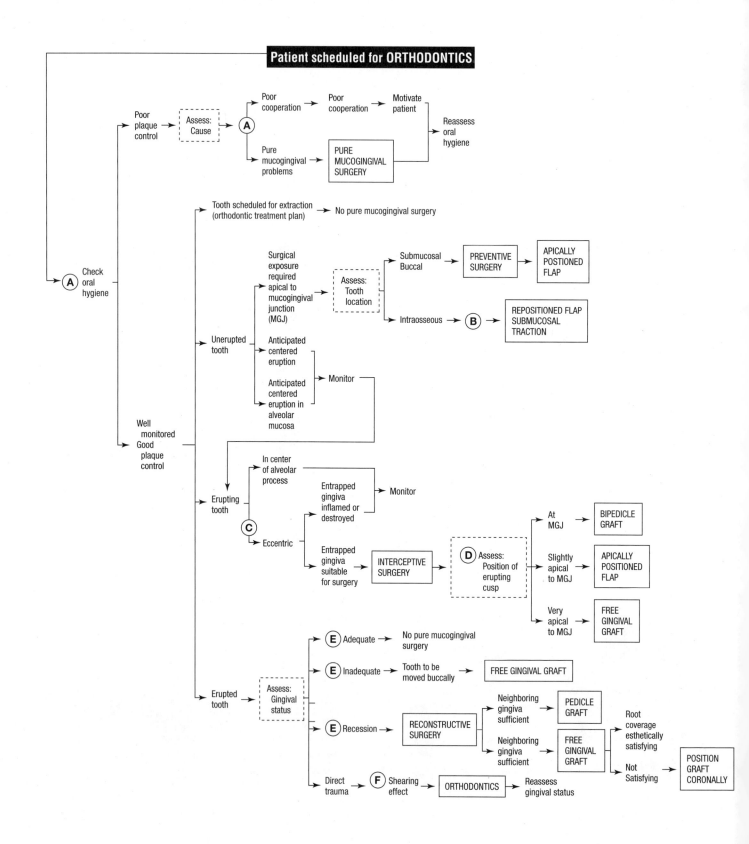

Patient scheduled for ORTHODONTICS

F Direct mechanical trauma to the gingiva is most often observed in Class II, division 2 malocclusion. It cannot be cured by means of periodontal surgery and requires orthodontic treatment before any mucogingival procedure.

References

Agudio G et al: Mucogingival interceptive therapy, *Int J Periodont Restor Dent* 5:49, 1985.

Coatoam GW, Beherents RG, Bissada N: The width of keratinized gingiva during orthodontic treatment: its significance and impact on periodontal status, *J Periodontol* 52:307, 1981.

Crescini A, Pini-Prato GP: Trattamento combinato del canino incluso: tecnica del doppio arco, *Dental Cadmos* 56:19, 1988.

Hall WB: Gingival augmentation/mucogingival surgery. In American Academy of Periodontology: *Proceedings of the world workshop in clinical periodontics*, Chicago, 1989, American Academy of Periodontology, pp VII-1.

Maynard G, Ochsenbein C: Mucogingival problems: prevalence and therapy in children, *J Periodontol* 46:543, 1975.

86 Treatment Planning the Restoration of the Partially Edentulous Dentition

W. Eugene Roberts

Restoration of optimal esthetics and function, consistent with a favorable long-term prognosis, are the principal goals for management of partial edentulousness. Because many patients needing comprehensive treatment have a poor history of timely dental care, the residual teeth may have extruded and drifted into a severe, unrestorable malocclusion. Cost-effective conservation of healthy teeth usually requires adjunctive orthodontic therapy, integrated into a comprehensive treatment plan. In the absence of orthodontics, poorly positioned teeth must be extracted, or endodontically treated and severely reduced to serve as prosthetic abutments. For substantial malocclusions, preprosthetic orthodontics is often the most cost effective and reliable option.

Alignment of abutments, management of edentulous space and enhancement of soft tissue contours are important preprosthetic objectives. Osseointegrated dental implants provide occlusal stops to correct the vertical dimension of occlusion (VDO) and serve as rigid anchorage for three-dimensional orthodontic alignment of the residual dentition. Carefully coordinated preprosthetic treatment to establish bilateral posterior occlusion (molars or implants) is an important goal for achieving a biomechanically-optimized restoration of occlusion (Fig. 86-1).

A Adequacy of the residual dentition is the initial consideration in planning the restoration of oral esthetics and function. If the health and prosthetic potential of the remaining dentition is inadequate to support fixed prostheses, the expecta-

tions of the patient must be reconciled with a more realistic treatment plan such as full dentures or overdentures. If fixed prostheses are the patient's preference, implants can be used to augment natural abutments. Adequate support (natural teeth and implants) and acceptable restorable spaces must be present or attainable in all four quadrants.

B If the residual dentition is adequate, the next issue is the alignment of the teeth relative to the edentulous spaces. In the event the teeth are adequately aligned and residual spaces are appropriate, proceed with conventional prosthetics. If the alignment of the teeth and pontic spaces are inadequate, adjunctive orthodontics is indicated (see Fig. 86-1).

C In considering the orthodontic option, determine if there is adequate intraoral or realistic extraoral anchorage in all three dimensions to achieve an appropriate preprosthetic alignment. If so, proceed with an orthodontic treatment plan. If not, consider the use of osseointegrated implants for supplemental orthodontic anchorage or for restoration of the VDO (Fig. 86-2).

D Once adequate anchorage is in place and the VDO is restored, consider if the abutments (implants and natural teeth) are adequately positioned. If so, proceed to conventional prosthetics. If not, an adjunctive orthodontic treatment plan is indicated.

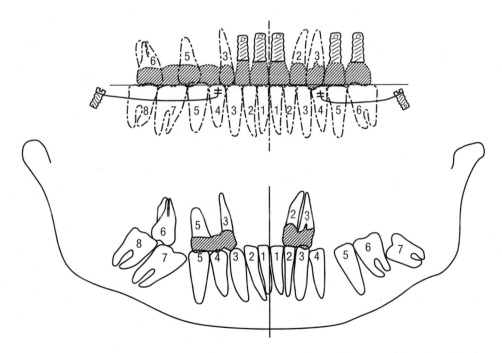

Fig. 86-1 The panoramic visual treatment objective (top) is a schematic drawing of the projected occlusion resulting from orthodontic alignment of the residual dentition and construction of desired prostheses. A tracing of the pretreatment panoramic radiograph is shown below.

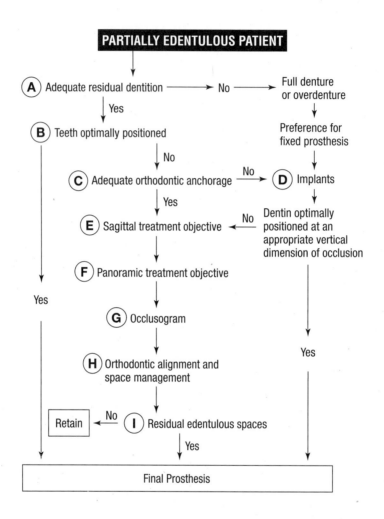

PARTIALLY EDENTULOUS PATIENT

A Adequate residual dentition — No → Full denture or overdenture

Yes ↓

B Teeth optimally positioned

No ↓

C Adequate orthodontic anchorage — No → **D** Implants

Yes ↓

E Sagittal treatment objective ← No — Dentin optimally positioned at an appropriate vertical dimension of occlusion

↓

F Panoramic treatment objective

↓

G Occlusogram

↓

H Orthodontic alignment and space management

↓

Retain ← No — **I** Residual edentulous spaces

Yes ↓

Yes

Final Prosthesis

E The sagittal treatment objective—to determine the VDO and desired position of the incisors—is derived from a cephalometric tracing. The facial profile and intermaxillary relationship of the jaws can be modified with orthognathic surgery, orthodontics, orthotics ("splints"), or prostheses. For this discussion, the most common problem is overclosure of the mandible, secondary to loss of posterior occlusal stops. As illustrated in Fig. 86-2, optimization of lip morphology (competence and protrusion) is the guide for "hinging" the mandible open to the desired VDO. For the case illustrated, a maxillary (Mx) anterior implant-supported prosthesis is positioned in the desired relationship with the mandibular (Md) incisors to establish a VDO consistent with adequate support for the lips. The incisal edge of Mx incisors is usually approximately 3 mm below the Mx lip. However, most Mx anterior fixed prostheses are more esthetic with an incisal exposure of only 0 to 1 mm. Before committing to the final prosthesis, the VDO is opened with reversible procedures (temporary fixed prostheses, occlusal orthotics).

F The panoramic treatment objective is derived from tracings of the pretreatment panoramic radiograph (see Fig. 86-1). Relative to the midline and a flat occlusal plane, the residual dentition is diagrammatically aligned to plan interdigitation, implant placement, pontic positions, and anchorage control (see Fig. 86-1). Because of the inherent distortion of panoramic films, these tracings are of limited usefulness for assessing the direction and distance that teeth are to be moved.

G Occlusograms are an occlusal treatment objective based on 1:1 tracings of all teeth and prostheses in the occlusal plane (Fig. 86-3). The occlusal view of all teeth are traced with standard cephalometric acetate from photographs or photocopies of the pretreatment casts at 1x magnification. The desired intermaxillary arch form is constructed through the most buccal-centric occlusal stops for the mandible (labial of the incisors and buccal cusp tips) and maxilla (lingual of the incisors and central fossae). For anterior-posterior reference, transverse lines (perpendicular to the midline) are drawn through the cusp tips of the cuspids and the mesial surface of the first molars. All natural and prosthetically restored teeth are traced in optimal position along the arch form for each arch. The best estimate of the direction and distance teeth must be moved is derived from superimposed cephalometric (see Fig. 86-2) and occlusogram (Fig. 86-3) tracings, comparing the original with the optimal positions.

H Orthodontic alignment in three dimensions is accomplished according to the planned objectives. Periodic monitoring of orthodontic progress with panoramic and cephalometric radiographs is indicated.

I At the end of active treatment, if all spaces are closed with the teeth in an optimal finished occlusion, routine orthodontic retention is indicated. If restorable (residual) spaces are anticipated at the end of orthodontic treatment, finishing is directed at optimizing pontic spaces and abutment alignment. Following termination of active therapy, construction of the final prosthesis or prostheses is indicated.

References

Roberts WE: Adjunctive orthodontic therapy in adults over 50 years of age, *Indiana Dent Assoc J* 76(2):33, 1997.

Roberts WE, Hartsfield, Jr, JK: Multidisciplinary management of congenital and acquired compensated malocclusions, *Indiana Dent Assoc J* 76(2):42, 1997.

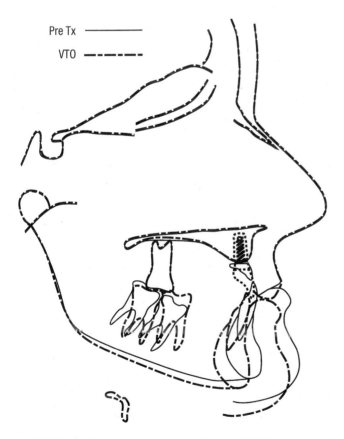

Fig. 86-2 The sagittal visual treatment objective (VTO) is constructed by tracing the pretreatment cephalometric radiograph (Pre Tx) and rotating the mandible open or closed to establish the desired vertical dimension of occlusion (lower facial height) consistent with planned prostheses. The actual VTO is the composite projection of craniofacial form with the mandible, teeth, and prostheses in the desired position.

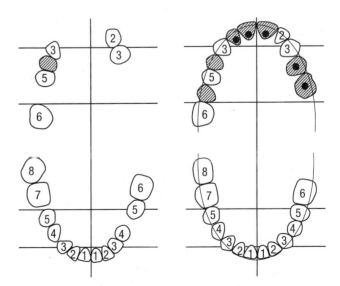

Fig. 86-3 The occlusogram is constructed from photocopies of the occlusal view of the casts. The original positions of the teeth are shown on the left, and the projected restored dentition is shown on the right.

87 Orthodontics and Pure Mucogingival Problems in the Transitional Dentition

Neal Murphy

A A distinction must be made between the growing and the nongrowing patient when evaluating the clinical significance of mucogingival problems for planning orthodontic treatment. Frank skeletal dysplasia (jaw malalignment) can exacerbate the pernicious effects of pure mucogingival orthodontic problems (i.e., a developing deep bite introduces the effects of direct gingival impingement by food and incisor contact on preexisting inadequately attached gingiva).

B Development of mucogingival problems can be anticipated in the primary dentition. If generalized spacing is evident throughout the anterior sextants, the chance of crowding is minimal. Interproximal contact of the primary teeth without crowding (arch length deficiency) may indicate anterior crowding, and crowded primary teeth will evolve into a crowded permanent dentition.

C Extraction of a deciduous tooth when the succedaneous tooth demonstrates 75% or more root formation can accelerate the permanent tooth eruption. Less than a 75% root formation on a succedaneous tooth suggests a delayed eruption of the permanent tooth if the primary mate is extracted. When 75% of the root is formed and the eruption trajectory leads to alveolar mucosa, the primary tooth should be extracted to allow the permanent tooth to erupt into gingiva.

D The mixed dentition, particularly at the transition stage, marks a critical opportunity to ameliorate or preempt a developing malocclusion. When patient cooperation is optimal, functional appliances can produce marked changes at this time. Indolent mucogingival pathoses may develop into clinical entities.

E Judicious serial extraction allows developing crowding in the mandibular anterior sextant to realign distally, relieving stress on the mandibular anterior attached gingiva.

F Nonextraction therapy may consist of movement of mandibular teeth anteriorly or interproximal enamel reduction (stripping) to gain space for the realignment of teeth. Prophylactic or therapeutic gingival augmentation is difficult if an overbite (vertical overlap of the anterior teeth) impinges on the mandibular anterior gingival margin.

G Overbite is not an encumbering factor if sufficient overjet (horizontal overlap of the anterior teeth) is sufficient to allow the surgeon adequate room to operate and place protective periodontal surgical dressing. Generally, 2 mm is sufficient overjet to preclude incisor impingement on the mandibular surgical site.

The secondary dentition in the growing patient presents greater necessity for extraction therapy in the repositioning of lower incisors lingually, away from a stressed labial attached gingiva. If extraction therapy is used to reduce labial protrusion, additional salutary effects are often seen as the thin attached gingiva becomes thicker and more resistant to insult.

References

American Academy of Periodontology: *Proceedings of world workshop in clinical periodontics,* Chicago, 1989, American Academy of Periodontology.

Coatoam GW, Behrents RG, Bissada NF: The width of traumatized gingiva during orthodontic treatment: its significance and impact on periodontal status, *J Peridontol* 52:307, 1981.

Dorfman HS: Mucogingival changes resulting from mandibular incisor tooth movement, *Am J Orthod* 74:286, 1978.

Hall WB: *Pure mucogingival problems,* Berlin, 1984, Quintessence Publishing, pp 44, 68, 178.

Maynard JG, Ochsenbein C: Mucogingival problems, prevalence and therapy in children, *J Periodontol* 46:543, 1975.

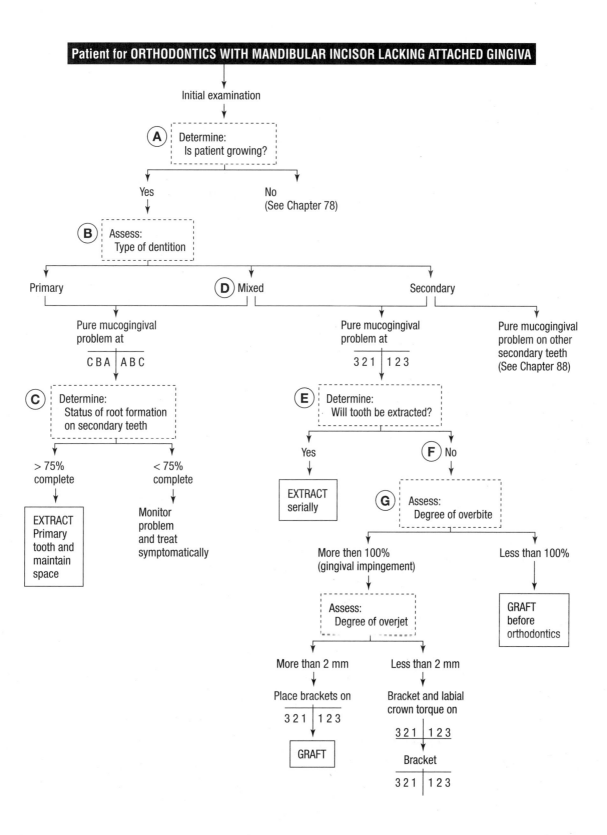

Patient for ORTHODONTICS WITH MANDIBULAR INCISOR LACKING ATTACHED GINGIVA

Initial examination

(A) Determine:
Is patient growing?

Yes

No
(See Chapter 78)

(B) Assess:
Type of dentition

Primary

(D) Mixed

Secondary

Pure mucogingival
problem at

C B A | A B C

Pure mucogingival
problem at

3 2 1 | 1 2 3

Pure mucogingival
problem on other
secondary teeth
(See Chapter 88)

(C) Determine:
Status of root formation
on secondary teeth

(E) Determine:
Will tooth be extracted?

> 75%
complete

< 75%
complete

EXTRACT
Primary
tooth and
maintain
space

Monitor
problem
and treat
symptomatically

Yes

(F) No

EXTRACT
serially

(G) Assess:
Degree of overbite

More then 100%
(gingival impingement)

Less than 100%

Assess:
Degree of overjet

GRAFT
before
orthodontics

More than 2 mm

Less than 2 mm

Place brackets on

3 2 1 | 1 2 3

Bracket and labial
crown torque on

3 2 1 | 1 2 3

GRAFT

Bracket

3 2 1 | 1 2 3

88 Pure Mucogingival Problems in Adult Orthodontic Cases

Neal Murphy

A Extraction of teeth to eliminate crowding keeps the remaining teeth within the confines of the existing alveolar bone and gingiva. If nonextraction techniques of space gaining are used (except for interproximal enamel reduction), stress on the dentogingival unit follows, presenting a potential for bony dehiscence and gingival recession. This occurs if the osteoblastic activity of fibroplasia does not compensate by accommodating the new tooth position space. If less than 1 mm of attached gingiva is present, grafting should precede tooth movement.

B Generally, a slower expansion of the dental arch transversely or anteriorly allows the attachment apparatus sufficient time to accommodate the teeth in their new positions. This occurs if (1) the new position lies within the phenotypical potential of the attached gingiva and alveoli, and (2) infection is controlled. If active recession occurs, however, grafting is needed.

C Rapid expansion generally results in more tooth movement than scalable expansion, greater tipping movement of the teeth, and greater relapse potential, in addition to the increase in dehiscence potential.

D If esthetic demands dictate that roots be covered with gingiva, the histologic attachment to the treated tooth surface may be epithelial. The only histologic continuity between soft tissue and root is hemidesmosomal with a thin coating of mucopolysaccharides. The possibility of new connective tissue attachment to new cementum using Sharpey's fibers is conjectural; thus if no esthetic imperative dictates root coverage, a submarginal free gingival graft should be used to increase the attached gingiva.

E One of the limitations of root coverage in providing a predictable new attachment is that the adjacent donor site does not present sufficient dense fibrous connective tissue to use a pedicle grafting technique. In such a case a free connective tissue graft must be used in conjunction with a marsupialized adjacent mucosa.

F If interproximal enamel reduction or tooth extraction gains sufficient room to treat arch length deficiency, attached gingiva can prove inadequate to resist the destructive forces of bacterial infection and mechanical orthodontic tooth movement.

Where the existing attached gingiva is less than 1 mm, close monitoring by the dentist and patient should meet the demands of both professional and legal imperatives. The potential for precipitous gingival dehiscence in an area of adequate attached gingiva (greater than 1 mm) is rare enough to justify monitoring by the dentist and the orthodontist during professional visits (usually every 4 to 6 weeks).

References

Carranza FA: *Clinical periodontology,* ed 7, Philadelphia, 1990, WB Saunders, p 875.

Corn H: Reconstructive mucogingival surgery. In Goldman HM, Cohen DW, editors: *Periodontal therapy,* ed 6, St Louis, 1980, Mosby, p 795.

Hall WB: *Pure mucogingival problems,* Berlin, 1984, Quintessence Publishing, p 63.

Hall WB: Gingival augmentation/mucogingival surgery. In American Academy of Periodontology: *World workshop in clinical periodontics,* Chicago, 1989, American Academy of Periodontology, VII-1.

Schluger S, Yuodelis R, Page RC, Johnson RH: *Periodontal disease,* ed 2, Philadelphia, 1990, Lea & Febiger, p 458.

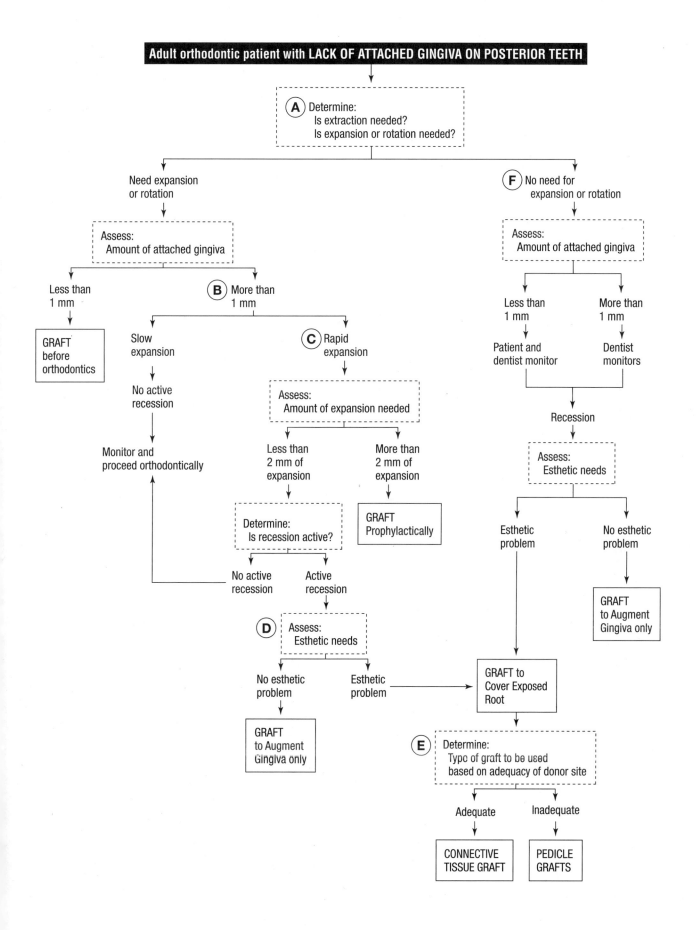

Adult orthodontic patient with LACK OF ATTACHED GINGIVA ON POSTERIOR TEETH

A Determine:
Is extraction needed?
Is expansion or rotation needed?

Need expansion or rotation

Assess:
Amount of attached gingiva

Less than 1 mm

GRAFT before orthodontics

B More than 1 mm

Slow expansion

No active recession

Monitor and proceed orthodontically

C Rapid expansion

Assess:
Amount of expansion needed

Less than 2 mm of expansion

More than 2 mm of expansion

GRAFT Prophylactically

Determine:
Is recession active?

No active recession

Active recession

D Assess:
Esthetic needs

No esthetic problem

Esthetic problem

GRAFT to Augment Gingiva only

F No need for expansion or rotation

Assess:
Amount of attached gingiva

Less than 1 mm

Patient and dentist monitor

More than 1 mm

Dentist monitors

Recession

Assess:
Esthetic needs

Esthetic problem

No esthetic problem

GRAFT to Augment Gingiva only

GRAFT to Cover Exposed Root

E Determine:
Type of graft to be used
based on adequacy of donor site

Adequate

Inadequate

CONNECTIVE TISSUE GRAFT

PEDICLE GRAFTS

199

PART FOUR

Prosthodontics

Eugene E. LaBarre, Editor

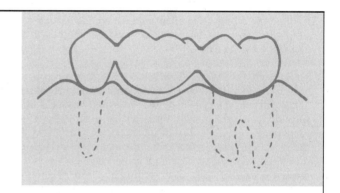

89 Prosthodontic Implications of a Hopeless Tooth

Eugene E. LaBarre

A common clinical situation is that of a single problem tooth in an otherwise intact dental arch. The problem may be the result of chronic inflammatory processes, trauma, or mechanical failure. If the most predictable and logical treatment for the tooth is extraction, the tooth is considered hopeless.

A A severe problem with a tooth is usually recognized as such by the patient and is frequently the cause of an emergency office visit. Patients may have already thought of extraction before the appointment and may be more interested in discussing replacement options. Occasionally, a patient with a hopeless tooth insists that the tooth be salvaged rather than extracted. Such a request must be balanced by the dentist's professional judgment regarding the feasibility of heroic treatment. To help the patient make a well-informed decision, the cause of the problem must be diagnosed and explained by the dentist.

B The majority of isolated, hopeless teeth have problems that are readily identified: severe periodontitis, unresolved periapical pathology, failed root integrity caused by cracks or resorption, or severe fracture of coronal structure (Fig. 89-1). All of these conditions are difficult and expensive to treat, and the short-term prognosis may be uncertain. Particular attention must be given to situations in which bone loss is progressive because this can compromise support of neighboring teeth and adversely affect replacement options in the future. The dentist must have a frank discussion with the patient so that costs and the potential for failure are fully disclosed.

C If the patient has no interest in pursuing heroic treatment or if salvage of the tooth is attempted and fails, the tooth is extracted. Short-term replacement possibilities include a provisional removable partial denture (RPD) or provisional fixed partial denture (FPD). Definitive replacement therapies are highly predictable, although the criteria that are used to select the most appropriate one for a patient are haphazard. The following statements about each treatment option may guide the clinician:

- An RPD can be used universally and has the lowest cost but is the most obtrusive and least functional prosthesis; it is the most esthetic approach when a significant ridge defect exists in the appearance zone.
- An FPD can be used for most single missing teeth, particularly when abutment teeth have significant coronal damage or existing crowns. However, preparations required for porcelain-metal retainers are not conservative for intact abutment teeth that have no secondary or reparative dentin. In situations where abutment teeth are virgin, an adhesive FPD should be considered.
- An implant is most similar to actual replacement of a missing tooth in that the neighboring teeth are not involved. Sufficient bone is required for implant placement, and the appearance of the implant-supported crown as it emerges from the soft tissue can be an esthetic challenge. Patients should be informed about the possibility of implant rejection.

D If the patient has opted for heroic treatment and the dental problem has been stabilized by preliminary therapy, restoration of the tooth itself is necessary. With a mobile tooth, some form of reversibility is desirable in the splinting prosthesis so that future problems with the tooth can be managed without sacrifice of the restoration. Telescopic restorations may be appropriate because the possibility exists for removing the outer prosthesis from cemented copings. However, the patient must understand that future events may necessitate replacement of a prosthesis and that regular recall is essential for maintenance.

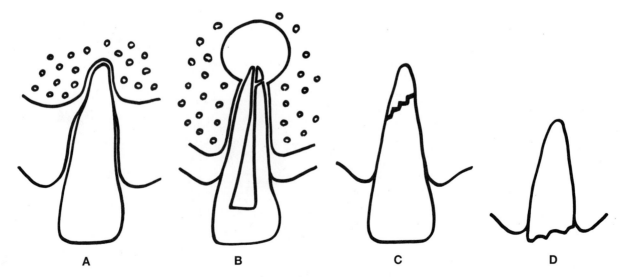

| A | B | C | D |

Fig. 89-1 Most frequent causes of individual tooth failure. **A,** Localized periodontitis. **B,** Failing endodontic seal. **C,** Root fracture. **D,** Coronal destruction.

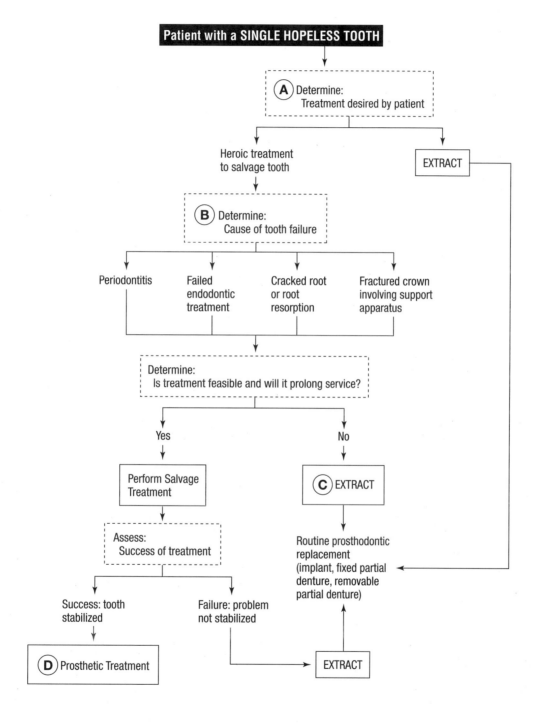

Patient with a SINGLE HOPELESS TOOTH

(A) Determine:
Treatment desired by patient

Heroic treatment
to salvage tooth

EXTRACT

(B) Determine:
Cause of tooth failure

Periodontitis | Failed endodontic treatment | Cracked root or root resorption | Fractured crown involving support apparatus

Determine:
Is treatment feasible and will it prolong service?

Yes

No

Perform Salvage
Treatment

(C) EXTRACT

Assess:
Success of treatment

Success: tooth
stabilized

Failure: problem
not stabilized

Routine prosthodontic
replacement
(implant, fixed partial
denture, removable
partial denture)

(D) Prosthetic Treatment

EXTRACT

References

Cohen S, Burns RC: *Pathways of the pulp,* ed 6, St Louis, 1994, Mosby, p 690.

Enquist B et al: Single tooth replacement by osseointegrated Brane-mark implants: a retrospective study of 82 implants, *Clin Oral Implants Res* 6:238, 1995.

Geurtsen W: The cracked-tooth syndrome: clinical features and case reports, *Int J Periodont Restor Dent* 12:395, 1992.

90 Prosthodontic Aspects of the Extensively Damaged Dentition

Eugene E. LaBarre

A patient who suffers from generalized advanced dental pathology, such as periodontitis, caries, or occlusal wear and collapse, may require extraction of some or all teeth. The patient may have neglected dental health, or, even if regular treatment has been received, the patient's problems may have become so advanced that treatment is no longer effective or predictable. The "downhill" oral health phenomenon has been described extensively, including a study by Nyman and Lindhe of the successful long-term periodontal and prosthetic rehabilitation of a carefully controlled population of patients with terminal or hopeless dentitions. More recently, endosseous dental implants have been developed that provide a predictable treatment alternative for partially and completely edentulous individuals. The patients for whom dental disease and damage have become a significant liability can be placed in one of the following categories:

- *Maintenance:* salvage of most or all teeth
- *Fixed prosthodontics:* selective extractions and restore with cast restorations and fixed partial dentures (FPD)
- *Removable prosthodontics:* extract most or all teeth; rehabilitate with removable partial dentures (RPD) or complete dentures (CD)
- *Implant prosthodontics:* any number of teeth are replaced by implants

In my experience, the majority of cases fall into the maintenance or removable prosthodontic categories. Planning and executing the rehabilitation that best suits the individual patient are great challenges in dentistry.

A The examination and diagnosis must be thorough. In particular, the success or failure of previous and prospective treatment must be determined. The patient must demonstrate a willingness and determination to participate in the treatment before any extensive rehabilitation is attempted. If there is any question about this important phase of treatment, it may be desirable to stabilize the dental pathology with interim restorations until satisfactory results are demonstrated. If the interim phase of treatment is a failure, it is possible to move on to extractions and removable prostheses without major sacrifice of time and energy.

B Maintenance treatment, such as root planing and operative dentistry, is effective in slowing or arresting pathology in a compliant patient and may be all that is required if tooth mobility is not advanced and if tooth migration has not occurred. If there are unreplaced missing teeth or if the teeth are in poor repair, maintenance will not prevent the arch and occlusal collapse that will progress inevitably. In cases of multiple missing teeth and advanced disrepair, following a patient's request to "only maintain the teeth for a while" has limited value and may commit the dentist to an inordinate number of patchwork procedures and emergency appointments.

C The salvage of teeth by extensive periodontal, endodontic, and prosthetic treatment has been shown to stabilize dental health in patients who learn effective home care regimens. Not all patients are capable of outstanding hygiene year after year. The telescopic prosthesis permits fixed splinting and tooth replacement by an outer prosthesis that can be removed from individually cemented copings for maintenance and repair and is a technique for providing fixed prosthodontic service to groups of patients with unpredictable long-term stability. However, any fixed prosthesis placed over teeth with guarded prognosis must be regarded as heroic, high risk treatment.

D A common treatment involves salvaging strategic abutments for prosthesis support and extracting noncritical or problematic teeth (Fig. 90-1). This approach has the advantage of simplifying treatment and maintenance while providing satisfactory denture support. Primary strategic teeth are well-supported canines and molars. At a minimum, a full-arch FPD or a tooth-supported RPD require four abutments; a distal extension RPD requires two abutments. The best locations for abutment teeth are the anterior and posterior corners of the arch.

E Full-mouth extraction is the most drastic treatment in terms of tooth loss but also the simplest and most predictable in eliminating dental pathology. The maxillary complete denture is a comfortable and functional prosthesis for many patients, and after an adaptation period during the transition from natural to artificial teeth, the average patient is satisfied with a maxillary denture (Fig. 90-2). By contrast, the mandibular CD is a poor substitute for natural teeth.

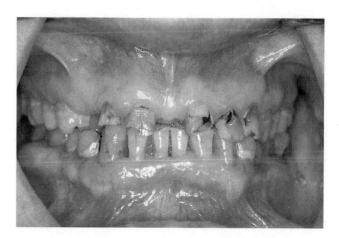

Fig. 90-1 In addition to severe coronal damage of the maxillary anterior teeth, including wear, caries, and fracture, tooth 6 is missing, and there is a large midline diastema. If the anterior teeth are extracted, the lack of interarch space (between the mandibular incisors and the palate) will become a primary concern.

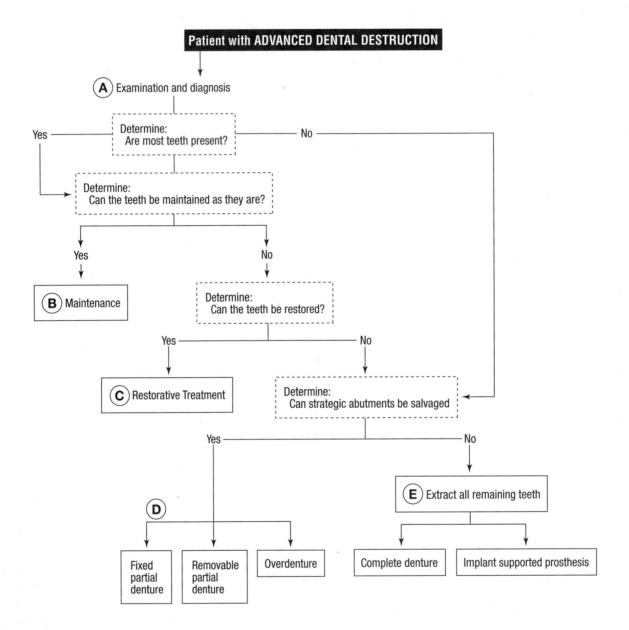

Patient with ADVANCED DENTAL DESTRUCTION

A Examination and diagnosis

Determine:
Are most teeth present?

Yes — No

Determine:
Can the teeth be maintained as they are?

Yes   No

B Maintenance

Determine:
Can the teeth be restored?

Yes — No

C Restorative Treatment

Determine:
Can strategic abutments be salvaged

Yes — No

D

E Extract all remaining teeth

| Fixed partial denture | Removable partial denture | Overdenture | Complete denture | Implant supported prosthesis |

Most patients will complain of the looseness and instability of a lower denture. For this reason, exceptional measures to preserve strategic teeth, even as passive overdenture abutments, are justifiable. There are close correlations between nutritional intake, general health, self-image, and dental status, particularly in the aged population. It is my opinion that all patients with edentulous mandibles are candidates for implant-supported overdentures, unless medical or psychologic frailties make the procedures impossible. Implants are effective and should be discussed with patients who are confronted with the realities of a hopeless dentition.

References

Diehl RL et al: Factors associated with successful denture therapy, *J Prosthodont* 5:84, 1996.

Joshipura KJ et al: The impact of edentulousness on food and nutrient intake, *J Am Dent Assoc* 127:459, 1996.

Nyman S, Lindhe J: A longitudinal study of combined periodontal and prosthetic treatment of patients with advanced periodontal disease, *J Periodontol* 50:163, 1979.

Owall B, Kayser AF, Carlsson GE: *Prosthodontics: principles and management strategies*, London, 1996, Mosby-Wolfe, p 49.

A 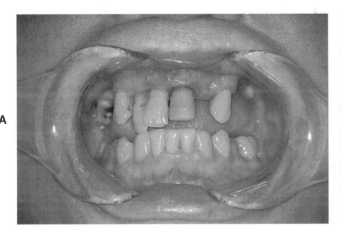 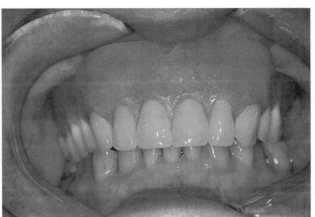 B

Fig. 90-2 The hopeless condition may be restricted to one arch. **A,** The maxillary teeth have severe periodontitis. **B,** The maxillary teeth have been extracted, and an immediate denture has been placed.

91 Transition to Dentures for the Patient with a Hopeless Dentition

Eugene E. LaBarre

Full-mouth extraction and transition to complete dentures represent a treatment option for patients with severely compromised natural teeth. Most often, this option must be chosen because of extreme neglect or financial considerations. Also, for patients in whom periodontal or restorative therapy has failed, complete dentures (CD) may be the final treatment or may be used as a transition into implant therapy. The decision to proceed with dentures is often difficult for patients with hopeless natural teeth because of the irreversibility of the treatment and because it represents a culturally negative life transition (end of youth, beginning of old age). The decision can be further complicated by the necessity to salvage strategic teeth for removable partial denture (RPD) or overdenture support, particularly in the mandible. The clinician should be aware that maintaining teeth for "psychologic" reasons may include emergency and patchwork dentistry and usually only delays the inevitable. Patients who are interested in beginning implant treatment should be advised that the first step is removal of all problem teeth, requiring the use of a transitional denture during residual ridge and implant healing periods.

A The first decision that should be made concerning a patient with a hopeless dentition is whether the teeth should be removed immediately, before a transitional prosthesis is fabricated. Conditions that warrant this approach include severe dental infection, pain, or teeth that are so mobile or malposed that impression making is impossible. In these situations the substantial health risk overrides esthetic or oral function considerations. Denture fabrication should be delayed 4 to 6 weeks postoperatively to permit healing and initial residual ridge remodeling. A conventional technique then can be used to fabricate dentures.

B The number and condition of the teeth to be extracted determine the sequence of surgical procedures. The classical technique for immediate dentures involves removing the posterior teeth, waiting for suitable ridge remodeling, and then fabricating the dentures and delivering them when the anterior teeth are extracted. This technique requires that the anterior teeth are present and able to withstand several months of function between surgical phases. The advantage of the technique is that it permits placement of the denture on a mature posterior ridge, reducing the need to reline at insertion and making the initial service of the denture more predictable.

C The most common way of managing the transitional denture is to fabricate the prosthesis first, often by a simplified technique, and to insert it when all teeth are removed in a single surgery. Temporary resilient denture liners make this possible because the fit of the immediate transitional denture can be easily customized. Typically, the patient is maintained with temporary reliners until the ridge has remodeled (3 to 6 months); the denture is then permanently relined.

D It is recommended that a second, definitive denture is fabricated after the ridge remodeling period. The transitional denture then becomes the emergency or spare denture, and any changes that are requested by the patient can be incorporated in the definitive prosthesis. On the other hand, if the patient desires to begin implant treatment, the transitional denture is used throughout the various healing periods until the implant supported prosthesis is completed. In either case the transitional denture serves as an immediate training prosthesis and is helpful in determining whether a patient will be able to tolerate dentures.

References

Weintraub GS: Provisional removable partial and complete prostheses, *Dent Clin North Am* 33:399, 1989.

Zarb GA: *Boucher's prosthodontic treatment for edentulous patients,* ed 10, St Louis, 1990, Mosby, p 534.

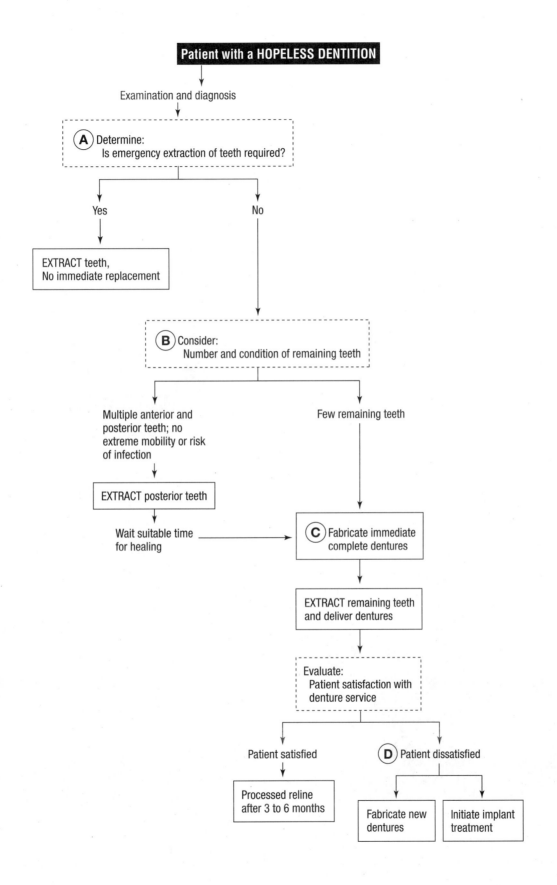

Patient with a HOPELESS DENTITION

Examination and diagnosis

A Determine:
Is emergency extraction of teeth required?

Yes

No

EXTRACT teeth,
No immediate replacement

B Consider:
Number and condition of remaining teeth

Multiple anterior and
posterior teeth; no
extreme mobility or risk
of infection

Few remaining teeth

EXTRACT posterior teeth

Wait suitable time
for healing

C Fabricate immediate
complete dentures

EXTRACT remaining teeth
and deliver dentures

Evaluate:
Patient satisfaction with
denture service

Patient satisfied

D Patient dissatisfied

Processed reline
after 3 to 6 months

Fabricate new
dentures

Initiate implant
treatment

92 Oral Conditions that May Require Preprosthetic Surgery

Alex McDonald

A patient needing prosthetic treatment must be examined carefully to assure that the residual ridges are or will be in an optimal condition to support dentures. A variety of hard and soft tissue conditions interfere with intimate fit between oral tissue and prosthesis and may require surgical repair. Any existing dentures should be examined to indicate whether and how the new prostheses might fit around the problem.

A In cases that require extraction, soft tissue recontouring, and minor osseous reduction the denture may be placed as an immediate restoration, using a temporary soft reliner to establish intimate fit and a seal, if necessary. Occasionally, extraction is followed by reduction of facially prominent bone or smoothing of interproximal bone spicules, although this should be minimized in favor of preserving the residual ridge. Impacted teeth may be left in place provided there is no clinical or radiographic sign of abnormality (Fig. 92-1). If the patient has an existing prosthesis that is fitted over the impaction site without difficulty, it is likely that a new prosthesis will be tolerated as well. Several minor preprosthetic soft tissue procedures can be accomplished with laser surgery, which is both safe and effective (Fig. 92-2).

B Residual ridge resorption (RRR) is a particular problem for edentulous patients. In the past, surgical treatment of RRR has included deepening the soft tissue vestibule or grafting ceramic or osseous materials to augment the ridge (Fig. 92-3). These procedures are still performed but they are as invasive as implant placement and do not ensure significantly improved denture service. For this reason, augmentation procedures are more important to create adequate bone support for implants, rather than to increase the denture-bearing area. Surgical augmentation for implant placement in RRR cases is now commonplace. While grafting of bone is a significant additional procedure, it permits predictable implant use that would be impossible otherwise. The need for bone grafting and the type of procedure that is most appropriate are surgical decisions that are made after a careful examination of the patient and a discussion of treatment objectives.

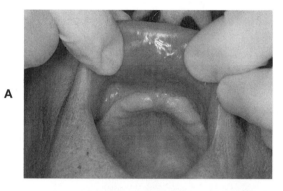

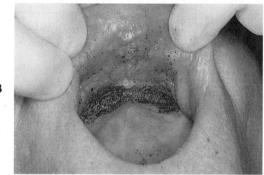

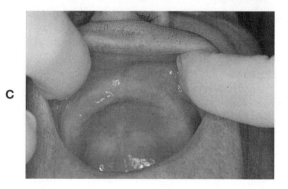

Fig. 92-1 As the patient is evaluated for extraction of the remaining maxillary teeth, the right third molar will be left in place. It is a partial bony impaction, there are no radiographic or clinical abnormalities, and the patient has an existing removable partial denture (RPD) that fits over the site.

Fig. 92-2 **A,** Preoperative view of excess soft tissue on anterior maxilla. **B,** Operative view of laser reduction. **C,** Postoperative status at 2 weeks.

Patient requiring a REMOVABLE PROSTHESIS

Determine:
Are there hopeless teeth or root tips present?

Yes → **(A) EXTRACT**

No → Determine:
Are there tori or other interfering bony features?

Yes → OSSEOUS REDUCTION

No →

Determine:
Is there redundant soft tissue?

Yes → SOFT TISSUE REDUCTION

No →

Determine:
Are there prominent frena?

Yes → FRENECTOMY

No →

Determine:
Is there adequate residual ridge?

Yes → Immediate or conventional complete denture service

No → **(B) RIDGE AUGMENTATION** or implant → Prosthetic treatment after surgical healing

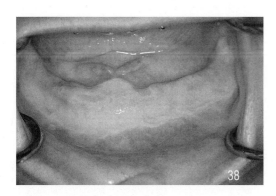

Fig. 92-3 The mandibular ridge has been augmented with a section of the patient's own rib, followed by a skin graft vestibuloplasty.

References

Fonseca RJ: *Reconstructive preprosthetic oral and maxillofacial surgery,* Philadelphia, 1986, WB Saunders.

Hopkins R: *Preprosthetic oral surgery,* Philadelphia, 1987, Lea & Febiger.

Pedersen GW: *Oral surgery,* Philadelphia, 1988, WB Saunders, p 119.

Zarb GA: *Boucher's prosthodontic treatment of edentulous patients,* ed 10, St Louis, 1990, Mosby, p 123.

93 Tooth-Supported Overdentures

Robert Sarka

When diagnosis and treatment planning dictate a transition from partial edentulism to complete dentures, the remaining teeth should be evaluated for possible use as overdenture abutments. It is not unusual to find two, three, or four strategically located natural teeth that can be used for overdenture abutments. Following the appropriate endodontic and periodontal treatment and dramatic reduction of the crown-to-root ratio, these teeth become desirable abutments. Overdenture abutments are "nature's implants" that preserve the residual ridge. They retain proprioception and load and tactile sensation residual in the periodontal ligament, enhancing the physiologic health of the periodontal ligament. They provide a firm, hard foundation for the denture base and a generally improved denture service.

Research has shown that an immediate overdenture is preferable to an immediate complete denture (CD) because there is less attrition of the supporting ridge with overdenture treatment. Patients with CDs lose *twice* as much bone in all parts of the mandible with most of the change occurring in the first year. Even teeth with a poor periodontal prognosis contribute to the retention of alveolar bone. The premise that the alveolar bone exists to invest and support the natural teeth is valid; loss of these natural teeth leads to rapid destruction of the alveolar ridge. Failure to present this treatment option to the patient may be a serious error of omission and may be a violation of the standard of care. While the mandibular immediate CD may be less expensive, it may also be a much less satisfactory treatment with long-term negative consequences for the maintenance of denture stability and retention.

In light of the earlier findings, several important decisions must be made before determining that this type of treatment can benefit the patient. Above all, patient selection, demonstrated patient motivation and understanding of the overdenture concept, and ongoing excellent plaque control are absolutely essential to overdenture success.

A Teeth selected for overdenture abutments should have a favorable prognosis, with 3 to 4 mm of attached gingiva and a minimum of 6 mm of alveolar bone support. CDs are indicated when the remaining teeth have a generally hopeless prognosis, but strategically located individual teeth may survive under the reduced mechanical demands of an overdenture. Treatable periodontal disease, feasibility of endodontic treatment, and restorability are critical factors. Crown-to-root ratio is improved when the coronal structure is amputated and domed and mobility is reduced (Fig. 93-1).

B Several other important prosthodontic factors should be evaluated. Typically, the need for denture support is greater in the mandible than in the maxilla because of reduced residual ridge and the difficulty in obtaining a satisfactory seal. The dramatically atrophic ridge warrants heroic measures to preserve remaining teeth and bone. In the interest of preserving well-developed ridges for long-term use, retention of several teeth should be considered (Fig. 93-2). The strategic value of teeth selected for overdenture abutments is determined by tooth position. Canines are the most desirable unless there are severe facial tissue undercuts. Consecutive abutments should have one tooth's width space between them. Other prosthodontic factors, such as lack of interocclusal space or the need to place implants in the future, may rule out an overdenture approach. The prosthodontic dentist must also determine whether the abutments will be active or passive, that is, whether they will be mechanically connected to the prosthesis by means of attachments or merely provide vertical support for the overdenture. Active abutments are under heavy stress and have more stringent requirements for root support than do passive abutments. The use of hemisected molars for additional overdenture support has been demonstrated (Fig. 93-3).

Typical restorations for endodontically treated passive abutments are the following:

- A Class I silver amalgam or composite restoration placed in the endodontic access opening, highly polished as a bearing area, with highly polished dentin treated with fluoride gel and fluoride rinse.

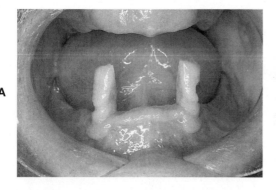 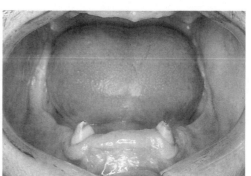

A
B

Fig. 93-1 **A,** Clinical indication for tooth-supported overdenture is the presence of canine abutments with poor crown-to-root ratio. **B,** The canines have been endodontically treated, the coronal tooth structure has been amputated, and the canal orifice has been sealed with amalgam.

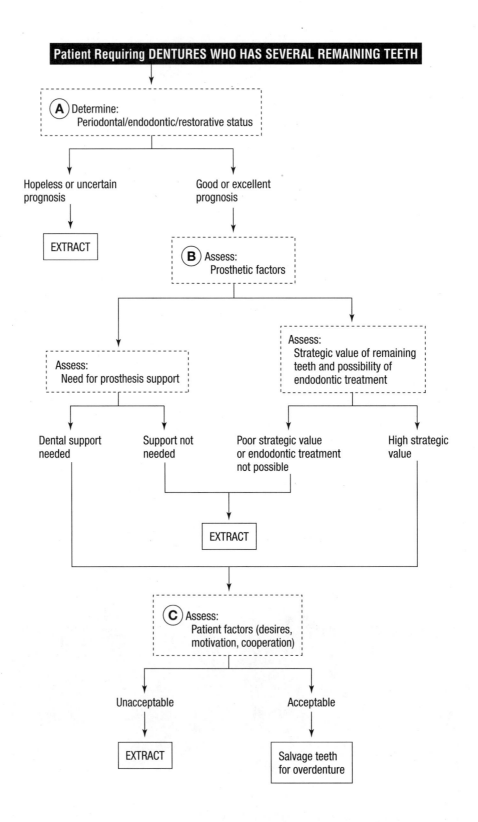

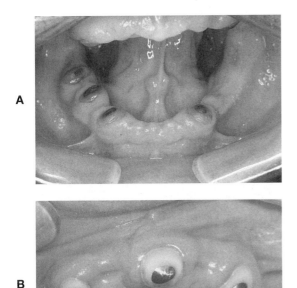

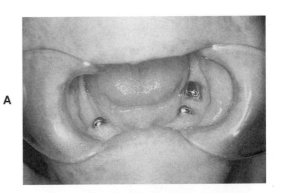

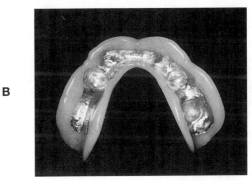

Fig. 93-2 **A,** Multiple interrupted overdenture abutments in the mandibular arch. **B,** Multiple interrupted overdenture abutments in the maxillary arch.

Fig. 93-4 **A,** Overdenture abutments with cast restorations. **B,** Mandibular overdenture with cast metal base.

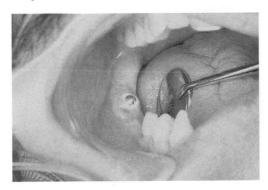

Fig. 93-3 A hemisected molar is used to support the distal extension base of a removable partial overdenture.

C Finally, the success or failure of overdenture treatment is dependent on the patient's willingness to take responsibility for the treatment, cooperate with follow-up care, and maintain the necessary level of plaque control. Initially, the patient must accept endodontic treatment and periodontal therapy, including gingival grafting if insufficient attached gingiva is present. A home care regimen of meticulous hygiene and daily fluoride treatment must be followed carefully. The patient needs to return to the dental office at regular intervals for evaluation and professional maintenance. Only patients with an obvious commitment to this type of dentistry should be selected.

- A cast gold post and coping that would protect the exposed tooth structure and provide retention from the post in the upper two thirds of the treated root canal. Doming should leave the abutment 1- to 2-mm maximum in height. Placement of a cast post and coping would dictate a cast base of similar metal to prevent abrasion and wear and maintain the vertical dimension of occlusion (Fig. 93-4).

References

Brewer AA, Morrow RM: *Overdentures,* St Louis, 1975, Mosby, pp 3, 24.

Castleberry DJ: Philosophies and principles of removable partial overdentures, *Dent Clin North Am* 34:589, 1990.

Sarka RJ, Richard GE, Arnold RM, Knowles KI: Hemisected molars for additional overdenture support, *J Prosth Dent* 38:16, 1977.

Zarb GA: *Boucher's prosthodontic treatment for edentulous patients,* ed 10, St Louis, 1990, Mosby, p 521.

94 Fixed Partial Denture Versus Removable Partial Denture Versus Implants

Eugene E. LaBarre

As a general rule, fixed tooth replacement is preferred over removable restorations because of greater patient convenience and acceptance. On the other hand, a removable partial denture (RPD) can be designed for virtually every partially edentulous patient; the fixed partial denture (FPD) requires adequate biomechanical support, whether from teeth or implants. Implants have the need for adequate bone volume for placement and also have a small but inherent risk of nonintegration with the bone. In addition, financial considerations may be compelling; a removable prosthesis may be chosen in a case where a fixed restoration is possible but is too expensive for the patient.

A A single missing tooth is best replaced by a conventional FPD or implant. Lateral and small central incisors have been replaced historically by a cantilevered pontic supported by a canine or central incisor. Although the simple FPD is predictable and successful, the presence of virgin abutments argues for a restorative approach that will conserve coronal tooth structure and pulpal health. In these situations an adhesive FPD or a single tooth implant are strongly recommended.

B In situations where multiple teeth are missing, several conditions should be met before a fixed replacement can be fabricated (Fig. 94-1). Mechanical considerations require an adequate number of sound abutments (roughly equal to the teeth being replaced) with controlled occlusal forces and sufficient occlusal gingival length to retain the restoration. The need for periodontal and endodontic health in tooth abutments is the same for fixed and removable restorations, but a complex FPD is much more of a commitment for a patient than its removable counterpart and has no reversibility or convertibility. Because a failing abutment can condemn a conventional FPD, a consideration should be given to over-engineering the final restoration. An RPD can often be modified to accommodate the loss of an abutment; a telescopic approach to tooth-supported FPD and placing extra implants for implant-supported restorations are both advisable when abutment longevity is uncertain.

C In situations where all posterior teeth are missing, the distal extension RPD has been the historic treatment of choice. If premolars are present and occlusion does not require replacement of both first and second molars, a cantilevered FPD using multiple abutments to support an undersized posterior pontic may be acceptable. Patients with intact dentitions posteriorly to the first molar have adequate occlusal function, as do many patients with second premolar occlusion. Implant replacement of premolars and molars is preferred, although implants in the posterior areas of both jaws can present significant problems with diminished bone volume, lack of access, and nonintegration with bone. Nonetheless, most patients with posterior implants regard them as a far superior service to a cantilever FPD or RPD.

D An important consideration in planning for tooth replacement in the esthetic zone is the appearance of the soft tissue. In situations where the tooth–soft tissue junction is visible, or where additional lip support is needed because of resorption of anterior edentulous ridge, an RPD has the greatest esthetic potential and may be the only choice if bone and soft tissue grafting can not be considered. It is advisable to perform diagnostic esthetic procedures, such as try-in of preliminary wax-up, or experimentation with provisional restorations, to evaluate the success of a particular approach before a commitment is made to treatment.

E In all matters related to implant placement, the primary consideration is whether sufficient bone quality and quantity exist to permit implant placement. As augmentation procedures become more common and predictable, implant replacement of missing teeth will be more universal. However, currently, a significant number of partially edentulous patients have only nonimplant prosthodontic options: conventional FPD or RPD.

References

Olsson M et al: Bridges supported by free-standing implants vs bridges supported by tooth and implant: a five-year prospective study, *Clin Oral Implants Res* 6:114, 1995.

Owall B, Kayser AF, Carlsson GE: *Prosthodontics: principles and management strategies*, London, 1996, Mosby-Wolfe, p 149.

Parel SM: Prosthesis design and treatment planning for the partially edentulous implant patient, *J Oral Implantol* 22:31, 1996.

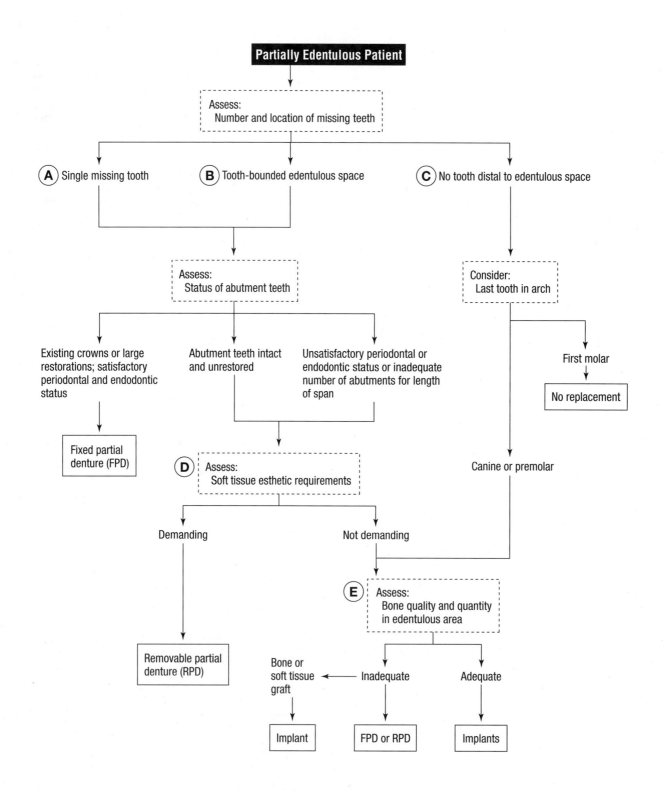

Partially Edentulous Patient

Assess:
Number and location of missing teeth

(A) Single missing tooth

(B) Tooth-bounded edentulous space

(C) No tooth distal to edentulous space

Assess:
Status of abutment teeth

Consider:
Last tooth in arch

Existing crowns or large restorations; satisfactory periodontal and endodontic status

Abutment teeth intact and unrestored

Unsatisfactory periodontal or endodontic status or inadequate number of abutments for length of span

First molar

No replacement

Fixed partial denture (FPD)

(D) Assess:
Soft tissue esthetic requirements

Canine or premolar

Demanding

Not demanding

(E) Assess:
Bone quality and quantity in edentulous area

Removable partial denture (RPD)

Bone or soft tissue graft ← Inadequate

Adequate

Implant

FPD or RPD

Implants

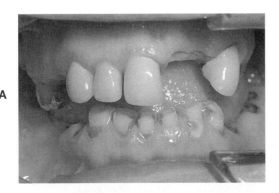

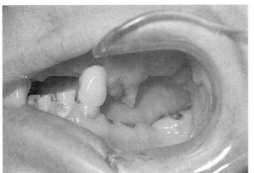

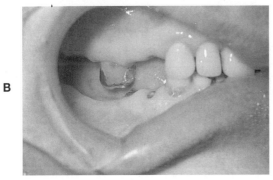

Fig. 94-1 A partially edentulous patient like the one pictured presents treatment planning dilemmas. The decisions regarding replacement of missing dentition must be made in the context of damaged and malposed remaining teeth, the patient's level of commitment to active and preventive therapy, and the clinician's estimation of future events. **A,** There are multiple retained posterior roots, teeth 9 and 10 were recently extracted, and the mandibular anterior teeth are severely worn by function against opposing porcelain surfaces. **B,** Tooth 3 is extruded almost to the crest of the opposing edentulous ridge. **C,** Teeth 12 and 13 have severely damaged crowns, and vertical overlap of the left canines (11 and 22) is extreme.

95 Selecting Fixed Prosthodontic Procedures

Casimir Leknius

In this time of rapidly developing alternative prosthodontic techniques, it is useful to review the indications for the use of fixed prosthodontics. These procedures include individual cast gold or porcelain fused-to-metal (PFM) crowns, splinted cast restorations, or fixed partial dentures (FPD) and constitute the bulk of fixed prosthodontic practice.

A The most obvious indication for crowns is to restore damaged teeth. Specific guidelines, such as isthmus width of existing intracoronal restorations exceeding certain intercuspal dimensions or missing cusps, have been suggested. Generally, it is advisable to restore any tooth weakened by existing restoration or caries where a significant risk of breakage exists. Published diagnostic criteria and indices are useful.

B Occlusal wear and missing teeth are often associated with severely compromised occlusal schemes, such as an exaggerated or reverse curve of Spee. This usually comes about as a result of extrusion following the extraction of antagonist teeth. Often it is further complicated by prostheses placed in a conforming manner without correction of the occlusal plane. These cases must be carefully analyzed before restoration and frequently require the disciplines of endodontics, orthodontics, and surgery for block resections and periodontics for crown lengthening before a predictably successful prosthesis can be placed. It is not prudent to perpetuate malocclusions or iatrogenic occlusal schemes simply because it is an expedient way to replace missing teeth.

It is desirable to match occlusal wear factors in the selection of restorative materials in such cases. PFM restorations have the potential for esthetic match or improvement of the natural teeth, but the increased hardness of porcelain compared with enamel makes this a destructive material choice in areas subjected to heavy parafunction. Currently, only cast gold alloys have wear properties similar to natural tooth structure, although softer porcelains and composite resins are emerging and may become as successful as gold for the occlusal surfaces.

C Replacement of missing teeth using fixed prosthodontic procedures is a predictable procedure. The possibility of replacing teeth with implants should also be explored. FPDs increase the occlusal load on abutment teeth, necessitating careful diagnostic review of bone support, mobility, crown length, edentulous span, and other factors related to restoration, durability, and strength. Ante's Law, which suggests that root surface area of abutments should equal that of the teeth being replaced is a good general guideline but is successfully violated on a routine basis in clinical practice. The classic argument against Ante's Law is exemplified by the canine-supported FPD, which replaces four incisors. Individual experience, rather than precise application of rules or guidelines, determines that this is an appropriate restoration for one patient and not for another.

D Splinting with cast restorations for periodontal or orthodontic stability is another routine application of fixed prosthodontic technology. The two main issues to be considered in splinting are whether it is physically possible to splint (in terms of alignment, number of teeth, cost) and whether the teeth are worth the extraordinary effort and difficulty in maintenance of splinting. If there is a possibility of implant placement, heroic restoration of marginal teeth is more difficult to defend now than in the past. Additionally, splinting reduces proprioception and reduces the physiologic occlusoapical movement of teeth. Therefore this treatment option should be used judiciously and mainly for mobile teeth that are already in jeopardy. Splinting of periodontally sound teeth should be done with extreme caution, if at all.

E Esthetic repair of damaged or discolored teeth is routinely done with PFM restorations and represents one of the major developments in dentistry during the last 30 years. However, tooth preparation for PFM is the least conservative of all designs and significant pulpal and periodontal consequences usually follow improper technique. The guidelines for tooth preparation are well established. The PFM is viewed by many clinicians as the universal restoration; however, risk versus benefit analysis suggests that the dentist should recommend the most conservative technique that achieves the desired result. In some cases bleaching, veneering, or restoration of defects with composite resin may be the treatment of choice. Porcelain laminate veneers have emerged as the most popular restoration for improving anterior esthetics. The glazed, nonporous surface of porcelain is abrasion resistant, esthetic, and biologically compatible with soft tissue. Silane coupling agents have increased bonding strength, and as much as 2 mm can be added to the incisal length without increasing the risk of fracture. The only limitation is that a sufficient amount of enamel remains for the bond. Ceramic inlays and onlays have been emerging as satisfactory posterior restorations because of the latest generation of adhesives. Inlays are more predictable because onlays require a greater amount of tooth reduction to resist fracture. Composite inlays are gaining in popularity because of the ease of construction, but longitudinal evaluations are limited as to their wear resistance and longevity.

References

Shillingburg HT, Hobo S, Whitsett LD: *Fundamentals of fixed prosthodontics,* ed 3, Chicago, 1997, Quintessence Publishing, p 16.

Smith BGN: *Dental crowns and bridges: design and preparation,* ed 2, Chicago, 1990, Mosby.

Stockstill JW, Bowley JF, Attanasio R: Clinical decision analysis in fixed prosthodontics, *Dent Clin North Am* 36:569, 1992.

Patient with UNSERVICEABLE RESTORATIONS, MISSING TEETH, OR ESTHETIC COMPROMISE

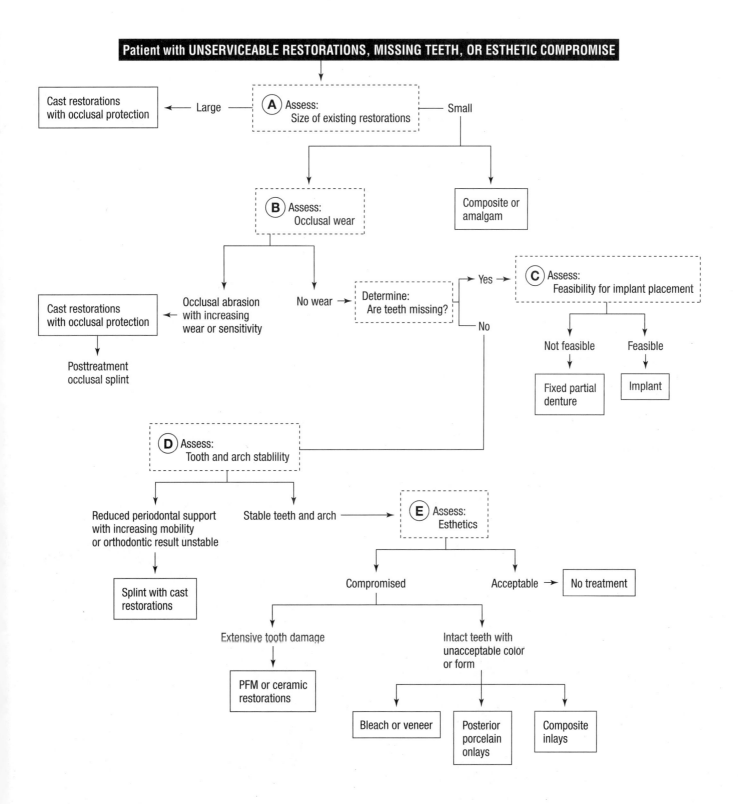

96 Treatment Decisions for Fixed Partial Dentures

Chi Tran

The tooth-supported fixed partial denture (FPD) is a standard form of treatment for partially edentulous patients. The techniques are well established, universally applied, and clinically successful. The FPD is not a conservative technique, and there is increasing recognition of implant treatment as appropriate for cases where an FPD was previously the only fixed option. Because the indications for the various tooth replacement therapies overlap and because planning decisions can profoundly affect the prognosis for an FPD, a careful, logical assessment of the patient's condition and desires is always needed.

A The initial assessment is of the edentulous area and its functional requirements. Ante's Law states that the root surface area of the supporting teeth should equal or exceed that of the teeth to be replaced, placing practical limits on span length in a fixed prosthesis. This law is violated regularly and successfully, depending on the location of the restoration. Three to four consecutively missing teeth are the maximum that can be replaced by a conventional FPD. Longer spans or distal extension edentulous areas should be restored by a removable partial denture (RPD) or implants (Fig. 96-1). Carefully evaluate the functional burden in the area of treatment because parafunctional habits, disrupted occlusal schemes, or replacement of guidance teeth increase the load on an FPD as well as demand for mechanical strength and abutment support (Fig. 96-2).

B The teeth adjacent to the edentulous area must be evaluated for their potential as abutment teeth. Factors related to mobility, length of crown, axial alignment, and restorative status must be reviewed before a prognosis can be determined for the prospective treatment. In situations where the abutment teeth have adequate support but are improperly aligned or are coronally too short, adjunctive therapy such as orthodontics and surgical crown lengthening can make an unfavorable situation acceptable. When abutment teeth lack adequate bone support or are mobile, the approach must be to reinforce the abutment by splinting it to neighboring teeth. The most ideal FPD abutments have preexisting crowns or large coronal restoration so that secondary and reparative dentin are present and there will be less risk to the pulp during tooth preparation. The presence of virgin teeth on either side of an edentulous space is a dilemma for dentists because of the reluctance to irreversibly cut away sound tooth structure. In these situations, pulpal trauma can be avoided entirely by planning an adhesive restoration (indicated for single missing teeth) or implants. In a borderline situation the dentist should determine risk-versus-benefit to help the patient decide whether to proceed with a fixed prosthesis or alternative treatment.

C The esthetic possibilities of restoring an anterior edentulous space must be evaluated before deciding upon an FPD. If long pontic teeth are visible, either because of severely resorbed anterior ridge or high lip line, the result may be unacceptable to the patient. If a situation like this can be corrected by soft tissue augmentation of the ridge, an FPD may still be indicated. Otherwise, another approach that permits prosthetic soft tissue to be incorporated in an RPD or implant-supported prosthesis should be selected.

References

Owall B, Kayser AF, Carlsson GE: *Prosthodontics: principles and management strategies,* London, 1996, Mosby-Wolfe, p 141.

Shillingburg HT et al: *Fundamentals of fixed prosthodontics,* ed 3, Chicago, 1997, Quintessence Publishing, p 85.

Studer S et al: Maxillary anterior single-tooth replacement: comparison of three treatment modalities, *Pract Periodontal Aesthet Dent* 2:51, 1996.

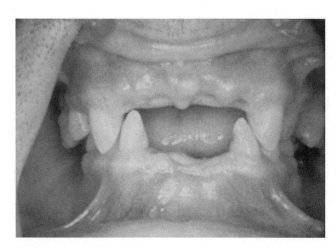

Fig. 96-1 **A,** The span of a fixed partial denture should be restricted to posterior edentulous areas of three teeth or less. **B,** A removable partial denture can be designed to restore any edentulous space but is particularly useful for long spans involving three or more posterior teeth.

Fig. 96-2 Fixed partial dentures would have an uncertain prognosis for this patient because the canines are intact and because of the extreme vertical overlap of the anterior occlusion.

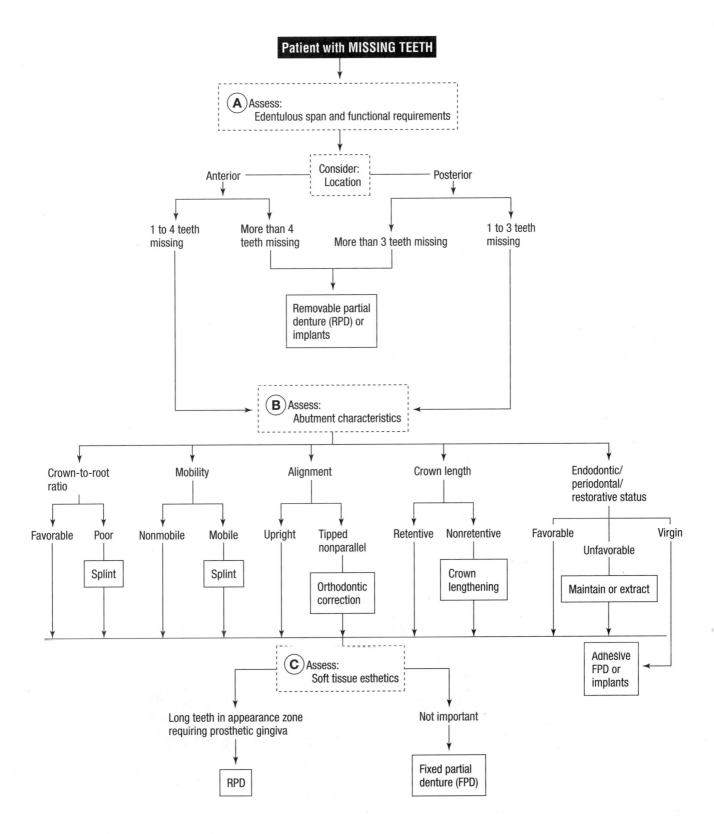

Patient with MISSING TEETH

(A) Assess:
Edentulous span and functional requirements

Consider:
Location

Anterior — Posterior

1 to 4 teeth missing | More than 4 teeth missing | More than 3 teeth missing | 1 to 3 teeth missing

Removable partial denture (RPD) or implants

(B) Assess:
Abutment characteristics

Crown-to-root ratio | Mobility | Alignment | Crown length | Endodontic/ periodontal/ restorative status

Favorable | Poor | Nonmobile | Mobile | Upright | Tipped nonparallel | Retentive | Nonretentive | Favorable | Virgin

Splint | Splint | Orthodontic correction | Crown lengthening | Unfavorable

Maintain or extract

(C) Assess:
Soft tissue esthetics

Long teeth in appearance zone requiring prosthetic gingiva | Not important

RPD | Fixed partial denture (FPD)

Adhesive FPD or implants

97 Adhesive Fixed Partial Denture Versus Conventional Prosthetics

Eugene E. LaBarre

Adhesive fixed partial dentures (A-FPDs) differ from conventional fixed partial dentures (FPDs) in that tooth preparation and retainer design are more conservative, mechanical or chemical adhesive mechanisms are required for both tooth structure and the internal aspect of the retainers, and an adhesive resin is used as a luting medium. Clinical research has demonstrated that A-FPDs are associated with an extremely low incidence of recurrent caries and periodontal inflammation, and patient satisfaction is high. The main problem with an A-FPD is partial or complete debonding of the restoration from the abutment teeth; the incidence varies from study to study but is significantly greater than that for a conventional FPD (Fig. 97-1).

A The A-FPD is a simple restoration and should be used to replace single missing teeth only (two mandibular incisors may be acceptable). Replacing multiple missing teeth or using multiple abutments should be avoided. The abutment teeth should be intact and sturdy. The strength of the bond is determined by surface area of retainer coverage; mobility in abutments significantly increases fatigue of the bond. For this reason, adhesive splints involving multiple mobile teeth are discouraged because they have shown high incidence of debonding, and it is difficult or impossible to repair a partially debonded splint.

B Patients with parafunctional habits have lower success rates with A-FPDs. Constant and forceful clenching or bruxing cause fatigue failure of the bond. For similar reasons, restoration of lateral guidance (e.g., replacement of a maxillary canine) should be avoided. The ideal patient for the A-FPD has uniform nondeflective centric contacts and effective anterior guidance.

C For anterior restorations, centric and guiding contacts should be located in the incisal third, permitting the gingival two thirds to be covered by the retainer without interfering with occlusion. Deep anterior occlusion is the most common contraindication for anterior A-FPDs. The situation that most favors longevity of an A-FPD is the anterior open bite; however, in these cases the dental technician must be advised not to cover the incisal edge with metal to avoid creating a gray color in the abutment teeth. This phenomenon is notoriously difficult to predict and is best avoided by leaving the incisal edge uncovered. For the same reason, caution must be exercised when using thin incisors as abutments because they may appear much darker after luting the restoration. Once graying has occurred, the only solution is to remove the restoration, which involves tedious ultrasonic vibration or sectioning of each retainer.

Diminished width of tooth space is a common finding in adults who lost an anterior tooth during childhood. Many of these individuals have used an acrylic stayplate or flipper for many years. The appearance of these "temporary" restorations is a good indication of whether a ceramic pontic can satisfy the individual's esthetic demands. In cases of slightly diminished width the abutment teeth can be narrowed during tooth preparation. Solutions for moderately reduced space include lapping the pontic facially over one or both abutments or conventional FPD. Severely reduced spaces may require orthodontic correction.

D Finally, the patient should be informed about the potential for debonding occurring within the first 5 years of service and should be willing to accept the consequences of a partial debonded restoration. The patient should also be informed about alternative approaches.

References

Creugers NH et al: An analysis of clinical studies on resin-bonded bridges, *J Dent Res* 70:146, 1991.

Simonsen R, Thompson V, Barrack G: *Etch cast restorations: clinical and laboratory techniques,* Chicago, 1983, Quintessence Publishing.

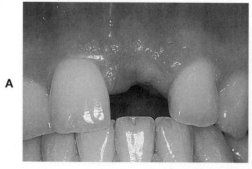
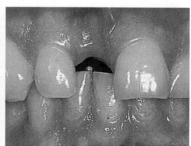

Fig. 97-1 Preoperative presentation of candidates for A-FPDs. **A,** Good indications for an A-FPD: centric occlusion in incisal one third, unblemished abutment teeth, edentulous ridge, and space within normal limits. **B,** Poor indications for an A-FPD: excessive vertical overlap and edentulous space that is narrow mesiodistally.

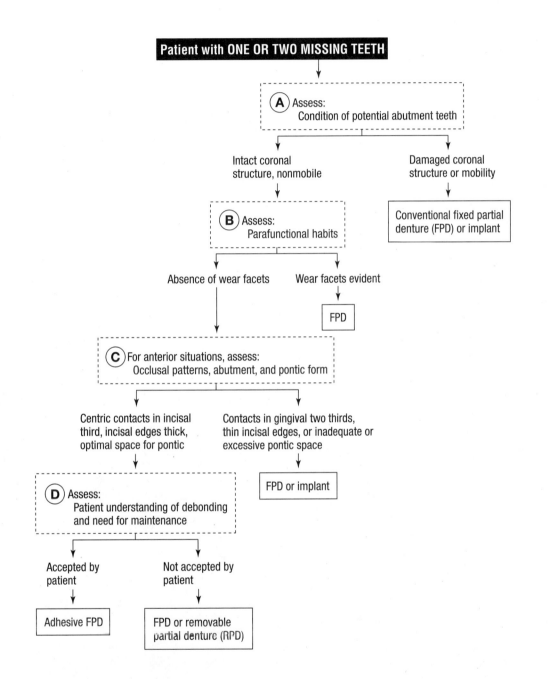

Patient with ONE OR TWO MISSING TEETH

A Assess:
Condition of potential abutment teeth

Intact coronal structure, nonmobile

Damaged coronal structure or mobility

Conventional fixed partial denture (FPD) or implant

B Assess:
Parafunctional habits

Absence of wear facets

Wear facets evident

FPD

C For anterior situations, assess:
Occlusal patterns, abutment, and pontic form

Centric contacts in incisal third, incisal edges thick, optimal space for pontic

Contacts in gingival two thirds, thin incisal edges, or inadequate or excessive pontic space

FPD or implant

D Assess:
Patient understanding of debonding and need for maintenance

Accepted by patient

Not accepted by patient

Adhesive FPD

FPD or removable partial denture (RPD)

98 Determining the Need to Splint

Chi Tran

There are various clinical situations that may require groups of teeth to be reinforced by splinting them together. Teeth develop mobility or unstable positions as a result of periodontitis, occlusal trauma, or recent orthodontic treatment. If the patient is to have a fixed partial denture (FPD) or removable partial denture (RPD) placed on compromised abutment teeth, additional teeth may be needed to adequately support the prosthesis. Decisions regarding whether to splint, how many teeth to include, and the technique of splinting must be made on a regular basis in clinical practice.

A The initial evaluation should determine the periodontal status of the involved teeth. Soft tissue inflammation in an environment of reduced alveolar support and heavy functional demands leads to more bone loss, increasing mobility, and loss of teeth. If periodontal treatment is likely to fail, permanent forms of splinting should not be attempted because little advantage can be attained for the patient. However, arrested or successfully treated periodontitis lends itself to a variety of restorative options.

B Tooth mobility patterns must be evaluated in the context of past events and future expectations. Teeth with documented increasing mobility patterns are unstable and may be expected to continually worsen until they are no longer serviceable, known as the "downhill" sequence. In the absence of inflammatory process a good prognosis can be achieved in these cases by mechanically splinting mobile teeth to each other or to strong neighbors. Several splinting restorations are possible (e.g., removable appliances, intermediate techniques using composite resin with reinforcement [Fig. 98-1], and definitive procedures such as soldered cast gold or porcelain fused to metal crowns). Splinting techniques embody a wide range of technical difficulty and expense. They should be selected following a deliberate analysis of risk versus benefit.

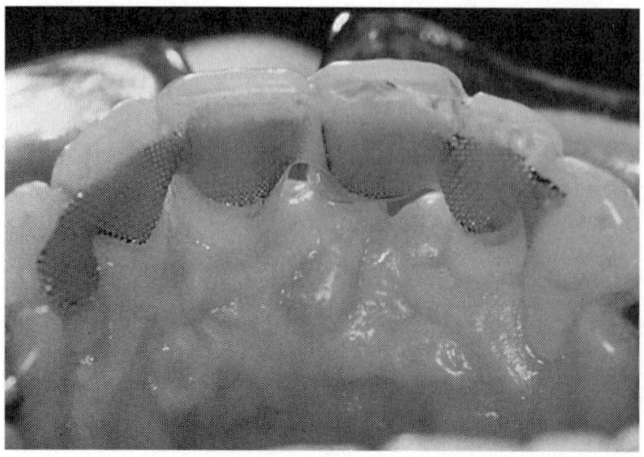

C Uncontrolled drifting and migration of teeth may be caused by a number of factors, including periodontal disease, tooth loss, unstable orthodontic results, or occlusal trauma. Instability of anterior teeth is highly noticeable to patients, and they often point out the problem. Posterior tooth movement usually must be deduced from patterns of extrusion, drifting, and collapse. In most situations splinting can only intercept tooth movement patterns; definitive realignment must be accomplished orthodontically or surgically. The clinician should also be aware of the limitations of splinting to secure the positions of a few remaining teeth (Fig. 98-2).

D Occasionally, teeth must be reinforced because of exceptional occlusal demands or because they must support fixed or removable prostheses. In these situations the restorative dentist must accurately predict the number of reinforcement teeth that are required to withstand the load. Double abutting and cross-arch splinting are acceptable techniques for increasing the support of long span restorations (Fig. 98-3). However, the use of implants to support weak nat-

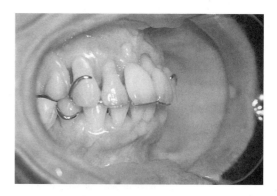

Fig. 98-2 In spite of a lingual cast gold, pin-retained splint that has been in place for 30 years, the combination of supporting a distal extension removable partial denture and progressive bone loss has resulted in facial migration of the maxillary anterior teeth.

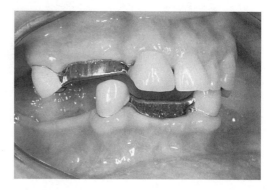

Fig. 98-3 Splinting for the removable partial denture abutment teeth is accomplished by joining porcelain fused-to-metal-crowns to cross-arch bars.

Fig. 98-1 The maxillary anterior teeth are splinted with composite resin reinforced with titanium mesh.

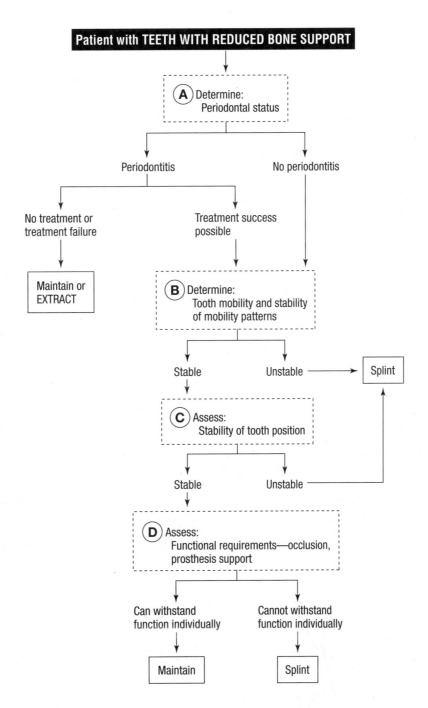

Patient with TEETH WITH REDUCED BONE SUPPORT

(A) Determine:
Periodontal status

Periodontitis — No periodontitis

No treatment or treatment failure — Treatment success possible

Maintain or EXTRACT

(B) Determine:
Tooth mobility and stability of mobility patterns

Stable — Unstable → Splint

(C) Assess:
Stability of tooth position

Stable — Unstable

(D) Assess:
Functional requirements—occlusion, prosthesis support

Can withstand function individually — Cannot withstand function individually

Maintain — Splint

ural teeth is not well established. Several problems unique to implant–tooth combinations have been observed, due in part to dissimilar mobilities and the effect of creating cantilever forces on the restoration. A simpler solution is to extract the weak teeth and to construct a fixed prosthesis that is supported solely by implants.

References

Dawson PE: *Evaluation, diagnosis, and treatment of occlusal problems,* St Louis, 1989, Mosby, p 483.

Ramfjord S, Ash MM: *Occlusion,* ed 3, Philadelphia, 1983, WB Saunders, p 481.

Smith BGN: *Dental crowns and bridges: design and preparation,* ed 2, Chicago, 1990, Mosby, p 211.

99   Telescopic Prostheses Versus Conventional Approaches

Eugene E. LaBarre

A telescopic prosthesis is a two component restoration where the outer prosthesis is detachable from the abutments. Many implant-supported restorations are telescopic by virtue of the stack of screws that assemble the components. In tooth-supported cases the prepared teeth are restored with metal copings that provide marginal seal and ideally tapered axial surfaces. A fixed partial denture (FPD) or removable overdenture is supported by the copings (Fig. 99-1).

A In a patient with misaligned abutment teeth, copings can be placed to realign axial surfaces to a common path of insertion. Examples of conditions that may be difficult to correct orthodontically include atypical dental development associated with severe cleft palate or partial anodontia associated with dentinogenesis imperfecta. Fabrication of parallel coping surfaces makes it possible to place an FPD or overdenture without the risk to pulpal integrity that can occur when tipped teeth are aggressively prepared.

B The most common application of telescopic restorations is in periodontal prostheses. In these cases periodontal support is compromised, and teeth with uncertain long-term prognosis may be required as abutments. The telescopic FPD is considered a reversible restoration because it is luted with provisional cement. This permits removal by the dentist for periodic maintenance or when an abutment must be repaired or extracted. Telescopic periodontal prostheses are demanding procedures requiring substantial tooth reduction to permit reasonable restoration contours. Each abutment tooth has two restorations and two margins that may present a challenge in the appearance zone.

C If the patient profile permits and there is bone of sufficient quantity and quality to support implants, heroic salvage of periodontally compromised teeth may be less predictable and less satisfactory to the patient than implant treatment. The telescopic approach has been used successfully in cases with combinations of tooth and implant abutments. However, the dentist is urged to use caution in planning such hybrid prostheses because of the differences in mobility between teeth and implants and the unequal support that may be provided to the prosthesis. The patient should understand the heroic nature of the

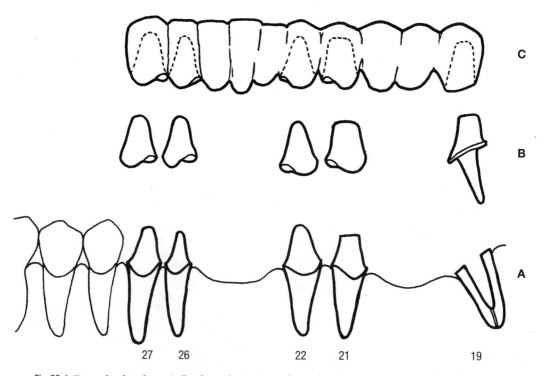

Fig. 99-1 Example of a telescopic fixed prosthesis. **A,** Teeth 19 (distal root), 21, 22, 26, and 27 have been prepared to receive copings. **B,** Copings are fabricated with a common tapering axis and are luted permanently to the individual teeth. **C,** The external prosthesis is a fixed partial denture and is retained passively by friction or with a temporary luting agent.

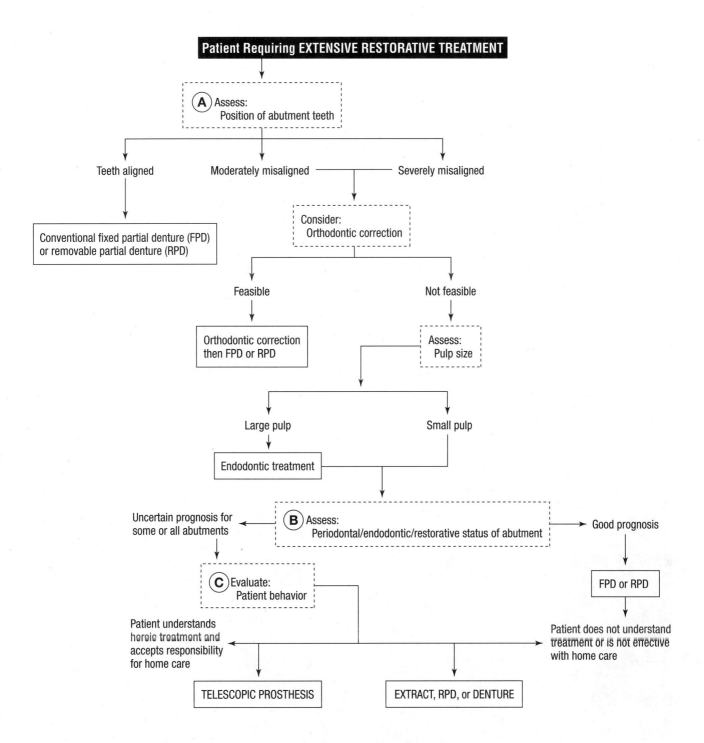

Patient Requiring EXTENSIVE RESTORATIVE TREATMENT

(A) Assess:
Position of abutment teeth

Teeth aligned → Conventional fixed partial denture (FPD) or removable partial denture (RPD)

Moderately misaligned / Severely misaligned → **Consider:** Orthodontic correction

Feasible → Orthodontic correction then FPD or RPD

Not feasible → **Assess:** Pulp size

Large pulp → Endodontic treatment

Small pulp

(B) Assess: Periodontal/endodontic/restorative status of abutment

Uncertain prognosis for some or all abutments

Good prognosis → FPD or RPD

(C) Evaluate: Patient behavior

Patient understands heroic treatment and accepts responsibility for home care → TELESCOPIC PROSTHESIS

EXTRACT, RPD, or DENTURE

Patient does not understand treatment or is not effective with home care

telescopic approach and should demonstrate adequate home care. As always, patient cooperation with home care is the most critical determinant of success in these complex treatment modalities, and frequent recall is highly recommended.

References

Owall B, Kayser AF, Carlsson GE: *Prosthodontics: principles and management strategies,* London, 1996, Mosby-Wolfe, p 155.

Shillingburg HT et al: *Fundamentals of fixed prosthodontics,* ed 3, Chicago, 1997, Quintessence, p 99.

100 Occlusion

Eugene E. LaBarre

Occlusion is an important topic in dentistry because of its role in transmitting stress to individual teeth and throughout the stomatognathic system. Excessive occlusal stress can be harmful, and the dentist is often required to manage and restore the damage caused by occlusal dysfunction. Reconstruction of major portions of a patient's occlusion is a demanding and unforgiving procedure. The well-established principles of simultaneous nondeflective centric contacts and anterior group or canine guidance in eccentric movements should be incorporated in every restoration.

A If a patient has the signs and symptoms of temporomandibular dysfunction (TMD), such as painful muscles and joints, loud noise in the joint, limited opening of the mouth, and history of locked jaw, comprehensive evaluation is necessary. A dental problem, such as improperly occluding restorations or bruxism, may be a cofactor in TMD. Conservative therapy should be attempted first; if occlusal rehabilitation is necessary, it should be delayed until the symptoms have been eliminated or reduced by reversible procedures. Because TMD patients are more likely to respond adversely to changes in occlusion caused by restorative dentistry, the dentist is advised to work with health professionals knowledgeable about TMD.

B Patients with missing teeth can be placed in two general categories: (1) Those with teeth missing from the posterior ends of the jaw so that the dental arch remains intact but is shortened and (2) those with teeth missing from mid-arch so that the integrity of the dental arch is interrupted. Posteriorly shortened dental arches are stable and functional for most patients when there are at least two opposing pairs of posterior teeth on each side of the arch (i.e., second premolar occlusion). Patients may elect to have missing molars replaced for esthetics or added function or to stabilize unopposed molars, in which case the prosthesis must be either a distal extension removable partial denture (RPD) or an implant-supported fixed partial denture (FPD). Mid-arch missing teeth should be replaced with a tooth- or implant-supported FPD or an RPD to prevent the eventual occlusal collapse caused by extrusion and tipping of neighboring and opposing teeth into edentulous areas.

C Premature centric or eccentric contacts can cause problems ranging from individual tooth wear and mobility to temporomandibular joint and neuromuscular symptoms. Mild disharmony can be corrected by selective grinding, while more substantial problems require occlusal coverage restorations or orthodontic and surgical correction. Articulated diagnostic casts can help to determine the severity of the disharmony. In cases requiring multidisciplinary treatment there are no rules governing which specialist performs the equilibration or the timing of the procedure in the overall treatment sequence. However, the restorative dentist should have an idea of the final occlusal scheme and reserves the right to direct the steps in achieving this.

D Worn functional surfaces of teeth may be caused by abrasion, attrition, or erosion (Fig. 100-1). The range of the problem should be identified and corrected, if possible. Conservative and reversible therapy, such as occlusal splints and biofeedback, can reduce the rate of tooth wear but cannot permanently replace missing structures. Conservative therapy is indicated for mild wear cases or for maintaining restored occlusions. More severe tooth wear, involving thermal or contact sensitivity or esthetic compromise, must be restored with occlusal protecting restorations such as onlays and crowns. The most extreme situations require a decision between heroic treatment, including endodontic treatment and surgical crown lengthening, or extraction followed by prosthetic treatment. In patients with occlusal wear there is an assumption the vertical dimension is lost along with tooth structure.

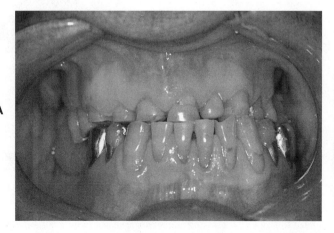
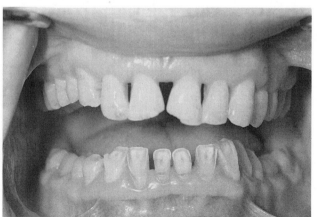

Fig. 100-1 Examples of extreme occlusal wear that would require reconstruction or extraction. **A,** Horizontal flattening of the maxillary teeth has been caused by bruxing and a Class III malocclusion. **B,** Angular wear is caused by bruxing and a severely overlapping anterior occlusion.

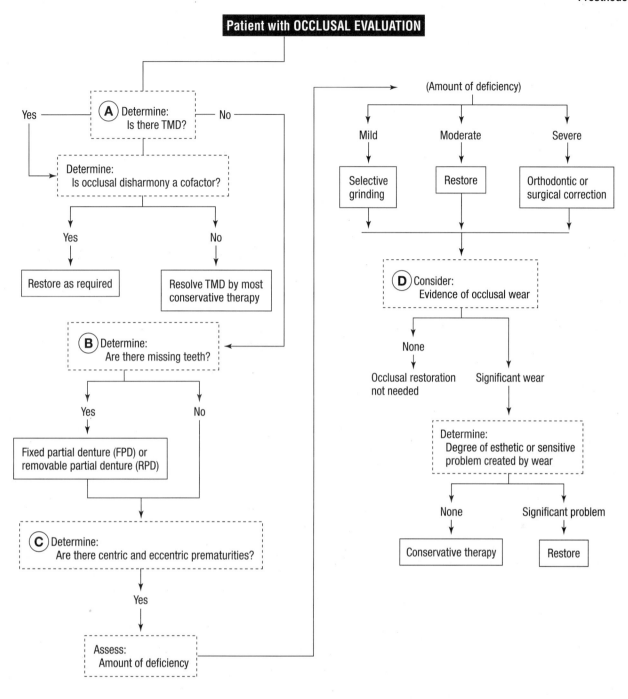

Patient with OCCLUSAL EVALUATION

However, even in the most severe cases, compensatory eruption occurs as the teeth wear, resulting in maintenance of freeway space and closest speaking space. It is important for restorative dentists to evaluate these functional parameters because the reflex to increase vertical dimension beyond physiologic limits can cause severe and chronic problems.

References

Allen PF et al: Shortened dental arch therapy: views of consultants in restorative dentistry in the United Kingdom, *J Oral Rehabil* 23:481, 1996.

Kampe T et al: Ten-year follow-up study of signs and symptoms of craniomandibular disorders in adults with intact and restored dentitions, *J Oral Rehabil* 5:416, 1996.

NIH Consensus Program: *Management of temporomandibular disorders,* Technology assessment conference statement, Kensington, Md, 1996, NIH Consensus Program.

Owall B, Kayser AF, Carlsson GE: *Prosthodontics: principles and management strategies,* London, 1996, Mosby-Wolfe, p 97.

Shillingburg HT et al: *Fundamentals of fixed prosthodontics,* ed 3, Chicago, 1997, Quintessence, p 11.

101 Endodontic Effects of Cast Restorations

Eugene E. LaBarre

Pulpal sensitivity is a common complaint following fixed prosthodontic procedures on vital teeth. Except for obvious situations, such as preparing virgin teeth with large pulps or over-preparing because of occlusal or path of insertion demands, development of pulpal symptoms is difficult to predict and may seem to occur in random patterns in prosthodontic practice. The clinician should be familiar with possible etiologies of pulpal trauma and exercise universal precautions to reduce its occurrence.

A During tooth preparation for full coverage restorations, potential for significant damage to the pulp exists. The enamel is removed, and all of the dentinal tubules in the coronal aspect of the tooth are cut. Overheating is the most common source of postoperative sensitivity, and the clinician should always monitor the amount of water spray and cutting efficiency of diamonds and burs. Clogged or worn rotary instruments should be replaced. Other contributing factors include: excessive pressure during grinding, vibration from asymmetric rotary instruments, and desiccation to aid visibility and impression making. Routine use of a dentin bonding agent or unfilled resin is recommended immediately following completion of tooth preparation to seal dentinal tubules and to protect the pulp from further trauma.

The provisional restoration must be managed with care, also. If large amounts of acrylic resin are polymerized directly on the prepared teeth, the exothermic setting reaction can cause a substantial increase in intrapulpal temperature. Frequent pumping and cooling of the provisional restoration are necessary during polymerization. Attention to fit is also important to minimize the effects of microleakage and occlusal trauma.

The cementation process has been shown to irritate a vital pulp. A barrier in the form of copal varnish or bonding agent is recommended. Cements differ in their capacities to elicit pulpal response. This has proven difficult to evaluate through clinical trials. As with tooth preparation, the clinician should realize that the luting procedure is a critical step for the health of the vital pulp and universal precautions should be exercised to minimize trauma to the pulp.

Thermal shock continues to be a significant problem following cementation of cast restorations. General recommendations include placing a base on deep areas of tooth preparation and advising patients that the situation is usually transient.

A tooth restored by a cast restoration may develop symptoms after long periods of comfort. Such cases usually suggest a chronic inflammatory response in the pulp that is clinically unremarkable until an exacerbation initiates symptoms. The pulpal status may result from the cumulative insult of previous caries and several restorative procedures. If obvious factors (e.g., occlusal trauma, recurrent decay, or fractures) are not found, no treatment is indicated until symptoms warrant endodontic therapy.

B Mild pulpal symptoms (e.g., thermal sensitivity that disappears when the stimulant is removed) indicate reversible pulpitis. No treatment is indicated in these situations until symptoms worsen.

C Severe symptoms (e.g., unprovoked pain, throbbing that interrupts sleep, or pain that lingers after the stimulus is removed) are more ominous and suggest irreversible pulpitis. Endodontic therapy is indicated.

D Restored teeth with severe pulpal symptoms should be evaluated for vertical periodontal defects to rule out a cracked root. If a crack is detected, heroic treatment involving endodontic therapy and periodontal maintenance of the defect area is unpredictable. In many cases extraction is the only effective treatment for the pain associated with these teeth.

References

Cohen S, Burns RC: *Pathways of the pulp*, ed 6, St Louis, 1994, Mosby.
Shillingburg HT et al: *Fundamentals of fixed prosthodontics*, ed 3, Chicago, 1997, Quintessence Publishing.

Patient with PULPAL SYMPTOMS FOLLOWING RESTORATION OF A VITAL TOOTH

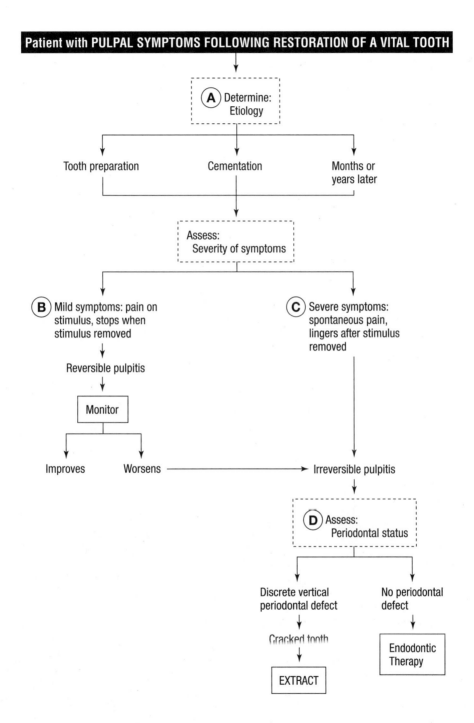

102 Rapid Extrusion Versus Crown Lengthening Surgery

Kathy I. Mueller, Galen W. Wagnild

Salvage of teeth severely compromised by caries, fracture, or large defective restorations often depends on the extent of damage below the free gingival margin. A tooth lengthening procedure is required when significant structural degradation has occurred. Periodontal crown lengthening surgery is a one-step tooth lengthening procedure that can expose most defects for restorative correction. This approach removes soft and hard supporting tissues and moves the attachment level apically. The tooth position remains unchanged; however, this surgery may affect esthetics or the maintenance potential of adjacent teeth. Rapid orthodontic extrusion is an alternative tooth lengthening method that also facilitates restoration of compromised teeth. This procedure moves the residual tooth structure coronally while the soft and hard supporting tissues remain in their pretreatment locations. Orthodontic rapid extrusion is indicated when esthetic considerations are critical or when adjacent tooth anatomy and adjacent coronal restorations would be jeopardized by the surgical apical repositioning of periodontal tissues.

A To be successful over time, restorative procedures must not invade the attachment apparatus. There must be adequate sound tooth structure between the lesion and the coronal extent of the junctional epithelium to place a restorative margin. The margin generally requires 2 mm of sound tooth structure coronal to the attachment. Operative invasion of the attachment often results in gingival recession, periodontal pocket formation, or chronic gingival inflammation (Fig. 102-1).

B Retention of the severely damaged tooth requires critical pretreatment evaluation. Accurate prediction of posttreatment crown-to-root ratio is mandatory. Sufficient periodontal attachment for the tooth to withstand functional forces must remain after the procedure. With all other variables equal, rapid orthodontic extrusion provides a more favorable posttreatment crown-to-root ratio than does periodontal crown lengthening surgery.

Cylindrical root form greatly enhances the functional and esthetic components of tooth lengthening. A tapered root form compromises the remaining periodontal ligament attachment after either procedure. Likewise, gingival embrasures are exaggerated when either orthodontics or surgery is performed on a tapered root (Fig. 102-2).

C Esthetic variables have a great impact on the modality selection between rapid orthodontic extrusion and periodontal crown lengthening surgery. Patients with great esthetic expectations and a high lip line may not tolerate the deformity produced by surgery. This defect will be apparent on the damaged tooth as well as adjacent teeth, in most cases.

Maintenance of free gingival margin symmetry could dictate that surgery be expanded to include the entire anterior sextant. This surgical expansion exposes root structure on all included teeth. These significant sequelae may be avoided by using orthodontics to correct the defect (see Fig. 102-2).

D The selected modality should not solve one problem while creating others. Short root trunks or significant developmental grooves on adjacent teeth may be exposed by surgery and therefore require the damaged tooth to be extruded. These anatomic findings render a tooth more difficult to maintain if the attachment level is moved apically by a surgical technique (see Fig. 102-2).

E Existing coronal restorations on adjacent teeth also influence the selection of extrusion or surgery. Intracrevicular margins on adjacent teeth are exposed by conventional periodontal surgical techniques to lengthen the tooth. Restorations that do not need replacement and demand intracrevicular margins for esthetics are indications for orthodontic rapid extrusion of the damaged tooth (see Fig. 102-2).

References

Biggerstaff R, Sinks J, Carazola J: Orthodontic extrusion and biologic width realignment procedures: Methods for reclaiming nonrestorable teeth, *J Am Dent Assoc* 112:345, 1986.

Kozlovsky A, Tal H, Lieberman M: Forced eruption combined with gingival fiberectomy: a technique for crown lengthening, *J Clin Periodontol* 15:534, 1988.

Pontoriero R, Celenza F, Ricci G, Carnevale G: Rapid extrusion with fiber resection: a combined orthodontic-periodontal treatment modality, *Int J Periodont Restor Dent* 5:30, 1987.

Rosenberg E, Garber D, Evian C: Tooth lengthening procedures, *Compend Contin Educ* 1(3):161, 1980.

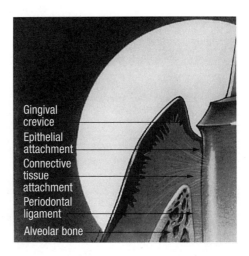

Gingival crevice
Epithelial attachment
Connective tissue attachment
Periodontal ligament
Alveolar bone

Fig. 102-1 The restorative margin must terminate on sound tooth structure coronal to the epithelial attachment. Mutilated teeth require alteration of the tooth-attachment relationship before restoration. This modification will allow margin placement while maintaining the integrity of the attachment apparatus.

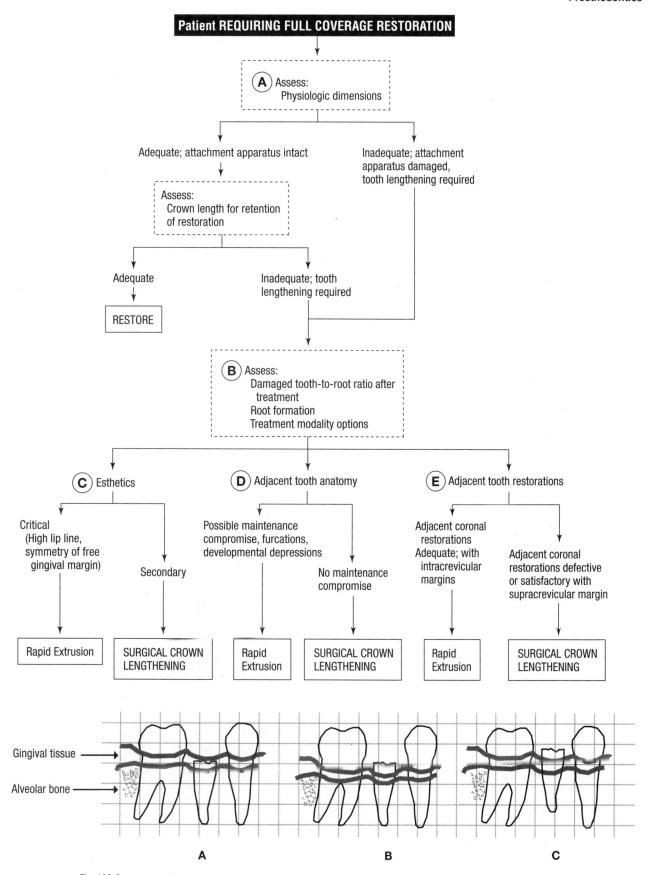

Patient REQUIRING FULL COVERAGE RESTORATION

A Assess:
Physiologic dimensions

Adequate; attachment apparatus intact

Inadequate; attachment apparatus damaged, tooth lengthening required

Assess:
Crown length for retention of restoration

Adequate

Inadequate; tooth lengthening required

RESTORE

B Assess:
Damaged tooth-to-root ratio after treatment
Root formation
Treatment modality options

C Esthetics

D Adjacent tooth anatomy

E Adjacent tooth restorations

Critical
(High lip line, symmetry of free gingival margin)

Secondary

Possible maintenance compromise, furcations, developmental depressions

No maintenance compromise

Adjacent coronal restorations
Adequate; with intracrevicular margins

Adjacent coronal restorations defective or satisfactory with supracrevicular margin

Rapid Extrusion

SURGICAL CROWN LENGTHENING

Rapid Extrusion

SURGICAL CROWN LENGTHENING

Rapid Extrusion

SURGICAL CROWN LENGTHENING

Gingival tissue

Alveolar bone

A

B

C

Fig. 102-2 **A,** A mutilated second premolar requires restoration; there is insufficient coronal structure for margin placement without damage to the attachment mechanism. **B,** Surgical crown lengthening exposes sufficient sound tooth structure; the periodontal tissues are apically repositioned, and the root position is unchanged. **C,** Orthodontic extrusion exposes sufficient sound tooth structure; the periodontal tissue position is unchanged but the root has been repositioned coronally.

103 Supragingival Versus Intracrevicular Margin Placement

Kathy I. Mueller, Galen W. Wagnild

The marginal periodontium operated on daily by restorative dentists requires definitive, logical decisions regarding margin location. Literature supports placement of margins slightly into the crevice or coronal to the free gingival margin. Restorations located deep in the sulcus risk irreversible damage, to the supporting structures.

A Esthetic requirements may dictate intracrevicular margin location despite other clinical findings that would allow a supragingival location. It is important to determine esthetic margin placement using factors such as tooth position, visibility of the margin area during normal function, and the patient's understanding of the objectives of the restorative therapy. The margin of a porcelain fused-to-metal restoration often can be placed 0.5 to 1.0 mm into a healthy gingival crevice. In a thin, scalloped gingival architecture, it may be impossible to conceal a metal collar margin at this depth. This problem may be resolved by use of a porcelain shoulder margin or a margin supported by metal that does not display a visible collar. When esthetics are secondary and structural features permit, restorative margins can be located outside of the gingival crevice. Supragingival margins are more accurately prepared, more predictably recorded, and more accessible for evaluation, finishing, and patient maintenance.

B Adequate preparation length to retain the final restoration must be planned. In cases with marginally adequate coronal structure an additional 1 mm of axial wall can often be obtained by preparing within the gingival crevice. The physiologic zone or biologic width must be maintained intact (Fig. 103-1). Attempts to increase coverage by apically positioning the restorative margin are limited by this fragile complex. Violation of this width may result in chronic gingival inflammation, recession of the free gingival margin, loss of crestal bone, and pocket formation (Fig. 103-2). If adequate retention and resistance cannot be obtained within the parameters of a healthy periodontium, surgical crown lengthening or rapid orthodontic extrusion may be indicated. Patients requiring restoration after periodontal therapy pose additional complexities. The gingival attachment is often positioned more apically, and postsurgical cases may have shallow gingival sulci. Attempts to place margins within the sulcus may lead to breakdown of the tissue complex. The elongated clinical crown in the periodontally compromised case requires additional axial wall reduction to achieve intracrevicular margins. This preparation may encroach on the pulp and threaten the vitality of the tooth. When possible, postsurgical margins should be placed above the free gingival margin.

C Preparation of margins should extend beyond existing restorations and lesions onto sound tooth structure. This sound structure should be a minimum of 2 mm in height. Placement of the margin in the gingival crevice will often accomplish these goals. However, defects deep in the crevice or into the attachment apparatus should be treated with surgical crown lengthening or orthodontic extrusion.

D Root sensitivity may be controlled or eliminated by conservative means. In severe cases endodontic treatment may be required. Supragingival margin placement is suggested if root sensitivity has been resolved before restoration.

References

Nevins M, Skurow H: The intracrevicular restorative margin, the biologic width, and maintenance of the gingival margin, *Int J Periodont Restor Dent* 3:31, 1984.

Schluger S, Yuodelis R, Page R, Johnson R: *Periodontal diseases: basic phenomena, clinical management and occlusal and restorative interrelationships,* Philadelphia, 1990, Lea & Febiger.

Shillingburg H, Hobo S, Whitsett D: *Fundamentals of fixed prosthodontics,* ed 2, Berlin, 1981, Quintessence Publishing, p 79.

Wilson R, Maynard G: Intracrevicular restorative dentistry, *Int J Periodont Restor Dent* 4:35, 1981.

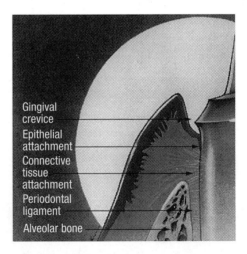

Fig. 103-1 The restorative margin must terminate above the level of the epithelial attachment. Potential operative damage and greater maintenance difficulty can occur as the margin approaches the base of the gingival crevice.

Gingival crevice
Epithelial attachment
Connective tissue attachment
Periodontal ligament
Alveolar bone

Patient with a TOOTH REQUIRING A FULL COVERAGE RESTORATION

(A) Consider:
Esthetics

Esthetics secondary

Esthetics critical → Intracrevicular margin

(B) Assess:
Retention and resistance form of coronal structure

Adequate

Inadequate

Grossly inadequate

Intracrevicular margin

Coronal buildup, surgical crown lengthening, or orthodontic extrusion

(C) Assess:
Location of lesions and old restorations

Supragingival

At the free gingival margin

In close proximity or within the attachment apparatus

Intracrevicular margin

Surgical crown lengthening or orthodontic extrusion

(D) Assess:
Root sensitivity

None

Sensitivity present because of exposure with no resolution following conservative therapy

Supragingival margins

Intracrevicular margins

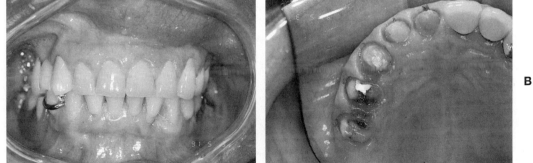

A   **B**

Fig. 103-2 Violation of the biologic width creates problems for the patient and the dentist. **A,** Preoperative view. All maxillary teeth are restored with individual porcelain fused-to-metal crowns. The interdental papillae are enlarged, and the patient reports chronic gingival pain. **B,** Crowns have been removed from teeth 4, 5, 6, 7, and 8, and the proximal areas with deeply subgingival margins show redness, swelling, and spontaneous bleeding of chronic inflammation. Surgical crown lengthening is now required to create a healthy gingival crevice.

104 Removable Partial Denture Considerations for the Periodontally Compromised Patient

Eugene E. LaBarre

Although the fixed partial denture (FPD) is the restoration of choice for restoring missing teeth, the removable partial denture (RPD) becomes necessary when the edentulous span is too long or when there is no end tooth (distal extension).

A The need for tooth replacement is first assessed according to the patient's esthetic or functional disability. Not all partially edentulous patients require restoration; when all molars are missing, a well-integrated second premolar occlusion is satisfactory for many people.

B When an RPD is fabricated for a periodontally compromised patient, the prosthesis should fit well, be rigid, and result in minimal coverage of marginal gingiva by the metallic portion. Open major connector designs placed at least 3-mm apical to marginal tissue in the mandible (6 mm in the maxilla) are preferred over plated designs, which cover the lingual surfaces of multiple teeth.

C Edentulous areas that are capable of supporting occlusal loads are covered fully, particularly in distal extension situations. The altered cast impression technique provides soft tissue contact simultaneous with seating of the rests, minimizing rocking of the restoration in function. A variety of mechanical clasping systems have been described to reduce functional leverage-type forces on distal extension RPD abutments (Fig. 104-1). If precision attachments are desirable esthetically, resilient designs that permit tissue-ward movement and rotation are necessary for periodontally compromised abutments.

D Splinting is required to reinforce mobile RPD abutments and is strongly recommended for free-standing premolar pier abutments. Double abutting also may be necessary for nonmobile abutments adjacent to severely resorbed distal

extension residual ridges because of the potential for increased movement of the restoration and consequent damage to the abutment teeth (Fig. 104-2). The presence of six or fewer anterior teeth as the only support in the arch for an RPD is a common occurrence. In this situation splinting all the teeth offers excellent support for the RPD. Highly mobile teeth have little value as RPD abutments and should be extracted. There must be at least two strategic nonmobile abutments or abutment groups to support an RPD; otherwise, a complete denture is indicated.

E The optimal occlusion for the reduced support RPD involves uniform posterior centric contacts without significant laterally displacing forces. Natural tooth guidance, if it exists and is nondestructive, should be maintained. Prosthetic tooth materials should have wear properties compatible with those of opposing dentition to preserve occlusal contact patterns: acrylic opposite acrylic; metal opposite enamel, metal, or porcelain fused to metal; and porcelain opposite porcelain denture teeth.

The success of any restoration in a compromised oral scheme depends on effective home care and regular recall. Removable restorations should be kept scrupulously clean and should be removed from the mouth for a minimum of 8 hours each day.

References

Carranza FA: *Glickman's clinical periodontology,* ed 7, Philadelphia, 1990, WB Saunders, p 945.

Gomes BC, Renner RP: Periodontal considerations of the removable partial overdenture, *Dent Clin North Am* 34:653, 1990.

Renner RP, Boucher LJ: *Removable partial dentures,* Chicago, 1987, Quintessence Publishing, p 53.

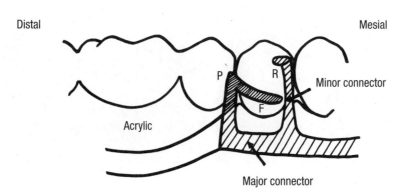

Distal — Mesial

P — R — Minor connector

Acrylic — F

Major connector

Fig. 104-1 Illustration of a stress-releasing clasp (RPF). *R,* Mesial rest, *P,* distal guide plane; *F,* Circumferential clasp placed at or gingival to the tooth height of contour. The minor connector provides bracing action and is designed to cover the soft tissue minimally. The major connector is placed apical to the free gingival margin.

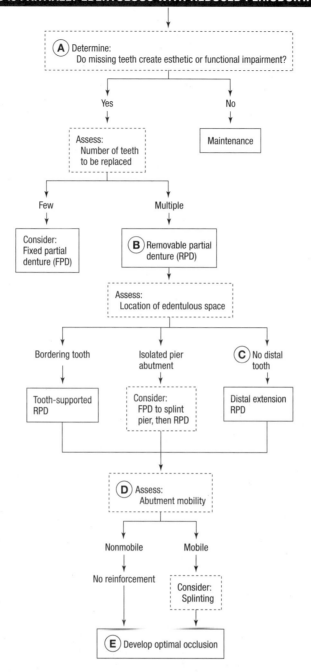

(A) Determine:
Do missing teeth create esthetic or functional impairment?

Yes → **Assess:** Number of teeth to be replaced

No → Maintenance

Few → Consider: Fixed partial denture (FPD)

Multiple → **(B) Removable partial denture (RPD)**

Assess: Location of edentulous space

Bordering tooth → Tooth-supported RPD

Isolated pier abutment → Consider: FPD to splint pier, then RPD

(C) No distal tooth → Distal extension RPD

(D) Assess: Abutment mobility

Nonmobile → No reinforcement

Mobile → Consider: Splinting

(E) Develop optimal occlusion

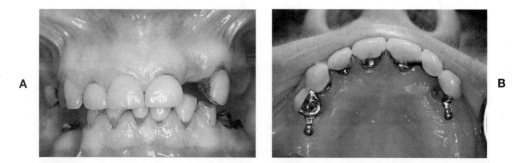

Fig. 104-2 In a combination treatment, fixed restorations are used to optimize removable partial denture (RPD) service in partially edentulous patients with periodontally compromised abutment teeth. **A,** Preoperative view showing that tooth 10 is missing and tooth 11 is a free-standing distal abutment. **B,** Postoperative view. The maxillary teeth are restored with porcelain fused-to-metal restorations. Teeth 5 and 6 are double abutted, and a fixed partial denture restores teeth 9, 10, and 11. The extracoronal attachments permit rotation and tissue-ward movement of the distal extension RPD.

105 Osseointegrated Implants for the Edentulous Mandible

I. E. Naert

The rehabilitation of the edentulous mandible may be achieved by means of a fixed prosthesis or an overdenture supported by endosteal root form implants. The cumulative failure rate for prosthesis stability of Branemark implants in the mandibular symphyseal area is low (1%). Other implant systems also report good results in this area, at least for intermediate term observations. Two to six fixtures usually are placed in the interforaminal region unless the mandible is resorbed.

A In general, an orthopantomograph and a profile radiograph suffice for evaluation of osseous structures. When the anterior mandible height is only 7 mm and its width is limited, the use of a small number of fixtures is advised so as not to weaken the mandible and to prevent a fracture of the jawbone. In the severely resorbed mandible a predictable procedure is the installation of two widely spaced fixtures connected above the alveolar crest by a cast bar oriented parallel to the mandibular hinge axis. The overdenture should be resilient. When loading the distal saddles of the overdenture, the fixtures should be subjected to axial loading only.

B If there is sufficient bone volume and the patient is young, the primary choice should always be a fixed full prosthesis (for Angle Class I and II relationships). With a fixed prosthesis, bone resorption in the anterior mandible is limited to physiologic amounts. In areas distal to the fixtures, alveolar bone resorption also is minimal.

With an Angle Class III relationship, the shortened arch destabilizes the upper denture and increases the resorption rate of the anterior maxilla. The ideal treatment is surgical correction of the Class III malocclusion by means of an osteotomy before a full fixed prosthesis is installed. A more conservative option is the placement of an overdenture, which can transfer load to the posterior area and limit overload of the anterior maxilla.

With overdenture therapy, resorption of the posterior ridge may continue and can exceed that which occurs with a complete denture because of the greater chewing forces associated with overdentures. Implant-supported overdentures are indicated primarily for older patients who do not object to a removable denture and only seek increased denture retention. To limit the harmful effects of continuous resorption of the posterior mandible, regular relining of the overdenture is indicated. This also decreases torquing forces on the fixtures.

In the fabrication of a mandibular fixed prosthesis opposing a maxillary complete denture, the occlusal forces should be distributed over the entire maxillary arch to lower the risk of further resorption of the anterior maxilla. However, "clearing" anterior centric contacts is not recommended because this practice may lead to overload of the distal fixtures from excessive pressure on the extension pontics.

C It is important to distinguish between the "physiologic" patient, who desires only better retention of the lower denture, and the "psychologic" patient, who is not only dissatisfied with the function of the denture but also wants to be freed from "removable teeth." The clinician should carefully determine which therapy objectives are reasonable; desires for dramatically youthful appearance or social problem solving may not be realistic, and the patient may be extremely disappointed in treatment results.

References

Adell R, Eriksson B, Lekholm U: A long-term follow-up study of osseointegrated implants in the treatment of totally edentulous jaws, *Int J Oral Maxillofac Implants* 5:347, 1990.

Albrektsson T, Zarb G, Worthington P: The long-term efficacy of currently used dental implants, *Int J Oral Maxillofac Implants* 1:11, 1986.

Jemt T, Stalblad PA: The effect of chewing movements on changing mandibular complete dentures to osseointegrated overdentures: a 4-year report, *J Prosthet Dent* 55:357, 1986.

Naert I, Quirynen M, Theuniers G et al: Prosthetic aspects of osseointegrated fixtures supporting overdentures: a 4-year report, *J Prosthet Dent* 65:671, 1991.

Quirynen M, Naert I, van Steenberghe D: Fixture design and overload influence marginal bone and fixture loss in the Branemark system, *Clin Oral Impl Res* 3:104, 1992.

Sennerby L, Carlsson GE, Bergman B et al: Mandibular bone resorption in patients treated with tissue-integrated prostheses and in complete-denture wearers, *Acta Odontol Scand* 46:135, 1988.

Patient who is EDENTULOUS AND HAS DIFFICULTIES WITH MANDIBULAR COMPLETE DENTURE

(A) Assess:
Bone height in anterior mandible

Less than 7 mm

More than 7 mm

(B) Determine:
Patient's age

Elderly

Young

Implant-supported
overdenture

Implant-supported
fixed prosthesis

(C) Assess:
Patient expectation for implant treatment

Secure denture

Eliminate denture

Implant-supported
overdenture

Assess:
Are expectations reasonable?

Yes

No

Implant-supported
fixed prosthesis

Avoid definitive
treatment

106 Osseointegrated Implants for the Totally Edentulous Maxilla

Joan Pi Urgell

When considering the restoration of the totally edentulous maxilla with a fixture-retained prosthesis, the first step is to evaluate the remaining bone by conventional assessment techniques.

A If there is enough residual bone for implant placement, the lip support and smile line are considered. If the lip is adequately supported by the existing ridge, and the lip is long enough to cover the implant-gingiva interface during smiling, then six to eight fixtures may be placed for a fixed bridge. If there is not enough lip support, an overdenture is the treatment of choice.

B In cases where there is not enough bone for implant placement consider the type of resorption that occurred in the maxilla.

C If the resorption has occurred on the facial aspect of the ridge, resulting in a thin maxilla, two surgical approaches are possible. In less severe resorption cases the fixtures are placed in a proper position with threads exposed, and a guided bone regeneration procedure is performed simultaneously with implant placement. In more severe resorption, an onlay bone graft is placed and allowed to heal for 6 to 8 months before placement of fixtures for a fixed bridge.

D When the maxilla resorbs by loss of crestal bone, the relationship between the residual ridge and the opposing arch is evaluated. For Angle Class I or II relationships, an onlay bone graft ("horse shoe" technique) should be performed simultaneously with implant placement to use the fixtures to secure and stabilize the graft. When the relationship is Class III, the best approach is to perform a LeFort I advancement of the maxilla, placing interpositional graft material and the implants simultaneously.

E If there is a severely resorbed maxilla with both horizontal and vertical bone loss, the patient may suffer physically and psychologically from the lack of prosthesis stability. The principal objective in these cases is to provide a retention system for the prosthesis. The patient's age, general health, and availability of bone locally for harvesting will determine the surgical approach. If there is not much bone available, or health conditions dictate a conservative approach, two block bone grafts can be harvested from the chin, hip, or calvaria and placed in the floor of the nasal cavity to enlarge the piriform rim. Four to six implants are placed simultaneously to stabilize the bone grafts. After integration, the implants are used to retain an overdenture. When local and health conditions are more favorable, an onlay bone graft may be performed simultaneously with two bone blocks inlayed in the floor of the nose and transfixed with fixtures. A fixed bridge may be placed if lip support is adequate and a majority of the grafts remain. In cases of less ideal surgical resolution or inadequate lip support, an overdenture is the final prosthetic treatment.

References

Lundquist S, Carlsson GE: Maxillary fixed prostheses on osseointegrated dental implants, *J Prosthet Dent* 50:262, 1983.

Misch CE, Sotereanos G, Dietsh F: *Autogenous bone grafts for endosteal implants: indications, success, and failures: contemporary implant dentistry,* St Louis, 1993, Mosby, p 599.

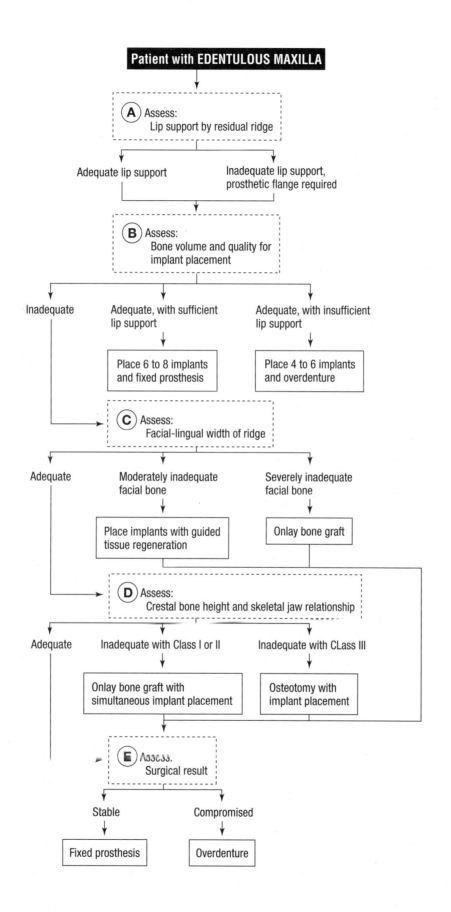

Patient with EDENTULOUS MAXILLA

(A) Assess:
Lip support by residual ridge

Adequate lip support | Inadequate lip support, prosthetic flange required

(B) Assess:
Bone volume and quality for implant placement

Inadequate | Adequate, with sufficient lip support | Adequate, with insufficient lip support

Place 6 to 8 implants and fixed prosthesis | Place 4 to 6 implants and overdenture

(C) Assess:
Facial-lingual width of ridge

Adequate | Moderately inadequate facial bone | Severely inadequate facial bone

Place implants with guided tissue regeneration | Onlay bone graft

(D) Assess:
Crestal bone height and skeletal jaw relationship

Adequate | Inadequate with Class I or II | Inadequate with CLass III

Onlay bone graft with simultaneous implant placement | Osteotomy with implant placement

(E) Assess:
Surgical result

Stable | Compromised

Fixed prosthesis | Overdenture

107 Single Tooth Implants

Larry G. Loos

A Healthy or predictably treatable teeth adjacent to the single edentulous space are more important to long-term implant success than the edentulous site itself. Adjacent teeth must be capable of carrying a greater incisal-occlusal load during function and parafunction to prevent implant overload. Crown-to-root ratio, root morphology, tooth mobility, and sulcus depths are critical periodontal considerations. The amount of parafunctional tooth wear must be correlated with patient age. Endodontically treated teeth with short dowels or large diameter cast dowels must be evaluated for their root fracture potential.

B If one or both of the teeth adjacent to the space are compromised or not predictably treatable to carry their share of loading, will splinting them to the adjacent tooth (or teeth) create adequate multiple abutments for a 4-5 unit fixed partial denture? Periodontal health, control of tooth mobility, and Ante's Law should be satisfied. If double abutting does not provide predictable abutment teeth adjacent to the space, then selective tooth extraction should be considered.

C Determine the result of extracting one or both teeth adjacent to the edentulous space. The new edentulous space will be larger. The new potential abutment teeth must be evaluated for their ability to sustain incisal-occlusal loading for each of the three treatment choices. The quantity of edentulous ridge must be evaluated for the vastly different requirements of a long-span, tooth-supported fixed partial denture (FPD), a removable partial denture (RPD), or multiple dental implants. The risk-benefit assessments will be different.

D When both teeth adjacent to the single space have sound clinical crowns with small or no existing restorations, then a single implant should be evaluated as the potential treatment of choice. If one or both adjacent teeth would benefit from a full coverage cast restoration, then a three-unit FPD solves both the missing tooth problem and the restorative needs of the abutment teeth. Full coverage cast restorations can improve tooth esthetics, function, and strength.

E The single edentulous space must be evaluated for the maximum length of an implant that it can safely accept. This is the most important feature of restored implant predictability. A 10-mm implant is the absolute minimum length. A 13-mm length is better, and longer than 13 mm is best. If 10 mm of bone are not present and cannot be obtained by guided tissue regeneration (GTR) or augmentation, then a three-unit FPD should be fabricated. The edentulous space must have adequate width to accommodate the desired implant diameter. Ridge augmentation may be used to create the acceptable width.

F Bone quality affects dental implant success. Type II quality is ideal for single tooth implants. Types I or III are frequently acceptable if the implant has good length. Type IV bone is poor quality and not recommended for single teeth. A three-unit FPD is more predictable.

G Evaluation of single tooth implant loading is more critical than loading of 4-6 splinted implants. An implant placed in posterior segments will receive greater forces than an identical implant in the anterior segment. Different functional positions and contours of the restored implant and its opposing teeth will produce variations in loading. Faciolingual forces created by steep occlusal morphology on posterior teeth are problematic. A single implant protected from parafunctional loading has a better future than one that is overloaded. Implants do not have the overload safety feature provided by a periodontal ligament so they are more susceptible to overload than teeth. Minimal loading of single tooth implants is highly recommended. Moderate to extensive loading may compromise success so a tooth-supported FPD would be more predictable.

References

Branemark PI, Zarb GA, Albrektsson T: *Tissue-integrated prostheses,* Chicago, 1985, Quintessence Publishing, p 201.

Engelman MJ: *Clinical decision making and treatment planning in osseointegration,* Chicago, 1996, Quintessence Publishing, p 169.

Jemt T, Lekholm U, Grondahl A: A 3-year follow up study of early single implant restorations ad modum Branemark, *Int J Periodont Restor Dent* 10(5):341, 1990.

Misch CE: *Contemporary implant dentistry,* St Louis, 1993, Mosby, pp 164, 175, 575.

Shillingburg HT, Hobo S, Whitsett LD, Jacobi R, Brackett SE: *Fundamentals of fixed prosthodontics,* ed 3, Chicago, 1996, Quintessence Publishing, p 85.

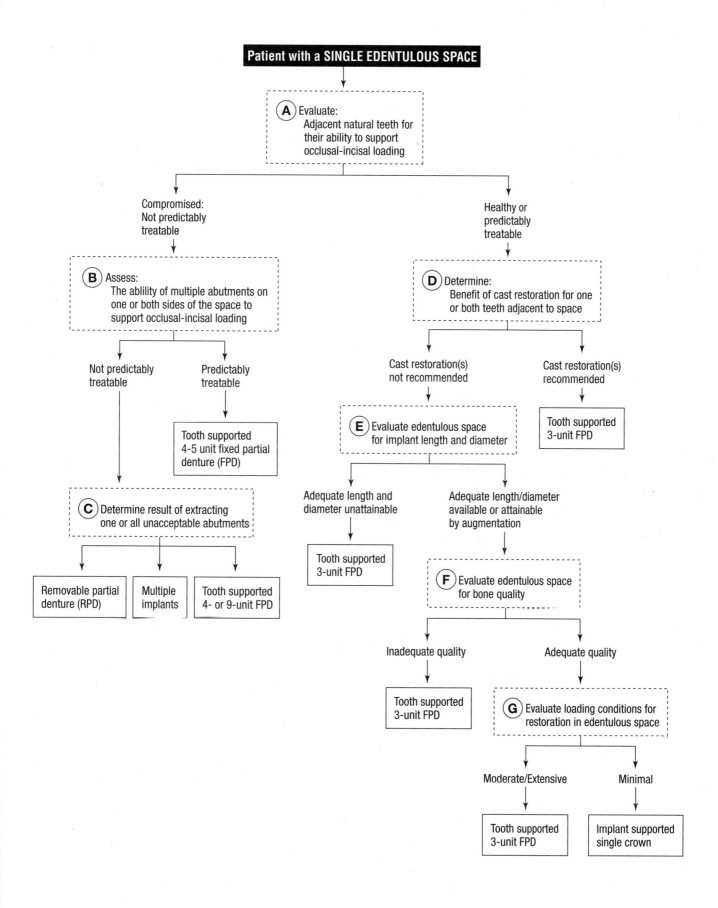

Patient with a SINGLE EDENTULOUS SPACE

(A) Evaluate:
Adjacent natural teeth for their ability to support occlusal-incisal loading

Compromised: Not predictably treatable

Healthy or predictably treatable

(B) Assess:
The ablility of multiple abutments on one or both sides of the space to support occlusal-incisal loading

(D) Determine:
Benefit of cast restoration for one or both teeth adjacent to space

Not predictably treatable

Predictably treatable

Cast restoration(s) not recommended

Cast restoration(s) recommended

Tooth supported 4-5 unit fixed partial denture (FPD)

(E) Evaluate edentulous space for implant length and diameter

Tooth supported 3-unit FPD

(C) Determine result of extracting one or all unacceptable abutments

Adequate length and diameter unattainable

Adequate length/diameter available or attainable by augmentation

Removable partial denture (RPD)

Multiple implants

Tooth supported 4- or 9-unit FPD

Tooth supported 3-unit FPD

(F) Evaluate edentulous space for bone quality

Inadequate quality

Adequate quality

Tooth supported 3-unit FPD

(G) Evaluate loading conditions for restoration in edentulous space

Moderate/Extensive

Minimal

Tooth supported 3-unit FPD

Implant supported single crown

108 Multiple Single Implants or Implants as Abutments

Larry G. Loos

A Decisions regarding implant placement in the partially edentulous patient must not be based solely on the edentulous site. The location, condition, and function of the remaining natural teeth are critical in determining the fixed prosthodontic treatment plan. Problematic teeth must be identified and included in the treatment. The mentality of "see a space, place an implant" does not contribute to predictable long-term success.

B The periodontal status of the remaining natural teeth is important whether they are being considered for tooth-supported fixed partial denture abutments, teeth opposing implants, teeth adjacent to implants, or teeth located remote distances from implants in the same or opposing arch. They will contribute directly or indirectly to the forces delivered to the implant(s). Crown-to-root ratio, root morphology, tooth mobility, and wear are necessary determinants for present restorative design and future prognosis.

C 1. Functional incisal loading can be categorized by the static anterior tooth position in maximum intercuspation and their contact relationship during right lateral, left lateral, and protrusive mandibular excursions. Ideally the functional horizontal overlap (i.e., distance between maxillary lingual surface and mandibular facial surface) should be less than 1 mm. Facial or lingual loading forces are then dependent on vertical overlap (i.e., distance between maxillary incisal surface of mandibular incisal surface). Minimal loading forces are created by vertical overlap of 0 to 2 mm. Moderate loading forces result from 3 to 5 mm vertical overlap and extensive loading forces by 6 mm or greater. Parafunctional incisal loading is potentially more damaging because the amount of force is greater and the duration of load is longer.

   2. Parafunctional loading of occlusal surfaces has even greater significance because maximum biting forces are much greater on posterior teeth than on anterior teeth. Minimum loading forces are produced by light centric contacts and absence of incline contact during excursive movements. Solid centric contacts and presence of incline contact on shallow occlusal morphology produce moderate loading forces. Extensive loading forces are created by heavy centric contacts and presence of incline contact on steep occlusal morphology.

D The mesio-distal dimension of the edentulous space is the first consideration in determining the number of implants. A minimum distance of 2 mm must exist between adjacent restored implants as they emerge through soft tissue in order for predictable soft tissue health. Knowing the diameter of each restored implant, one can calculate the "maximum" number of implants for a specific edentulous span. The "actual" number of implants recommended for the space can be determined by evaluating implant length and diameter, bone quality, and implant loading. Implant length is the single most predictable factor in success rates. Larger implant diameters may compensate for shorter length implants. Bone quality is determined from radiographs and surgical assessment. Types I and II are good quality, Type III is mediocre, and Type IV is poor bone quality. Implant loading is effected by the anteroposterior location of the restoration, functional contours of the restoration with its opposing surfaces, and the degree and duration of parafunction. A thorough evaluation of these loading conditions will produce categories of loading described as minimal, moderate, or extensive.

- *Unfavorable conditions* for implants would include short length implants (less than 10 mm), poor bone quality (Type IV), and extensive loading.
- *Neutral conditions* for implants are average lengths (10-13 mm), average bone quality (Type III), and moderate loading.
- *Favorable conditions* include long implants (15 mm or longer), good quality bone (Type I or II), and minimal loading.

References

Branemark PI, Zarb GA, Albrektsson T: *Tissue-integrated prostheses,* Chicago, 1985, Quintessence Publishing, p 201.

Engelman MJ: *Clinical decision making and treatment planning in osseointegration,* Chicago, 1996, Quintessence Publishing, p 169.

Kaukinen JA, Edge MJ, Lang BR: The influence of occlusal design on simulated masticatory forces transferred to implant-retained prostheses and supporting bone, *J Prosthet Dent* 76:50, 1996.

Misch CE: *Contemporary implant dentistry,* St Louis, 1993, Mosby, pp 164, 705.

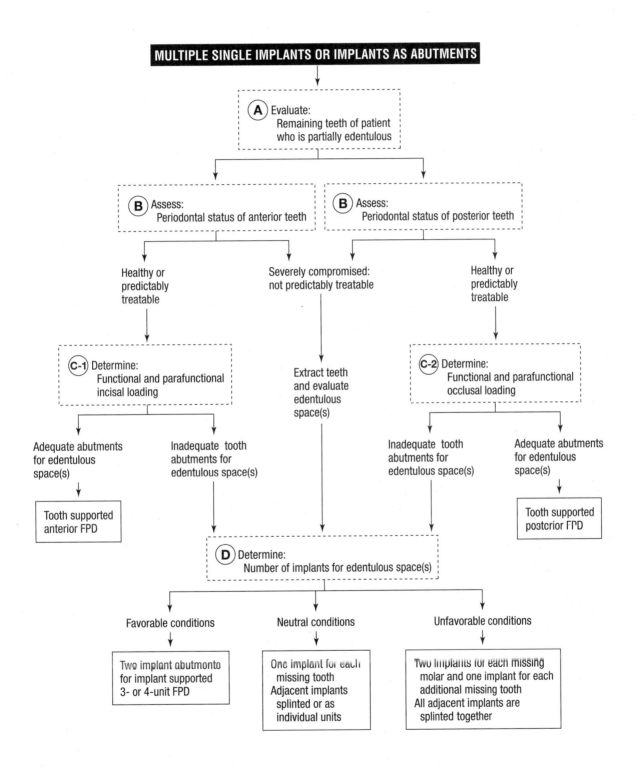

PART **FIVE**

Oral Surgery

James Garibaldi, Editor

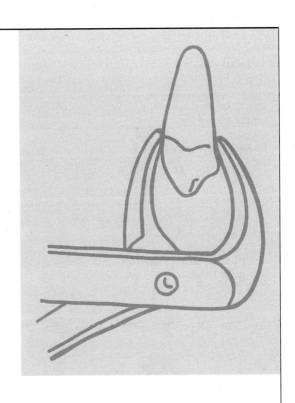

109 Patient with an Erupted Wisdom Tooth Who is Considering Extraction

James Garibaldi

When a patient has an erupted wisdom tooth, the first thing the dentist must ascertain is whether or not the tooth is symptomatic.

A If the tooth is asymptomatic, then factors such as whether the tooth is cleansable should be considered. If upon physical examination, the dentist notes that the distal of the wisdom tooth is against or close to the ramus, then it will be impossible for the patient to keep this area clean. Another consideration in an asymptomatic wisdom tooth that has enough space on the distal to be kept clean is the presence and adequacy of surrounding attached gingiva.

B After determining that the tooth is cleansable and free of both periodontal problems and caries, the dentist must make sure the tooth has erupted into normal occlusion, not to the buccal or lingual, which is common. Also, it should be noted whether the tooth has an opposing tooth, allowing it to be functional for the patient and preventing possible supereruption.

C However, if the wisdom tooth does not have an opposing tooth but is asymptomatic and periodontally sound, then it is up to the dentist and patient with regard to retention or extraction of the tooth. The question to answer is if this tooth could ever be used in a treatment plan in the future or if it could simply supererupt with time and cause problems, such as cheek biting.

D If the patient is symptomatic, then the first item to ascertain is the presence or absence of caries. If present and the tooth has periodontal problems, lack of attached gingiva, or is up against the ramus, extraction is indicated.

E On the other hand, if there are caries but the tooth is free of periodontal problems and can be kept clean, a determination should be made as to whether the tooth is functional or not (i.e., in occlusion with an opposing tooth). If this is the case it should be restored and maintained.

F Finally, if the wisdom tooth is cleansable without any periodontal or attached gingiva problems and has no caries (but is symptomatic) and if the tooth is in occlusion, the patient should be checked for cracked-tooth syndrome (see Chapter 5). If this can be ruled out, oral hygiene should be increased and symptoms further evaluated. This includes checking for sensitivity secondary to exposed cementum and prematurity in occlusal contact. If symptoms do not resolve after appropriate treatment, the tooth should be extracted if it is of no value in a future treatment plan.

References

Hooley JR, Whitacre RJ: *Assessment of and surgery for third molars: a self-instructional guide,* ed 3, Seattle, 1983, Stoma Press.

Lysell L, Rohlin M: A study of indications used for removal of the mandibular third molar, *Int J Oral Maxillofac Surg* 17:161, 1988.

Pedersen GW: *Oral surgery,* Philadelphia, 1988, WB Saunders, p 60.

Peterson LJ, Ellis E, Hupp JR, Tucker MR: *Contemporary oral and maxillofacial surgery,* ed 2, St Louis, 1993, Mosby, p 225.

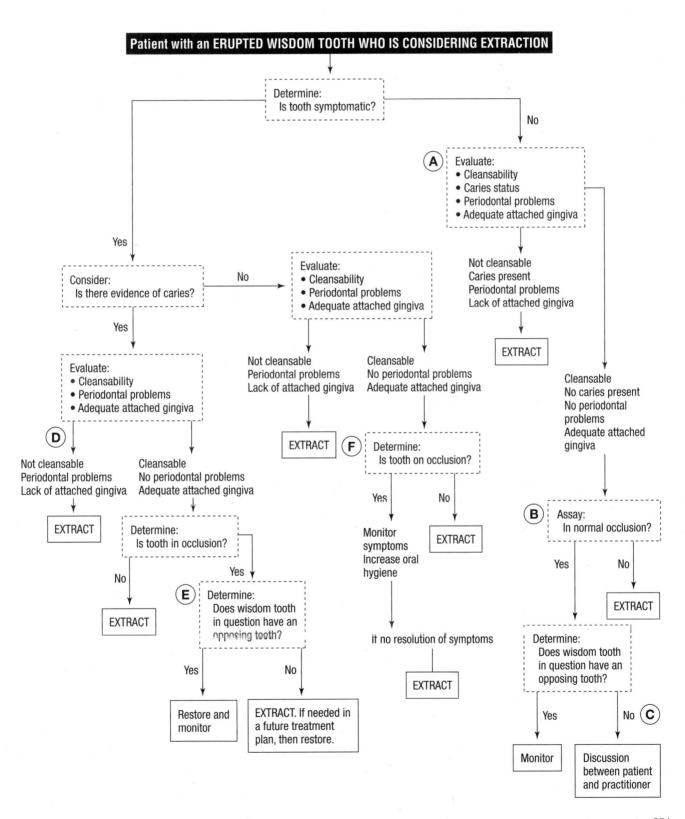

Patient with an ERUPTED WISDOM TOOTH WHO IS CONSIDERING EXTRACTION

Determine:
Is tooth symptomatic?

No

Yes

(A) Evaluate:
• Cleansability
• Caries status
• Periodontal problems
• Adequate attached gingiva

Consider:
Is there evidence of caries?

No

Evaluate:
• Cleansability
• Periodontal problems
• Adequate attached gingiva

Not cleansable
Caries present
Periodontal problems
Lack of attached gingiva

EXTRACT

Cleansable
No caries present
No periodontal
problems
Adequate attached
gingiva

Yes

Evaluate:
• Cleansability
• Periodontal problems
• Adequate attached gingiva

Not cleansable
Periodontal problems
Lack of attached gingiva

Cleansable
No periodontal problems
Adequate attached gingiva

EXTRACT

(F) Determine:
Is tooth on occlusion?

(D) Not cleansable
Periodontal problems
Lack of attached gingiva

Cleansable
No periodontal problems
Adequate attached gingiva

EXTRACT

Determine:
Is tooth in occlusion?

Yes

No

Yes

Monitor
symptoms
Increase oral
hygiene

EXTRACT

(B) Assay:
In normal occlusion?

Yes

No

No

EXTRACT

Yes

EXTRACT

(E) Determine:
Does wisdom tooth
in question have an
opposing tooth?

Determine:
Does wisdom tooth
in question have an
opposing tooth?

If no resolution of symptoms

Yes

No

EXTRACT

Yes

No (C)

Restore and
monitor

EXTRACT. If needed in
a future treatment
plan, then restore.

EXTRACT

Monitor

Discussion
between patient
and practitioner

110 Patient with a Soft Tissue Impacted Wisdom Tooth Who is Considering Extraction

James Garibaldi

When a patient has a symptomatic soft tissue impaction, the most likely cause is pericoronitis. The tooth begins to erupt somewhat but then, because of proximity to the ramus or adjacent second molar, is prevented from erupting fully. The overlying soft tissue operculum can often become the site for entrapment of food debris and proliferation of microorganisms leading to inflammation. Generally, this phenomenon is painful, involves the mandibular wisdom teeth, and progresses to a full-blown infection.

A Therefore the first thing assessed is whether the patient is symptomatic and if the cause is pericoronitis or not. If so, one should next consider the age of the patient, which generally correlates with the amount of root formation to some degree.

B The ideal time to remove an impacted wisdom tooth is when one third to two thirds of the root is formed, which generally corresponds with the middle to late teenage years. If it is removed too early, when no root is formed, the extraction is difficult because the tooth rolls around in its bony crypt (some root formation prevents this). If, on the other hand, the roots are completely formed, the tooth is anchored firmly in place.

C Hence, with *lack of full eruption potential*, symptoms of pericoronitis, which can subside and reoccur at any time, and one third to two thirds of the root formed, the tooth should be extracted. Other factors that also would indicate an extraction include associated pathology, not enough attached gingiva if the wisdom tooth could erupt, or the tooth cannot be kept clean on the distal if it were to erupt fully. The key is to remove a tooth with these factors when the patient is young so the chances of regeneration of periodontal structures on the distal of the second molar are good. The surgery itself is easier compared with later in life, and the recuperation is generally uneventful, with less potential for postoperative complications. If none of these factors are present, the tooth can be left and monitored.

D If the patient is asymptomatic, one should again consider the age of the patient. The ideal time for extraction is when one third to two thirds of the root is formed and no pathology is noted, especially if the potential for full eruption is improbable or impossible.

E If the patient is older, the status of the second molar should be considered. If no pathology or periodontal problems are noted, the situation should be monitored. However, if radiographs show that the wisdom tooth is abutted against the distal of the second molar, potentially compromising the distal of the second molar's periodontal structures and (1) there is not enough space for full eruption of the wisdom tooth, (2) there is pathology or inadequate attached gingiva, or (3) the patient is unable to keep it clean if the tooth were to erupt, it should be extracted, even if asymptomatic. Guided tissue regeneration may be considered.

References

Kugelberg CF, Ahlstrom U, Ericson S et al: The influence of anatomical, pathophysiological and other factors on periodontal healing after impacted lower third molar surgery, *J Clin Periodontol* 18:37, 1991.

Laskin DM: Indication and contraindications for removal of impacted third molars, *Dent Clin North Am* 13:919, 1969.

Pedersen GW: *Oral surgery*, Philadelphia, 1988, WB Saunders, p 60.

Robinson PD: The impacted lower wisdom tooth: to remove or to leave alone? *Dent Update* 21(6):245, 1994.

Tate TE: Impactions: observe or treat? *J Calif Dent Assoc* 22(6):59, 1994.

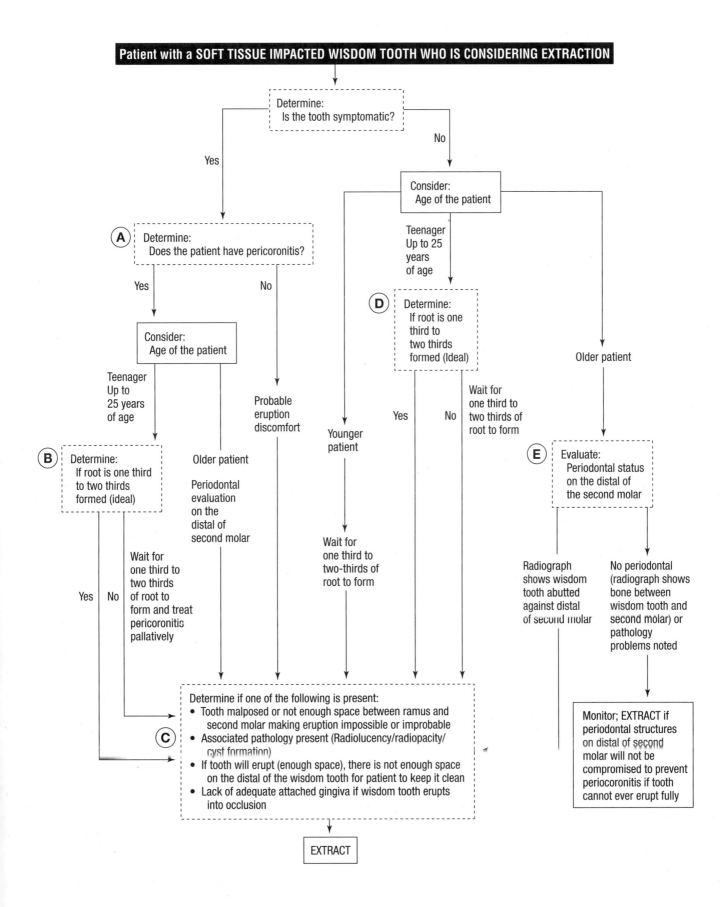

Patient with a SOFT TISSUE IMPACTED WISDOM TOOTH WHO IS CONSIDERING EXTRACTION

Determine:
Is the tooth symptomatic?

Yes

No

(A) Determine:
Does the patient have pericoronitis?

Yes

No

Consider:
Age of the patient

Consider:
Age of the patient

Teenager
Up to
25 years
of age

Teenager
Up to 25
years
of age

(D) Determine:
If root is one
third to
two thirds
formed (Ideal)

Older patient

(B) Determine:
If root is one third
to two thirds
formed (ideal)

Older patient

Probable
eruption
discomfort

Younger
patient

Yes

No

Wait for
one third to
two thirds of
root to form

(E) Evaluate:
Periodontal status
on the distal of
the second molar

Periodontal
evaluation
on the
distal of
second molar

Yes

No

Wait for
one third to
two thirds
of root to
form and treat
pericoronitis
pallatively

Wait for
one third to
two-thirds of
root to form

Radiograph
shows wisdom
tooth abutted
against distal
of second molar

No periodontal
(radiograph shows
bone between
wisdom tooth and
second molar) or
pathology
problems
noted

(C) Determine if one of the following is present:
• Tooth malposed or not enough space between ramus and
  second molar making eruption impossible or improbable
• Associated pathology present (Radiolucency/radiopacity/
  cyst formation)
• If tooth will erupt (enough space), there is not enough space
  on the distal of the wisdom tooth for patient to keep it clean
• Lack of adequate attached gingiva if wisdom tooth erupts
  into occlusion

Monitor; EXTRACT if
periodontal structures
on distal of second
molar will not be
compromised to prevent
periocoronitis if tooth
cannot ever erupt fully

EXTRACT

111 Patient with a Partial Bony Impacted Wisdom Tooth Who is Considering Extraction

James Garibaldi

Probably the most common complaint of a patient with a partial bony impaction is pain secondary to pericoronitis. This results basically from the jaw, usually the mandibular, being too small to accommodate the full eruption of a wisdom tooth. Hence its complete eruption is prevented by the ramus or the adjacent second molar.

A The ideal time to remove a partially impacted wisdom tooth with not enough space between the ramus and the second molar for complete eruption is when one third to two thirds of the root is formed.

B If the patient is symptomatic but does not have pericoronitis the cause is most probably eruption discomfort. If the tooth possesses pathology, or is malposed or impacted under the ramus making complete eruption improbable or impossible, it should be removed.

C When the patient is asymptomatic, but on radiographs a partial bony impaction is noted, the patient, especially a teenager with one third to two thirds of the root formed, should be evaluated. The reason is that if pathology or other factors, such as impossible or improbable eruption of the tooth, are noted, this is the time for removal. The bone is elastic, and the roots are not completely formed to anchor the tooth. The surgery is then met with fewer postoperative complications, and the recovery is generally quicker than in an older patient. The elasticity of bone in the younger patient can be compared with the need for bone removal in the older patient with its potential for postoperative morbidity.

D In the asymptomatic patient, as with all patients, risk factors should be assessed in removing wisdom teeth. Sinus proximity and potential damage to the inferior alveolar nerve must be considered. In the older patient, where bone elasticity decreases, these risk factors can be of more concern than in the teenager. Therefore the status of the distal of the second molar should be evaluated periodically and, if no pathology or periodontal concerns are noted, the tooth should be monitored and followed closely.

References

Koerner KR: The removal of impacted third molars: principles, indications and procedures, *Dent Clin North Am* 38(2):255, 1994.

Mercier P, Precious D: Risks and benefits of removal of impacted third molars, *Int J Oral Maxillofac Surg* 21(1):17, 1992.

Peterson LJ, Ellis E, Hupp JR, Tucker MR: *Contemporary oral and maxillofacial surgery*, ed 2, St Louis, 1993, Mosby, p 225.

Tate TE: Impactions: observe or treat? *J Calif Dent Assoc* 22(6):59, 1994.

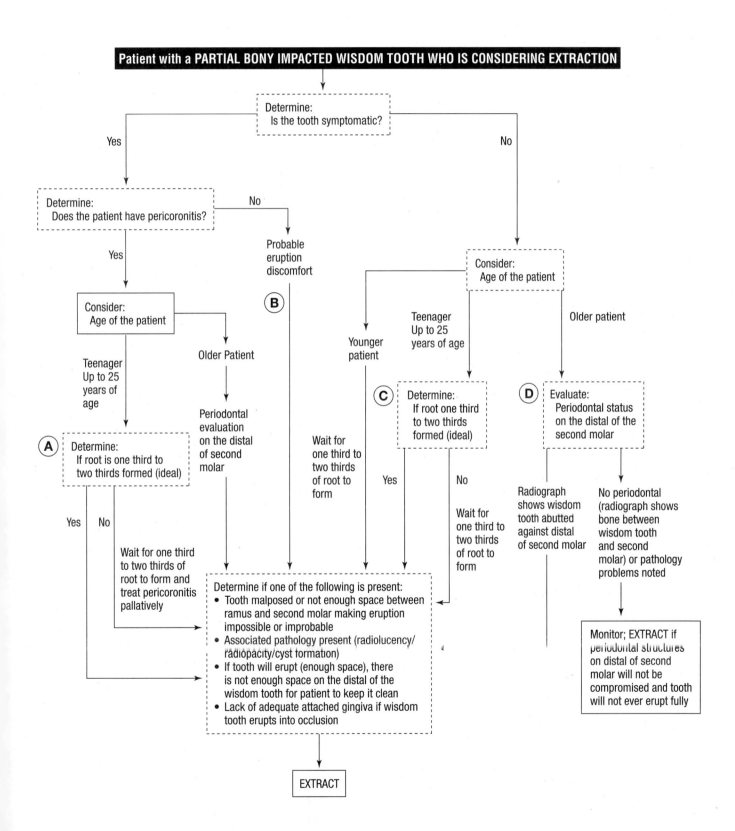

Patient with a PARTIAL BONY IMPACTED WISDOM TOOTH WHO IS CONSIDERING EXTRACTION

Determine:
Is the tooth symptomatic?

Yes

No

Determine:
Does the patient have pericoronitis?

No

Yes

Probable
eruption
discomfort

B

Consider:
Age of the patient

Consider:
Age of the patient

Teenager
Up to 25
years of age

Older patient

Older Patient

Younger
patient

Teenager
Up to 25
years of
age

Periodontal
evaluation
on the distal
of second
molar

C Determine:
If root one third
to two thirds
formed (ideal)

D Evaluate:
Periodontal status
on the distal of the
second molar

A Determine:
If root is one third to
two thirds formed (ideal)

Wait for
one third to
two thirds
of root to
form

Yes

No

Yes

No

Wait for
one third to
two thirds
of root to
form

Radiograph
shows wisdom
tooth abutted
against distal
of second molar

No periodontal
(radiograph shows
bone between
wisdom tooth
and second
molar) or pathology
problems noted

Wait for one third
to two thirds of
root to form and
treat pericoronitis
pallatively

Determine if one of the following is present:
• Tooth malposed or not enough space between
ramus and second molar making eruption
impossible or improbable
• Associated pathology present (radiolucency/
radiopacity/cyst formation)
• If tooth will erupt (enough space), there
is not enough space on the distal of the
wisdom tooth for patient to keep it clean
• Lack of adequate attached gingiva if wisdom
tooth erupts into occlusion

Monitor; EXTRACT if
periodontal structures
on distal of second
molar will not be
compromised and tooth
will not ever erupt fully

EXTRACT

112 Patient with a Fully Bony Impacted Wisdom Tooth Who is Considering Extraction

James Garibaldi

In the patient with a full bony impaction that is symptomatic, the *least* likely cause is pericoronitis. The reason is that a portion of the tooth must be erupted allowing for the development of an operculum, which can lead to entrapment of food debris and proliferation of microorganisms. However, there are times when an erupted maxillary wisdom tooth can supererupt and begins biting on the gingiva overlying the lower fully impacted wisdom tooth. This can create the same sort of symptoms, hence making the patient with a full bony impaction symptomatic.

A Therefore the first thing to consider in the symptomatic patient is age and if pathology is present or not. If pathology is present in the form of an enlarged follicle, presence of a cyst, or a radiolucency or radiopacity associated with the tooth, the tooth in question should be removed and the specimen sent to pathology for evaluation. The most common pathology noted with full bony impactions is the dentigerous cyst, which can continue to enlarge in time.

B Neoplasms, such as squamous cell carcinoma, can develop in the lining of cysts especially as the patient becomes older. Therefore if a third molar without pathology is left at an early age, the tooth needs to be followed with periodic radiographs. If it is found that the symptoms are caused by supererupted maxillary molar biting on the gingiva of a full bony mandibular impaction, the supererupted tooth should be removed.

C In the young asymptomatic patient with a full bony impaction, if no pathology is present, one should wait until at least one third to two thirds of the root is formed. The reason here is twofold: (1) usually the wisdom tooth will erupt more with time (i.e., not be as close to the maxillary sinus or inferior alveolar canal) and (2) if a tooth is re-moved without any root formation, it can roll around in its bony crypt, making the extraction more difficult than if some root structure is present to stabilize the tooth during extraction.

D If the patient is asymptomatic, one should again consider the patient's age. Generally, as the patient grows older, the health can decline and may necessitate the use of prescription drugs for such things as high blood pressure, arthritis, or chronic atrial fibrillation. The dentist needs to take into account this information before deciding on an extraction. At times, a medical consult, laboratory work, or even hospitalization may be required to complete the procedure. If the distal of the second molar is periodontally sound, the wisdom tooth cannot be felt with a periodontal probe, and no pathology is noted in association with the wisdom tooth, it should be monitored with periodic radiographic evaluation.

References

Braden BE: Deep distal pockets adjacent to terminal teeth, *Dent Clin North Am* 13:161, 1969.

Koerner KR: The removal of impacted third molars: principles, indications and procedures, *Dent Clin North Am* 38(2):255, 1994.

Laskin DM: Indication and contraindications for removal of impacted third molars, *Dent Clin North Am* 13:919, 1969.

Mercier P, Precious D: Risks and benefits of removal of impacted third molars, *Int J Oral Maxillofac Surg* 21(1):17, 1992.

Robinson PD: The impacted lower wisdom tooth: to remove or to leave alone? *Dent Update* 21(6):245, 1994.

Stanley HR, Alattar M, Collett WK et al: Pathological sequelae of "neglected" impacted third molars, *J Oral Pathol* 17:113, 1988.

Tate TE: Impactions: observe or treat? *J Calif Dent Assoc* 22(6):59, 1994.

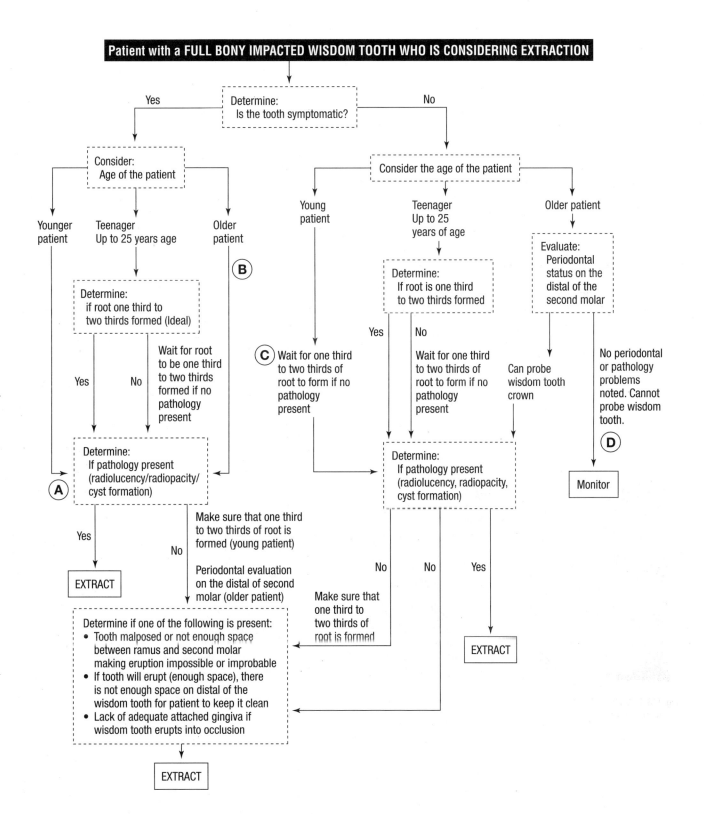

Patient with a FULL BONY IMPACTED WISDOM TOOTH WHO IS CONSIDERING EXTRACTION

Determine: Is the tooth symptomatic?

Yes

Consider: Age of the patient

Younger patient | Teenager Up to 25 years age | Older patient

B

Determine: if root one third to two thirds formed (Ideal)

Wait for root to be one third to two thirds formed if no pathology present

Yes | No

A — Determine: If pathology present (radiolucency/radiopacity/cyst formation)

Yes → EXTRACT

No

Make sure that one third to two thirds of root is formed (young patient)

Periodontal evaluation on the distal of second molar (older patient)

Determine if one of the following is present:
- Tooth malposed or not enough space between ramus and second molar making eruption impossible or improbable
- If tooth will erupt (enough space), there is not enough space on distal of the wisdom tooth for patient to keep it clean
- Lack of adequate attached gingiva if wisdom tooth erupts into occlusion

→ EXTRACT

No

Consider the age of the patient

Young patient | Teenager Up to 25 years of age | Older patient

Evaluate: Periodontal status on the distal of the second molar

C Wait for one third to two thirds of root to form if no pathology present

Determine: If root is one third to two thirds formed

Yes | No

Wait for one third to two thirds of root to form if no pathology present

Can probe wisdom tooth crown

No periodontal or pathology problems noted. Cannot probe wisdom tooth.

D

Determine: If pathology present (radiolucency, radiopacity, cyst formation)

No | No | Yes

Make sure that one third to two thirds of root is formed

→ EXTRACT

Monitor

113 Impacted Third Molars

Walter B. Hall

Impacted third molars often create serious periodontal problems on adjacent teeth or become involved with periodontal problems on adjacent teeth as they develop. Early extraction of developing third molars may prevent some of these problems from occurring; however, patients often hesitate over treatment of potential problems that are not symptomatic. As an impacted third molar develops, it may grow increasingly closer to the second molar root (Fig. 113-1). Once it is close, removal of the third molar may result in pocket depth distal to the second molar. Such surgically related pockets usually are accompanied by a three-walled residual osseous defect. If the defect is narrow, it may be amenable to a bone regeneration procedure. The decision as to residual pocked depth and the possibility of bone regeneration should be delayed for 6 months or more following extraction.

A If the impacted third molar is not close to the root of the second molar and the third molar is fully formed, the decision to retain or extract is not a periodontal one. If the third molar is still developing and appears unlikely to become close to the root of the second molar, the decision to retain or extract is not a periodontal one; however, if further development of the third molar is likely to result in its crown approaching the second molar root, the prompt extraction of the third molar is desirable periodontally.

B If the impacted third molar already is close to, or touching, the root of the second molar, the existing periodontal status of the second molar will influence decisions regarding the third molars.

C If the second molar is not periodontally involved, prompt extraction of the third molar is desirable periodontally. Do not probe the distal surface of the second molar for 6 months. Then, if a pocket exists, and the osseous defect appears to be a three-walled one, its narrow portion would be amenable to osseous regeneration (see Chapter 29). If the distal furcation of a maxillary second molar is involved significantly, the molar may be a good candidate for bone regeneration; however, ostectomy may be preferable if it is a shallow effect. Performing guided tissue regeneration (GTR) at the time of extraction should be considered (see Chapter 35).

D If the crown of an impacted third molar is close to a second molar root that is periodontally involved, the degree of bone loss on the second molar will influence treatment planning. If the bone loss is early to moderate and the third molar could erupt to replace the second molar, consider extraction of the second molar. If a probe placed in the distal defect on the second molar can touch the third molar crown (this requires especially careful probing), extract the second molar promptly. If the crown of the third molar cannot be touched, the extraction may be delayed but is still periodontally desirable. If the third molar is unlikely to erupt to adequately replace the second molar, extract the third molar promptly, if its crown can be touched, or later, if it cannot be touched. If the third molar is unlikely to erupt to replace the second molar, the patient may consider extraction of the third molar and GTR either at the time of extraction or following healing (see Chapter 35). Extraction of both molars may be considered.

References

Ash MM: Third molars as periodontal problems, *Dent Clin North Am* 8:51, 1964.

Ash MM, Costich ER, Hayward JR: Study of periodontal hazards or third molars, *J Periodontal* 33:209, 1962.

Friedman JW: The case for preservation of third molars, *J Calif Dent Assoc* 5:50, 1977.

Hall WB: Removal of third molars: a periodontal viewpoint. In McDonald RL, editor: *Current therapy in dentistry*, St Louis, 1980, Mosby, p 225.

Laskin DM: Indications and contraindications for removal of impacted third molars, *Dent Clin North Am* 13:919, 1969.

Fig. 113-1 An impacted third molar appearing to contact the root of the adjacent second molar.

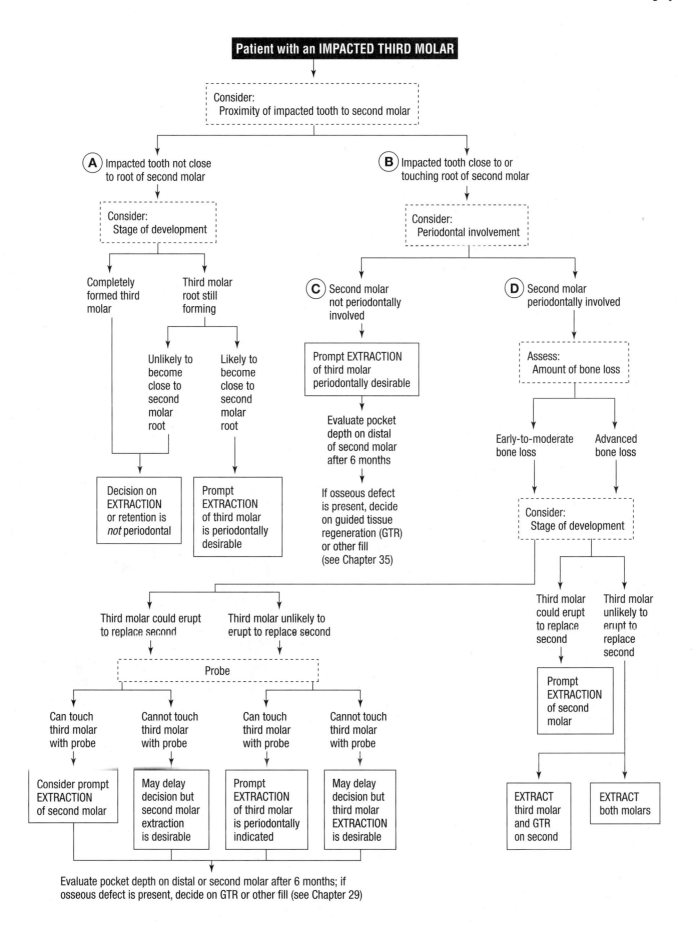

Patient with an IMPACTED THIRD MOLAR

Consider:
Proximity of impacted tooth to second molar

(A) Impacted tooth not close to root of second molar

Consider:
Stage of development

Completely formed third molar

Third molar root still forming

Unlikely to become close to second molar root

Likely to become close to second molar root

Decision on EXTRACTION or retention is *not* periodontal

Prompt EXTRACTION of third molar is periodontally desirable

(B) Impacted tooth close to or touching root of second molar

Consider:
Periodontal involvement

(C) Second molar not periodontally involved

Prompt EXTRACTION of third molar periodontally desirable

Evaluate pocket depth on distal of second molar after 6 months

If osseous defect is present, decide on guided tissue regeneration (GTR) or other fill (see Chapter 35)

(D) Second molar periodontally involved

Assess:
Amount of bone loss

Early-to-moderate bone loss

Advanced bone loss

Consider:
Stage of development

Third molar could erupt to replace second

Third molar unlikely to erupt to replace second

Prompt EXTRACTION of second molar

EXTRACT third molar and GTR on second

EXTRACT both molars

Third molar could erupt to replace second

Third molar unlikely to erupt to replace second

Probe

Can touch third molar with probe

Cannot touch third molar with probe

Can touch third molar with probe

Cannot touch third molar with probe

Consider prompt EXTRACTION of second molar

May delay decision but second molar extraction is desirable

Prompt EXTRACTION of third molar is periodontally indicated

May delay decision but third molar EXTRACTION is desirable

Evaluate pocket depth on distal or second molar after 6 months; if osseous defect is present, decide on GTR or other fill (see Chapter 29)

114 Partially Erupted Third Molars

Walter B. Hall

Partially erupted third molars present a rare set of periodontal problems. A partially erupted third molar has pocket depth at least to its cementoenamel junction. Although this is only a pseudopocket initially, it can lead to loss of attachment on the third molar and to pocket formation on the adjacent second molar. Extraction of the third molar before significant periodontal problems occur is desirable; however, if the third molar is impacted against the root of the second molar, a residual defect on the distal of the second molar is likely to occur following the extraction. This defect is more likely to occur than with fully impacted third molars because insufficient gingiva to permit primary closure of the wound following third molar extraction is more likely to exist around partially erupted than around fully impacted teeth.

A A third molar can be partially erupted but not in close proximity to the second molar (i.e., a vertical impaction in the ramus of the mandible). If the second molar is healthy or has had little bone loss, consider extraction of the third molar eventually. If the second molar has moderate-to-severe bone loss and the partially erupted third molar could be moved into good position following extraction of its neighbor, one may consider extracting the second molar and moving the third molar orthodontically into its position or uprighting it for use as an abutment.

B If the partially erupted third molar is close to, or touching, the second molar (Fig. 114-1), other options apply. If the third molar is close to, or touching, the crown of the second molar only and the second molar has little or no bone loss, prompt extraction of the third molar is periodontally advisable before significant pocketing occurs distal to the second molar. If the second molar has moderate-to-advanced bone loss and the third molar has adequate remaining support, the second molar should be removed and the third molar moved orthodontically into its place or uprighted for use as an abutment.

C If the partially erupted third molar is close to, or touching, the root of the second molar, several possibilities exist. If the second molar has little or no bone loss and the third molar has little remaining support, prompt extraction of

the third molar and evaluation of the pocket status distal to the second molars, no sooner than 6 months after the extraction, are indicated. A residual, narrow, three-walled defect may be amenable to bone regeneration surgery. If the third molar has little or no bone loss and the second molar has moderate-to-advanced bone loss, the second molar could be extracted and the third molar moved orthodontically either into its place or uprighted to serve as an abutment. If both molars are badly involved, both should be extracted; they are prone to abscess formation because of difficulty of cleaning by either the patient or the dentist. An alternative would be to extract one tooth and do guided tissue regeneration on the remaining one.

References

Ash MM: Third molars as periodontal problems, *Dent Clin North Am* 8:51, 1964.

Ash MM, Costich ER, Hayward JR: Study of periodontal hazards of third molars, *J Periodontal* 33:209, 1962.

Braden BE: Deep distal pockets adjacent to terminal teeth, *Dent Clin North Am* 13:161, 1969.

Hall WB: Removal of third molars: a periodontal viewpoint. In McDonald RL, editor: *Current therapy in dentistry*, St Louis, 1980, Mosby, p 225.

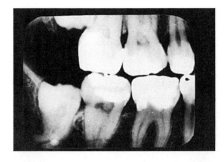

Fig. 114-1 Partially erupted third molar appearing to be in close contact with the second molar.

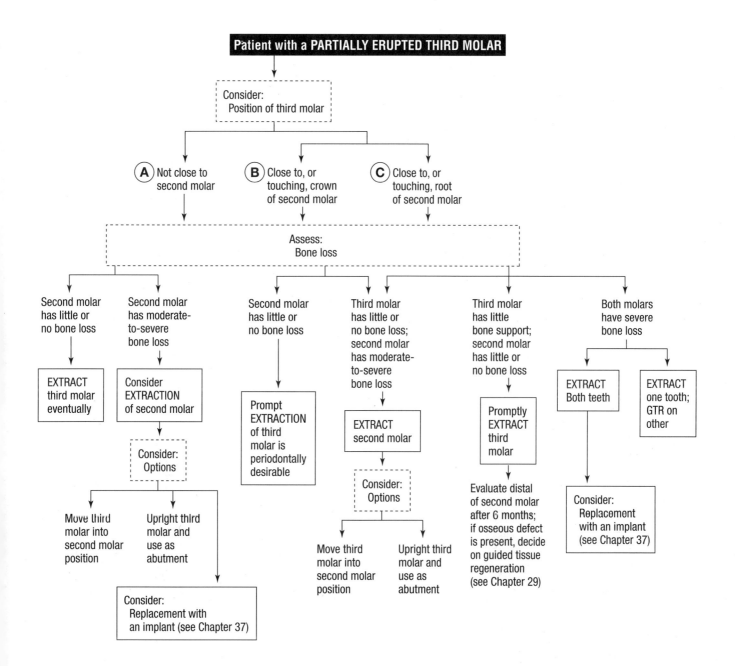

Patient with a PARTIALLY ERUPTED THIRD MOLAR

Consider:
Position of third molar

A Not close to second molar

B Close to, or touching, crown of second molar

C Close to, or touching, root of second molar

Assess:
Bone loss

Second molar has little or no bone loss

EXTRACT third molar eventually

Second molar has moderate-to-severe bone loss

Consider EXTRACTION of second molar

Consider:
Options

Move third molar into second molar position

Upright third molar and use as abutment

Consider:
Replacement with an implant (see Chapter 37)

Second molar has little or no bone loss

Prompt EXTRACTION of third molar is periodontally desirable

Third molar has little or no bone loss; second molar has moderate-to-severe bone loss

EXTRACT second molar

Consider:
Options

Move third molar into second molar position

Upright third molar and use as abutment

Third molar has little bone support; second molar has little or no bone loss

Promptly EXTRACT third molar

Evaluate distal of second molar after 6 months; if osseous defect is present, decide on guided tissue regeneration (see Chapter 29)

Both molars have severe bone loss

EXTRACT Both teeth

EXTRACT one tooth; GTR on other

Consider:
Replacement with an implant (see Chapter 37)

INDEX